HUMAN BIOCHEMICAL
GENETICS

HUMAN BIOCHEMICAL GENETICS

BY

H. HARRIS

WITH A FOREWORD BY

L. S. PENROSE, F.R.S.

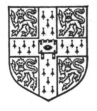

CAMBRIDGE

AT THE UNIVERSITY PRESS

1966

CAMBRIDGE UNIVERSITY PRESS
Cambridge, New York, Melbourne, Madrid, Cape Town, Singapore,
São Paulo, Delhi, Dubai, Tokyo, Mexico City

Cambridge University Press
The Edinburgh Building, Cambridge CB2 8RU, UK

Published in the United States of America by Cambridge University Press, New York

www.cambridge.org
Information on this title: www.cambridge.org/9780521093927

© Cambridge University Press 1959

This publication is in copyright. Subject to statutory exception
and to the provisions of relevant collective licensing agreements,
no reproduction of any part may take place without the written
permission of Cambridge University Press.

First published 1959
Reprinted 1962, 1966
First paperback edition 1966
Re-issued 2010

A catalogue record for this publication is available from the British Library

ISBN 978-0-521-05213-9 Hardback
ISBN 978-0-521-09392-7 Paperback

Cambridge University Press has no responsibility for the persistence or
accuracy of URLs for external or third-party Internet Web sites referred to in
this publication, and does not guarantee that any content on such Web sites is,
or will remain, accurate or appropriate.

FOREWORD

At the present time the science of human genetics is growing very rapidly. This development was predictable because of the increasing number of workers who are coming into the field and the new techniques which are being applied in the recognition of hereditary characters. In one special region, that concerned with biochemistry, however, advances have exceeded all expectations.

When Garrod produced the second edition of his *Inborn Errors of Metabolism* in 1923, he was able to describe in detail only some half dozen rare anomalies, and only a few discerning people had then realised that a revolution in the study of heredity was in progress. The new outlook was destined to be especially significant in human genetics and it altered eugenic philosophy. No longer could hereditary defects be attributed to the action of mysterious noxious influences, carried by degenerate germ plasm and perhaps engendered by parental vice. Under biochemical scrutiny, hereditary defects were repeatedly found to be quite specific inborn peculiarities. These individual chemical differences seem quantitatively very slight, like the substitution of just one aminoacid residue in an otherwise perfect chain. No stigma can be attached to such impersonal variations. If there are unfavourable effects connected with a chemical variant, these merely present a therapeutic challenge.

In his previous book, *Introduction to Human Biochemical Genetics*, published in 1953, Dr Harris reviewed the position of the subject and described all the well-established advances which had been made since Garrod's time. Now there is, again, much fresh information available and a larger book is required. It is extremely difficult to keep pace with the rate at which discoveries are being made. To present the very latest views in every detail cannot be a practical aim. Dr Harris has again minimised this disadvantage by devoting the book mainly to the description of well-authenticated material, leaving out speculative interpretations of anomalies which are, so far, not well understood. This plan does not involve neglect of dramatic discoveries such as acatalasaemia and analbuminaemia. How do people get on when their blood is deprived of such apparently essential substances as catalase or albumen? The answers are unexpected.

A book of this kind must necessarily include an account of the principles of human population genetics. It is now quite insufficient simply to describe an inherited condition and to demonstrate its mode of transmission in a few pedigrees. The human geneticist must ascertain the prevalence of each defect and must seek to determine why it occurs with the population frequency actually observed. When a trait has been identified in terms of a biochemical peculiarity, accurate incidence figures eventually can be obtained and the situation is favourable for the exploration of problems concerning mutation and natural selection.

In presenting this well-balanced and learned account of the subject, Dr Harris has done a valuable service to medicine, to biochemistry and to genetics. I have much pleasure in drawing the attention of workers in these subjects to this book, for it can open a new world to them.

L. S. PENROSE

GALTON LABORATORY
UNIVERSITY COLLEGE, LONDON
June 1958

CONTENTS

ACKNOWLEDGEMENTS

I would like to thank Professors C. E. Dent, L. S. Penrose, W. T. J. Morgan, and F. L. Warren for much helpful advice and discussion.

I would also like to thank those authors and publishers who have granted permission to reproduce figures from other publications. The names of the authors are quoted in the captions and the place of original publication in the lists of references at the end of each chapter.

I am extremely grateful to Mrs S. White and Mrs N. Myant for assistance in preparing the figures and index.

H. HARRIS

DEPARTMENT OF BIOCHEMISTRY
THE LONDON HOSPITAL MEDICAL COLLEGE

CHAPTER 1

INTRODUCTION

This book is about inborn differences between human beings. More particularly it concerns those differences which can be formulated in biochemical terms. These include differences in structures of macro-molecules such as proteins and mucopolysaccharides, differences in the formation of certain enzymes, differences in the composition of body fluids and secretions, and differences in excretory products. Ultimately, however, they must each depend on differences in the biochemical characteristics of the fertilised ova from which all individuals develop. The significant differences here probably lie in the structural organisation of the desoxyribose nucleic acid present in the cell nucleus.

The inborn errors of metabolism and biochemical individuality

The scientific study of inherited differences in human biochemistry began with the work of Garrod at the turn of the century. In 1902 he published a paper in the *Lancet* called 'The incidence of alkapto-nuria, a study in chemical individuality'[1], and in it he first drew attention to the biological significance of differences of this kind.

Alkaptonuria is a rare condition which is characterised by the excretion of large quantities of homogentisic acid (Fig. 1). Several grams of this substance may be passed daily in the urine, and its excretion is continuous and goes on throughout life. It is a very striking peculiarity because the urine goes black on standing, and the disorder is often recognised in early infancy by the characteristic staining of the napkins. The affected individuals are in other respects quite healthy, though as they get older they are rather more prone than other people to develop osteoarthritis.

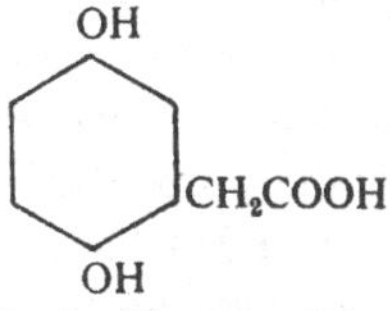

Fig. 1. Homogentisic acid.

Garrod made some fundamental points about the condition. He observed that a person is either frankly alkaptonuric or conforms to the normal type, that is, he either excretes several grams of

homogentisic acid a day, or none at all. Garrod pointed out that
the homogentisic acid must be largely derived from the aminoacid
tyrosine, and that the essential peculiarity of such people was an
inability to break down the benzene ring of this aminoacid in the
normal way. Instead they passed it intact in the urine. It seemed
more appropriate, he suggested, to regard the peculiarity as an aspect
of the person's inborn individuality rather than a disease process in
the ordinary sense.

The other striking feature of the condition to which he drew
attention was its familial distribution. It was often found among
several members of the same family. Frequently two or more of a
group of brothers and sisters would be affected, the parents being
quite normal as were other more distant relatives. Furthermore, the
parents of alkaptonurics were often blood relatives, usually first or
second cousins. The familial distribution of the condition showed a
highly characteristic pattern and Garrod had little hesitation in con-
cluding that it implied a hereditary or genetical basis for the disorder.
It was possible to take this conclusion further. Garrod consulted
Bateson, one of the earliest of British geneticists, who pointed out
that the situation might be readily explained in terms of the then
recently rediscovered laws of Mendel. The frequent occurrence of the
disorder among the brothers and sisters of an alkaptonuric, its rarity
among their antecedents or descendants, and the high incidence of
consanguinous marriage among the parents who were themselves
unaffected, was precisely the type of familial distribution to be
expected if alkaptonuria was inherited as a Mendelian recessive
character. This was in fact the first example of recessive inheritance
to be recognised as such in man.

Garrod therefore interpreted alkaptonuria as an inborn metabolic
variant inherited as a recessive Mendelian character. The metabolic
anomaly apparently lay in a peculiar inability to break down the
benzene ring of the aminoacid tyrosine, and he suggested that this
kind of genetically determined biochemical variation was not a unique
phenomenon, but was probably of general occurrence. He instanced
a number of other metabolic peculiarities which he thought might be
regarded as further examples of such 'chemical individuality'.

Concerning the biological significance of such conditions he made
the following remarks:

If it be, indeed, the case that in alkaptonuria and the other conditions
mentioned we are dealing with individualities in metabolism and not with

the results of morbid processes, the thought naturally presents itself that these are merely extreme examples of variations of chemical behaviour which are probably everywhere present in minor degrees and that just as no two individuals of a species are ever absolutely identical in bodily structure neither are their chemical processes carried out on exactly the same lines. Such chemical differences will be obviously far more subtle than those of form, for whereas the latter are evident to any careful observer the former will only be revealed by elaborate chemical methods.

This passage is remarkably modern in outlook. Alkaptonuria and the other metabolic peculiarities of which Garrod was then aware were all extremely rare. At that time and indeed until very recently such conditions have been regarded in medicine as little more than curiosities of no general importance. At a time when both the study of genetics and of human biochemistry were still in their infancy, Garrod showed singular insight in perceiving the biological interest of these disorders. He was probably alone among the physicians of his day in appreciating that the detailed study of these rare and peculiar conditions was likely to throw considerable light on the general nature of human variability.

Garrod developed the argument in his Croonian Lectures in 1908 [2] and in later works [3], with a detailed examination of a number of other analogous disorders such as cystinuria, porphyria, and pentosuria. He called them 'inborn errors of metabolism'. Since then many further examples of the same kind of thing have been discovered. These include phenylketonuria, galactosaemia, fructosuria, the glycogen storage diseases, and the various forms of goitrous cretinism. Although they represent a very diverse series of biochemical peculiarities and differ widely from one another in their clinical significance, they nevertheless have in common certain characteristic features which make it profitable to study them together.

They each occur much more frequently among the close relatives of affected individuals than in the general population. Munro [4], for example, found among 179 brothers and sisters of phenylketonuric patients thirty-eight further examples of the condition. In contrast he estimated that the incidence of the disorder in the general population from which they were drawn was something of the order of 1 in 40,000. This high familial concentration cannot in general be accounted for in terms of differences between environments in which different family groups live, because in each case the underlying biochemical peculiarity appears to be little influenced by ordinary environmental variations. The simplest explanation in fact is that the conditions are each genetically determined. The occurrence in some cases of an increased frequency of parental consanguinity, and the existence of highly characteristic types of pedigree configurations afford further evidence that the peculiarities are inborn and hereditary.

Characteristically, each of these peculiarities serves to divide human beings more or less sharply into separate groups differing metabolically from each other in some particular respect. The metabolic anomaly is in each instance highly specific. A fructosuric, for example, is unable to metabolise fructose completely, but his ability to deal with glucose and other sugars is not impaired. His brothers and sisters are more likely than an unrelated person to exhibit fructosuria. They are, however, no more likely than anybody else to manifest other quite different metabolic peculiarities. Even closely related disorders such as phenylketonuria and alkaptonuria, both of which represent abnormalities in the oxidation of the aromatic aminoacids, occur independently and are inherited quite specifically.

The effects on the viability of the individual and on his biological fitness, that is his capacity to reproduce, are very diverse. Fructosuria and pentosuria, for example, seem to confer no disadvantage at all on the affected individuals. They remain quite healthy and their reproductive ability is not curtailed; such conditions can only be regarded as normal variants. In other cases serious consequences are regularly associated with the metabolic abnormality. Galactosaemia, for example, if left untreated, usually results in severe liver damage, cataract formation, mental impairment, and retardation of growth. It is often fatal in early life. Phenylketonuria, while not usually leading to early death, is nevertheless always associated with some degree of mental defect. This usually amounts to idiocy or imbecility, and necessarily involves a gross curtailment of biological fitness. In practice it is difficult in these various conditions to draw any sharp line between what may be regarded as normal variations and what must be considered as pathological. Every degree of intermediacy may be encountered.

Thus the 'inborn errors of metabolism' can be regarded as genetically determined biochemical variations, which sharply characterise human beings. They are highly specific and represent many diverse metabolic phenomena, which result in very varied effects on the viability and fitness of the individual.

Garrod developed a simple hypothesis which he thought might explain in a general way the common features of the various 'inborn errors of metabolism'. He suggested that in each condition the body was unable to perform some particular step in the normal course of metabolism. This was presumably due to the congenital absence of the enzyme usually concerned in catalysing the step in question, and as a result a block occurred at this point in the metabolic processes. The unusual concentrations of metabolites in the body fluids and excretions, and the various clinical signs and symptoms with which they might be associated, could all ultimately be traced back to the inability to perform this single step in the metabolic sequence. Thus, if we consider a series of reactions which can be written

$$A \rightarrow B \rightarrow C \rightarrow D \rightarrow E$$
$$\alpha \quad \beta \quad \gamma \quad \delta$$

the congenital absence of the enzyme γ would be expected to result in a failure to form the metabolite D from its precursor C, and in consequence C would tend to accumulate and perhaps be excreted in unusual amount. The formation of C in excessive quantities or the failure to form D might result in diverse consequences for the organism. Their effect on its viability and fitness would depend on the character of the particular metabolites involved, and on the relative importance of the disturbed sequence of reactions in the overall biochemical economy of the body.

There is little doubt that this concept of an inborn metabolic block provides an accurate and useful way of understanding the biochemical disturbances to be found in many inherited abnormalities. For example, the sequence of reactions which are believed to take place during the normal oxidation of phenylalanine and tyrosine are shown in Fig. 2. The peculiar composition of the body fluids and urine in phenylketonuria can largely be accounted for in terms of a metabolic block at the point A, and it has now been demonstrated directly that the enzyme system necessary to carry out this step is indeed deficient in phenylketonuria. Similarly a block at point B would be expected to result in the kind of changes which are observed in alkaptonuria. Here again a specific deficiency of the relevant enzyme has been demonstrated directly.

However, it should be pointed out that not all the conditions which Garrod originally regarded as examples of metabolic errors can be explained in terms of abnormalities of intermediary metabolism. The excessive excretion of cystine and certain other aminoacids in classical cystinuria, for example, is now thought to be due not to a defect in the intermediary metabolism of cystine, but to a failure in renal tubular reabsorption from the glomerular filtrate. The abnormality is 'renal' rather than 'metabolic'. From the theoretical standpoint the discrepancy is probably only a superficial one. Transport of metabolites across the renal tubule cells, as across other membranes in the body, is in general an active and highly specific process. Although little is known about the detailed mechanisms involved, they are probably enzymically controlled. An inborn defect in the formation of a specific enzyme in the renal tubule cells concerned in the transport of cystine might well be the explanation of classical

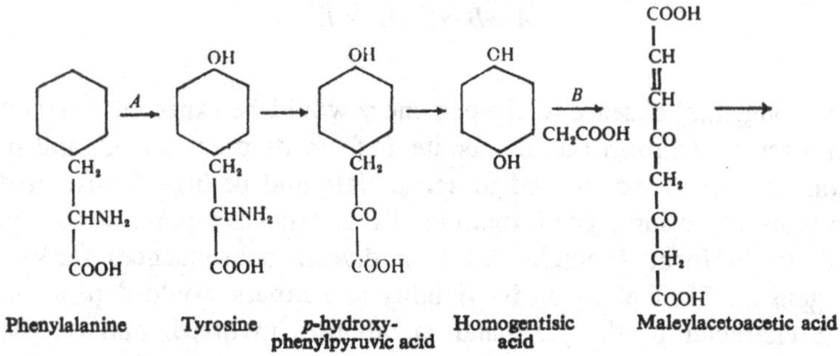

Fig. 2. Steps in the oxidation of phenylalanine and tyrosine.

cystinuria, and such an explanation would in principle be much the same as that advanced to account for the inborn abnormalities in intermediary metabolism.

The important implication of this general theory of the inborn errors of metabolism was that genetical factors could play a specific role in the formation of enzymes. The idea was later to be considerably extended and elaborated. In the form of the one gene–one enzyme hypothesis it became a key working hypothesis in experimental genetics. This was largely the result of the experimental production in large numbers of 'biochemical' mutants in certain organisms such as the bread mould, *Neurospora*. In essence these mutants exhibited specific blocks in metabolism of the kind originally envisaged by Garrod to explain the 'inborn errors of metabolism'.

Although all enzymes are probably proteins, not all proteins behave as enzymes. If it is true that inherited differences can lead to differences in enzyme formation, then it might be anticipated that inborn differences in the formation of proteins with other kinds of functional properties also occur. This, indeed, turns out to be the case. In some instances the inherited peculiarity results in a complete or almost complete failure to synthesise the particular protein or group of proteins. This is so, for example, in afibrinogenaemia, agammaglobulinaemia, and analbuminaemia. Perhaps of more fundamental significance, however, are those inherited differences which result not in the failure to form a particular protein, but in the formation of proteins similar in most respects to those usually encountered but differing from them in the finer details of their structural organisation and their physico-chemical properties. The most important example of this kind of phenomenon is provided by the series of different types of haemoglobin which have now been identified in human beings. The character of the haemoglobin or haemoglobins which an individual possesses appears to depend more or less directly on certain features of his genetical constitution.

Another example of inherited variation in protein synthesis is the differences which have been encountered between people in the properties of certain of their plasma proteins, the haptoglobins. Individuals may be divided quite sharply into three classes according to the type of haptoglobin they possess. In European populations these three classes of individual occur with a frequency of about 16 per cent, 48 per cent and 36 per cent respectively. In this situation it is clearly impossible to regard one type of haptoglobin as 'normal' and another as 'abnormal'. Each type represents a different version of 'normality', and in any one individual it reflects one particular facet of his biochemical individuality and genetical constitution.

In fact, the first demonstration that subtle chemical differences between human beings may be a common phenomenon was provided by Landsteiner's fundamental work on the blood groups, the first results of which were published at about the same time as were Garrod's. It was found that people could be classified into four groups according to whether they possessed one (A), another (B), both (AB), or neither (O) of two different antigenic substances on the surfaces of their red blood cells. These substances are now thought to be mucopolysaccharides. The differences in their immunological specificity imply differences in their chemical structures and hence in their biosynthesis. These differences are genetically determined.

Subsequently a number of other genetically determined systems of blood-group antigens such as the MN system and the Rh system were discovered. In general, each system is determined independently of the others, so that any single individual has a complex of antigenic substances present on the surface of his red cells which includes components belonging to each of these different systems. By using all the antisera which are available to characterise these different antigens, it is now possible to define more than a million different classes of people according to whether they possess in their red cells one or another combination of these antigenic substances. Many of these possible combinations are extremely rare, but the discriminative power of the technique is illustrated by the findings of Race and his colleagues(5) who, using seventeen different antisera, were able to classify 475 Londoners into 296 distinct types. Of these, 211 antigenic combinations occurred only once, and no more than ten individuals had the same combination. This affords some measure of the individual differentiation occurring in respect of what is only one relatively minor feature of the body's biochemical architecture.

The uniqueness of the biochemical make-up of the individual is further illustrated by the phenomena which occur when attempts are made to transplant skin or other tissues from one person to another. In general such transplants fail to take unless the individuals concerned are uniovular twins and therefore have the same genetical constitution, or unless the recipient of the graft has some defect in his capacity to form antibodies, as for example occurs in agammaglobulinaemia. The failure of a tissue transplant to take successfully can be attributed to an immunological reaction which develops in the recipient against foreign substances which are introduced. These foreign substances which induce the reaction must be macromolecules, and one can conclude that the transplanted tissue contains macromolecules different in structure from the equivalent ones present in the recipient's own tissues.

There is thus ample indication of inborn diversity in the biochemical make-up of human beings. This may be reflected in differences in the patterns of metabolic processes, or in differences in the structures of macromolecules. A particular kind of variant may be rare or common. It may result in pathological consequences for the individual or it may lead to no obvious effect on viability or biological fitness. It is probable that, with the exception of uniovular twins, no two human beings are exactly alike in their inborn biochemical potentialities. The analysis of this biochemical individuality forms the subject-matter of human biochemical genetics.

Chromosomes and genes

Modern genetics views heredity as an atomistic process. The genetical constitution of an individual is regarded as being composed of a large number of specific functional units which are directly inherited from his parents. Inborn differences between people are thought of as being due to specific differences in the character of these units, and differences in the combinations in which they occur.

This view is based on a vast amount of experimental evidence in animals, plants, and micro-organisms. The principles that have emerged appear to have a remarkable degree of generality, and although direct evidence for certain of them is not available in the human species, nevertheless there seems little doubt that they apply. An account of general genetics is outside the scope of this book. However, in order to facilitate the subsequent discussion some of the key concepts will be outlined somewhat dogmatically.

An individual arises from the fusion of two cells or gametes derived from his parents: the ovum from the mother, and the sperm from the father. The hereditary potentialities of the new individual or zygote formed by the fertilisation of the ovum by the sperm are derived from the characteristics of these two component cells. Most of the genetical character of these cells is determined by the particular properties of a series of thread-like structures present in their nuclei and known as chromosomes. Chromosomes are differentiated longitudinally into more or less discrete regions with genetically distinct properties. These chromosomal subdivisions are called genes, and they represent the specific units involved in Mendelian heredity. Each chromosome contains a large number of genes, possibly hundreds or even thousands. They are arranged in a characteristic order along its length, so that each gene can be said to have its own special position in any one particular chromosome. This is called its locus.

The nucleus of each human gamete is now thought to contain twenty-three chromosomes (6, 7). Each of them is different from the others in its genetical properties. When the ovum and sperm come together their nuclei fuse, so that the fertilised egg thus formed has a nucleus containing forty-six chromosomes, made up of twenty-three pairs. In general, each member of such a pair of homologous chromosomes is similar in its genetical properties to its fellow. Each member of the pair contains the same number of genes, and the gene loci are arranged in exactly the same order. There is, however, one pair of chromosomes that is exceptional in this respect. They are called the sex chromosomes. In males, the pair of sex chromosomes is made up of one long one (the X chromosome) and one short one (the Y chromosome). The X chromosome certainly contains genes not represented on the Y chromosome, and it is possible that the Y chromosome contains genes not represented on the X. The X chromosome is derived from the mother, and the Y from the father. In females there are two X chromosomes and they resemble one another in the same way as do the members of the other twenty-two pairs of so-called 'autosomal' chromosomes.

In the development of the individual from the fertilised egg a successive series of cell divisions takes place. Prior to each cell division the chromosomes are duplicated in such a way that each of the two daughter cells comes to contain a set of chromosomes exactly like the other and like those of the parent cells. Hence they possess the same complement of genes. Thus with a few exceptions every cell in the body is thought to possess the same content of genetical determinants in its nucleus as every other cell. The main exception occurs in the formation of the sex cells or gametes. Here a special type of cell division occurs (meiosis), the result of which is that only one member of each pair of chromosomes appears in each gamete. Thus the gametes contain twenty-three chromosomes each.

A gene is an extremely stable entity and its replication at each cell division is very exact. Occasionally, however, it may undergo a sudden change, called a mutation. The new form of the gene so produced is then duplicated at each cell division in the same way as the old one, so that the mutant form persists. As a result of past mutations a number of alternative forms of the same gene may occur at a particular chromosomal locus. These are called alleles. The same chromosomal locus will in general be represented twice in a fertilised ovum, once on each of a pair of homologous chromosomes. Thus only two alleles of the same gene can be present, one derived from the father and one from the mother. If these two alleles are the same the individual is said to be homozygous with respect to the genes present at that locus. If they are different he is said to be heterozygous. A heterozygous person will, with the rare exceptions resulting from further mutations, come to possess replicates of the same two alleles in the nucleus of each of his somatic cells. Since the sex cells or gametes only contain one member of each pair of chromosomes, half of them will contain one allele, and half the other.

An individual is likely to be heterozygous for genes at many different loci on many different chromosomes. Because only one gene from each pair of alleles is transmitted to any one of his offspring, the alleles at the various chromosomal loci are continually being reassorted into new combinations. The degree of possible reassortment is greatly extended by the phenomenon known as crossing over. This involves the exchange of material between two homologous chromosomes during meiosis. In general, the closer together two genes are on the same chromosome the less likely are they to be separated by crossing over. Gene loci on the same chromosome are said to be linked, and the analysis of the relative frequency with which different genes on the same chromosome are separated by crossing over allows an assessment to be made of the relative positions of the different loci. In this way it is possible to construct detailed 'maps' of the different chromosomes which indicate the order of the gene loci present. So far, however, only a very few examples of 'linked' genes have been identified in human beings.

Each gene can be regarded as having a specific functional role in the biochemistry of the cell, and hence in the biochemical economy of the body as a whole. A mutation presumably alters the structure of a gene in some way and this may be expected to be reflected in its functional behaviour. In practice we can only know anything at all about a particular gene if as a result of past mutations it occurs in more than one allelic form, and if the different possible combinations of allelic genes result in detectable differences between the individuals who carry them. The simplest situation which can be analysed occurs where in any population of individuals there exist at a particular chromosomal locus one or other of two allelic genes. If these are called A and a, then with respect to this particular chromosomal locus three genetically distinct types of individual will occur, and they can be designated AA, Aa, aa. Each of these three types of individual will be in some respect biochemically different from the others. If our techniques of investigation are adequate it may, in fact, be possible to distinguish each of these three types clearly from the others. Often, however, only two classes of individual may be recognised; one which we can designate ā, corresponding to the genotype aa, and the other designated as Ā, corresponding to the genotypes AA and Aa, which are indistinguishable. In such circumstances it may be said that the gene A is dominant to the gene a, and that a is recessive to A. The class Ā is called the phenotype corresponding to the genotypes AA and Aa.

The concept of the gene implies that this biological unit must have several remarkable properties. It must play a specific part in cell metabolism, it must be capable of exact duplication, and, although it must in general be an extremely stable structure, it must nevertheless be susceptible to occasional sudden change or mutation resulting in the formation of a new unit differing structurally from the original one but self-reproducing in its new form. In practice the precise definition of a gene in experimental terms proves to be rather difficult. This is because, in situations susceptible to very refined analysis, the gene defined as a unit of function turns out to be subdivisible in terms of crossing over, or of mutation. These difficulties are ultimately reflections of our imperfect understanding of the structural organisation of the hereditary material which makes up the chromosomes. For the present, however, the idea of genes as the inherited units of biochemical function forms an adequate working hypothesis in human genetics.

Nature and nurture

Differences between people may be due not only to differences in their inborn constitutions, but also to differences in the environments in which they developed and in which they live. Causes of 'environmental' differences (or nurture) can be said to be those which operate subsequently to the formation of the fertilised ovum. They include differences in intrauterine conditions as well as more obvious differences occurring after birth. Causes of inborn differences (or nature) are those which act prior to the fertilisation of the ovum. They include whatever factors may be responsible for gene mutation.

In some instances environmental factors or nurture appear to be of relatively little importance in determining why one person differs from another in some particular attribute. This is thought to be so, for example, in the case of the blood-group antigens. All the available evidence suggests that a given genetical constitution necessarily results, provided the organism is viable, in the appearance of a particular pattern of antigenic substances on the red-cell surface. This appears to be the same over a very wide range of possible environments. Put another way, we can say that differences in the biosynthesis of these substances determined by structural differences in certain genes are little if at all susceptible to modification by metabolic variations induced by external causes.

Often, however, the situation is not so simple. Both nature and nurture may play a significant part in determining the difference between people which one observes, and their respective roles can be very difficult to disentangle. This is the case, for example, with respect to the occurrence of the common disorder of carbohydrate metabolism known as diabetes mellitus. Environmental factors certainly influence the manifestation of this disease. The precise nature of these is still obscure, but among other things variations in the diet, both qualitative and quantitative, appear to be important. There was, for example, a marked fall in mortality rates and probably also the morbidity rates of diabetes mellitus in Europe during and in the years immediately following the two world wars. This seems to be closely related to food rationing, and it has been suggested that the most important factor was the restriction of fats[8]. Similarly differences in incidence between different social groups and different occupations may be roughly correlated with differences in dietary habits.

On the other hand, diabetes occurs very much more commonly among the close relatives of affected individuals than in the general population. Because there are usually no obvious environmental differences which might plausibly explain why one member of a family and not another should develop the condition, and why the abnormality should be particularly prevalent in some family groups and not in others living in rather similar environmental circumstances, this high familial concentration has been generally attributed to genetical factors. The simplest explanation is that some people are more predisposed to develop the condition than others. The predisposition is mainly determined by genetical factors, but whether or not the predisposed individual actually manifests the condition will depend on environmental factors, such as diet. The situation is complex and more detailed analysis suggests that in different cases nature and nurture probably vary in their relative importance.

The interaction of nature and nurture in its simplest form is perhaps most clearly illustrated by the situation in galactosaemia, a typical 'inborn error of metabolism'. This condition probably only occurs if an individual is homozygous for a particular abnormal gene. This results in a defect in the formation of a certain enzyme which normally plays an essential part in the conversion of galactose-1-phosphate to glucose-1-phosphate. In consequence, galactose cannot be properly metabolised. When galactose is present in the diet the blood galactose becomes elevated, galactose-1-phosphate accumulates in the tissues, and a series of diverse and rather serious pathological disturbances ensues. If, however, a diet entirely free from galactose but adequate in all other respects is provided, the abnormal accumulation of galactose and its phosphorylated derivatives does not occur, carbohydrate metabolism is not impeded and the various clinical consequences are not encountered. Now galactose in the form of the disaccharide lactose is the main carbohydrate constituent of milk, and so in the normal course of events all galactosaemic infants will be exposed to it. The recognition of the disorder and the prompt introduction of a galactose-free diet will stop the further development of tissue damage, and probably allow the infant to grow up in a normal manner. In a sense, then, galactosaemia can be regarded as a specific inherited inability to cope with one particular feature of the normal environment, namely galactose in the diet. If the environment is modified appropriately, the ill effects of this disability are minimised or even prevented. The individual will still differ biochemically from other individuals because he will continue to lack a particular enzyme. In his new environment, however, this will not incommode him. He will as it were be predisposed without being clinically affected. Galactosaemia is of course regarded as an inherited disease because the particular aspect of the environment to which such individuals are ill-adapted is virtually always present. It is, however, not difficult to visualise more complex situations where the feature of the environment to which the individual is poorly adapted is rather more variable. The resultant metabolic disturbance will then depend on the particular form of environment which the individual encounters, as well as on his genetical constitution.

Another important aspect of the nature-nurture problem emerges when one considers differences in the genetical structures of populations living in diverse environments, as well as differences in the genetical constitution of individuals. One of the most striking features of human genetics is the way in which particular genes occur with widely differing frequencies in different populations. This will be considered in rather more detail later, and it is sufficient here to point out that this phenomenon may often be a reflection of the fact that particular genotypes are better adapted to some environments than to others. From the point of view of viability and biological fitness, a particular inborn pattern of metabolic behaviour may be relatively advantageous in one set of environmental conditions and relatively disadvantageous in another. Natural selection would tend to increase the frequency of the more favoured genotypes in the different localities. Changes in the environment would tend to result in changes in the frequency of particular genes because the balance of selective pressures would be altered. Thus, paradoxically, differences in the genetical structures of different populations can be a function of the differences in the environments in which they live.

The exploration of these possibilities in terms of the biochemical effects of specific genes and their influence on biological fitness in different environments is still in its infancy. One of the complications is that a high frequency of one particular genotype in a population necessarily implies the occurrence of others which may be very different in terms of fitness. For example, it seems very probable that individuals heterozygous for the gene which determines the formation of one type of haemoglobin, haemoglobin S, are at some selective advantage in certain parts of Africa, compared with people not carrying this gene. However, a high frequency of this gene in a population necessarily means that a significant proportion of all children born will be homozygous for it. Such individuals develop a severe anaemia and frequently die in childhood or adolescence. Thus, while the gene in a single dose may be advantageous to the organism, the gene in double dose results in a drastic reduction of fitness. The particular frequency a gene assumes in a given population will reflect the fitness of all the different genotypic combinations in which it may occur. Where several alleles exist, the number of possible combinations at the one locus is increased and the situation becomes increasingly complex. Different genotypic combinations may in general be expected to differ from one another to a greater or lesser degree in any one environment, and their relative differences in fitness to vary from one environment to another.

REFERENCES

(1) Garrod, A. E. (1902). *Lancet*, **2**, 1616.
(2) Garrod, A. E. (1908). *Lancet*, **2**, 1, 73, 142, 214.
(3) Garrod, A. E. (1923). *Inborn Errors of Metabolism*, 2nd ed. Oxford University Press.
(4) Munro, T. A. (1947). *Ann. Eugen., Lond.* **16**, 282.
(5) Bertinshaw, D., Lawler, S. D., Holt, H. A., Kirman, B. H. and Race, R. R. (1950). *Ann. Eugen., Lond.* **15**, 234.
(6) Tijo, J. H. and Levan A. (1956). *Hereditas*, **42**, 1.
(7) Ford, C. E. and Hamerton, J. L. (1956). *Acta Genet.* **6**, 264.
(8) Himsworth, H. P. (1949). *Lancet*, **1**, 465.

CHAPTER 2

SOME ASPECTS OF MENDELIAN HEREDITY IN MAN

Gene frequency

In most animals and plants knowledge of the genetical basis of particular inborn differences is derived from the analysis of deliberate, and often highly elaborate, breeding experiments. In human beings this kind of evidence is not available. We are left only with the possibility of inferring the nature of the genetical processes involved by considering the manner in which certain characters, distinguished by one or more techniques, are distributed in human populations and more particularly within different family groups.

The central concept in the genetical analysis of human data is that of gene frequency. This leads to certain conclusions about the frequency with which different combinations of genes may be expected to occur among individuals in a given population, and the way particular combinations will be distributed in families.

If we consider a population where, at a particular locus on one of the autosomal chromosomes there may occur either the gene A or its allele the gene **a**, then, since this chromosome will be represented twice in each person, three genetically distinct types of individual will occur. They are AA, Aa and **aa**. If the numbers of individuals of the three genotypes are

Genotype	AA	Aa	aa
Number of individuals	x	y	z

then p, the gene frequency of the gene A in the population is given by

$$p = (x+y/2)/(x+y+z),$$

and q the gene frequency of the gene **a** in the population is given by

$$q = (z+y/2)/x+y+z.$$

so that $p+q = 1$.

Now it was pointed out independently by Hardy[1], and by Weinburg in 1908[2], that if the population is mating at random and the three genotypes are equally fit, then the relative proportions of the three types of individual in the population is

$$
\begin{array}{ccccc}
\textbf{AA} & : & \textbf{Aa} & : & \textbf{aa} \\
p^2 & : & 2pq & : & q^2
\end{array}
$$

In such a population six different types of mating may occur. Their relative frequencies and the expected frequencies of the different genotypes among their offspring can be readily calculated (Table 1). An important point is that both the gene frequencies and the genotype frequencies are the same in the population of offspring as in the parental population. In other words, the situation represents a form of genetical equilibrium. It is usually referred to as the Hardy-Weinberg equilibrium.

Table 1. *Frequencies of parental mating types and their offspring for an autosomal gene pair, where mating is at random*

Parents		Offspring		
Mating type	Frequency of mating type	AA	Aa	aa
AA × **AA**	p^4	p^4	—	—
AA × **Aa**	$4p^3q$	$2p^3q$	$2p^3q$	—
AA × **aa**	$2p^2q^2$	—	$2p^2q^2$	—
Aa × **Aa**	$4p^2q^2$	p^2q^2	$2p^2q^2$	p^2q^2
Aa × **aa**	$4pq^3$	—	$2pq^3$	$2pq^3$
aa × **aa**	q^4	—	—	q^4
All matings		p^2	$2pq$	q^2

Often the effect of one of the genes (**a**) cannot be recognised in the presence of the other (**A**). The heterozygotes **Aa** are indistinguishable by the available techniques from the homozygotes of genotype **AA**. Hence only two phenotypes will be observed. These are the so-called recessive phenotype ā corresponding to the genotype **aa**, and the so-called dominant phenotype Ā corresponding to individuals of genotypes **AA** and **Aa**. The mating table can be simplified appropriately. The frequencies of the different types of matings and the expected incidence of the two phenotypes among their offspring are shown in Table 2.

A typical application of this is the analysis of the familial distribution of the two gamma globulin types recently discovered by Grubb and Laurell [3]. These workers found that individuals could be divided quite sharply into two types according to whether or not their gamma globulins showed certain serological properties. They called these

Table 2. *Random mating table for an autosomal gene pair* A *and* a, *where only two phenotypes can be recognised. Phenotype* $\bar{A}$ *corresponds to genotypes* AA *and* Aa. *Phenotype* $\bar{a}$ *corresponds to genotype* aa

	Parents	Offspring	
Mating	Frequency of mating	$\bar{A}$	$\bar{a}$
$\bar{A} \times \bar{A}$	$p^2(1+q)^2$	p^2+2p^3q	p^2q^2
$\bar{A} \times \bar{a}$	$2pq^2(1+q)$	$2pq^2$	$2pq^3$
$\bar{a} \times \bar{a}$	q^4	—	q^4
All matings		p^2+2pq	q^2

types Gm (a+) and Gm (a−), and in a random series of 360 healthy Swedish adults they found that 59·7 per cent were Gm (a+) and 40·3 per cent were Gm (a−). The observed distribution of the two types among the progeny of the different types of mating occurring in twenty-eight families is shown in Table 3. Gm (a−) × Gm (a−) matings resulted only in Gm (a−) offspring. This suggests that Gm (a−) is inherited as a recessive character. If this is so, the gene frequency of the gene **Gm** for which Gm (a−) individuals are homozygous will be in this Swedish population 0·635, that is, $\sqrt{0\cdot403}$, and the frequency of the other allele **Gm**^{a} will be 0·365, that is, $1-0\cdot635$. From these gene frequencies the expected numbers of matings of the different types and the expected numbers of the two phenotypes among their progeny may be readily calculated. It will be seen that the agreement between the observed numbers and those theoretically expected is very good.

Table 3. *γ-Globulin types* (Gm (a+) *and* Gm (a−)) *in twenty-eight families. (After Grubb and Laurell, 1956)*

	Parents		Children				
	Number		Gm (a+)		Gm (a−)		
Mating	Obs.	Exp.	Obs.	Exp.	Obs.	Exp.	Total
Gm (a+) × Gm (a+)	9	10	30	28·0	3	5·0	33
Gm (a+) × Gm (a−)	14	13·5	25	22·6	12	14·4	37
Gm (a−) × Gm (a−)	5	4·5	—	—	24	24	24

Rare abnormalities

One important conclusion which follows from the Hardy-Weinberg principle concerns the frequencies with which heterozygotes and homozygotes for a relatively rare gene may be expected to occur in a given population. The point is illustrated in Table 4, from which it can be seen that when the gene a is relatively uncommon, the frequency of heterozygotes approximates to twice the gene frequency, that is, $2q$, and such individuals occur very much more commonly in the population than do the homozygotes **aa**, which have a frequency of q^2.

Table 4. *Incidence of heterozygotes and homozygotes at different gene frequencies*

Frequency of gene a q	Incidence of heterozygotes **Aa** $2pq$	Incidence of homozygotes **aa** q^2	Ratio heterozygotes to homozygotes $2pq:q^2$
0·5	0·5	0·25	2:1
0·2	0·32	0·04	8:1
0·1	0·18	0·01	18:1
0·01	0·0198	0·0001	198:1
0·001	0·001998	0·000001	1998:1
0·0001	0·00019998	0·00000001	19998:1

This accounts for some of the characteristic features of the familial distribution of rare 'recessive' abnormalities. Affected individuals (**aa**) will only be derived from matings in which both parents carry the gene **a**. The possible matings are

Father		Mother
Aa	×	**Aa**
Aa	×	**aa**
aa	×	**Aa**
aa	×	**aa**

Since **Aa** individuals will be so much commoner than **aa** individuals, the great majority of affected individuals will be derived from matings between two heterozygotes. In other words, both parents will be unaffected in most cases. Thus if affected individuals occurred in the population with a frequency of 1 in 40,000, the frequency of heterozygotes would be about 1 in 100, and the relative frequencies of the four types of mating from which affected individuals could arise would be

Father		Mother	
Aa	×	**Aa**	1
Aa	×	**aa**	1/400
aa	×	**Aa**	1/400
aa	×	**aa**	1/160,000

If the abnormality results in a diminished viability or fertility in the affected homozygotes, then the effect will be even more accentuated.

Approximately one-half of the uncles and aunts, one-quarter of the cousins and so on, of the affected individual **aa** will also be heterozygous for the gene **a**. The chance that any of these will mate with a homozygote **AA** is very much greater than the chance of mating with a heterozygote **Aa**. In the example given above it is about a hundred times greater. Consequently it will be rather unusual for any further cases of **aa** individuals to turn up in other branches of the family. In the same way it is much more likely that an affected individual will marry a normal homozygote **AA** than a heterozygote, so it will be uncommon for affected individuals to have affected offspring. On the other hand, the brothers and sisters of affected individuals (**aa**) will also be derived in the main from **Aa** × **Aa** matings. Consequently one in four of them may be expected to be affected.

Thus characteristically a rare recessive abnormality is usually only found in a single sibship in any one family. On the average, one in four of the brothers and sisters of affected individuals will be similarly affected, but the abnormality will be rare among the parents, children and other relatives of affected cases.

Abnormalities determined by a rare gene in single dose, that is occurring in the heterozygotes, show an entirely different type of familial distribution. If the rare abnormal gene is **a**, most of the affected individuals will be **Aa**. They are much more likely to marry normal individuals of genotype **AA** than affected individuals carrying the abnormal gene. On the average, therefore, one expects half their children to be **Aa** and show the abnormality, and half to be **AA** and be unaffected. Rather typical pedigrees result, in which the abnormality is found in several generations and in different branches of the same family. It appears to be transmitted directly from a parent to about half the offspring and so on.

Using the kind of arguments outlined above, it is usually possible to infer from pedigrees of families in which rare abnormalities are segregating whether or not the affected individuals are homozygous or heterozygous for a particular abnormal gene.

Parental consanguinity

The assumption of completely random mating is rarely entirely justified in human populations. There is, for example, usually some degree of inbreeding, which results in a significantly greater proportion of cousin marriages than would be expected in a random mating system. The general effect of this is to increase the proportions of homozygotes relative to heterozygotes. However, where the genes concerned are relatively common the effect in most human populations is too small to be detectable. On the other hand, in the case of rare genes the effect is important, and the incidence of the homozygotes is appreciably increased.

Garrod pointed out in 1902 that a high proportion of cases of alkaptonuria were derived from consanguineous matings and he and Bateson interpreted this as indicating that the affected individuals were homozygous for a rare recessive gene. The same effect has since been noted in many other rare abnormalities, and the finding of a significantly increased frequency of cousin marriage among the parents of patients with particular disorders has become recognised as an important diagnostic feature of homozygosity for a rare gene. This follows from the fact that the close relatives, that is the uncles, aunts, cousins, etc., of a heterozygous individual **Aa** are much more likely to carry the rare gene **a** than are unrelated individuals chosen at random from the general population. Therefore if such a heterozygous person marries his first cousin, the probability that his partner is also heterozygous for the same rare gene is relatively high, and hence the probability that one or more of his offspring will be homozygous (**aa**) is increased, compared with the probability of this if he marries an unrelated person. As a result the incidence of cousin marriage among parents of individuals homozygous for a rare gene may be expected to be higher than that in the general population. For similar reasons the occurrence of a parent and child both homozygous for a rare gene is much more likely to be found if the parent has married a close relation than if he has not.

The incidence of parental consanguinity to be expected in any particular homozygous condition in a given population will depend on the degree of inbreeding in the population as a whole and on the frequency of the particular gene concerned. Dahlberg's [4] formula

$$F = \frac{c(1+15q)}{16q+c(1-q)}$$

where $c =$ the incidence of first cousin marriages in the general population, and $q =$ the gene frequency of the rare gene **a**, gives an approximate estimate, F, of the incidence of first cousin marriages to be expected among parents of homozygous individuals **aa**. Estimates of F assuming different values for c and q are given in Table 5. It is apparent that the less frequent is the homozygous condition in the general population the higher is the incidence of cousin marriage expected among the parents of affected individuals.

Table 5. *Percentage of first cousin parentage (F) for rare 'homozygous' disorders*

Case frequency q^2	Gene frequency q	Frequency of first cousin marriages in general population (c)		
		0·1 % (F)%	0·5 % (F)%	1·0 % (F)%
1/400	1/20	0·2	1·1	2·2
1/10,000	1/100	0·7	3·5	6·8
1/40,000	1/200	1·3	6·3	11·9
1/1,000,000	1/1000	6·0	24·2	38·5

The formula may also be used to get a rough estimate of the gene frequency q from the observed values of F and c. Here

$$q = \frac{c(1-F)}{16F - 15c - cF}.$$

Typical of the kind of results which may be obtained are those of Munro on phenylketonuria [5]. He found that five out of forty-seven pairs of parents of sibships in which phenylketonuria occurred were first cousins. Thus here $F = 5/47 = 0.106$. The incidence of first cousin marriage in the population he was studying was thought to be about 8 per 1000 (that is, 0·008). Hence

$$q = \frac{0.008 \, (1 - 0.106)}{16 \, (0.106) - 15 \, (0.008) - (0.008)(0.106)}$$
$$= 0.0045.$$

He estimated independently that the incidence of phenylketonuria in the population was roughly 1 in 40,000. This implies a gene frequency of $\sqrt{(1/40,000)} = 1/200 = 0.005$. In view of the errors involved in the various frequency estimates, the agreement between the two values of q is remarkably good.

The precise application of this and similar, more exact, formulae which have been worked out, is in practice rather difficult in most situations in human genetics. This is largely because of uncertainties regarding the first cousin marriage rate, or of the coefficient of in-breeding which is a more precise measure of the inbreeding of a population. Large human populations tend to be composed of multiple subpopulations which may vary in their degrees of inter-connection with one another, and also in their degree of inbreeding. Consequently cases homozygous for a particular rare gene may be rather irregularly distributed. Another difficulty is that in many populations during the last fifty years there has been a marked relaxation of inbreeding reflected by a fall in the rate of first cousin marriages, consequent on social changes and increased population mobility. One effect of this has probably been to diminish the frequency of certain rare recessive conditions without making much appreciable difference to the gene frequency.

Heterozygotes and homozygotes

The distinction which is usually made in human genetics between 'dominant' and 'recessive' modes of inheritance of different un-common abnormalities depends essentially on whether or not the abnormality which is being studied is evident in individuals hetero-zygous or homozygous for the particular gene responsible. So-called 'dominant' inheritance occurs when the great majority of affected individuals are heterozygous for the gene, that is, possess it only in single dose. So-called 'recessive' inheritance refers to the situation when only individuals homozygous for the abnormal gene are affected and the heterozygotes are indistinguishable from the homozygotes for the normal allele. Both these terms require qualification and the distinction between the two types of situation is by no means as clear cut as is often suggested.

Strictly speaking the term dominance implies that the effects produced by a particular abnormal gene in single dose are the same as in double dose. The heterozygotes and the homozygotes exhibit the same peculiarity. In the case of many so-called 'dominant' abnormalities this point has not been established because the homozygote is evidently so rare that it has not been observed, or if it has been observed it has not been recognised for what it is. If, for example, heterozygotes showing a particular abnormality occurred with a frequency as high as 1 in 5000 of a population, the gene frequency of the abnormal gene would be about 1 in 10,000 and the expected frequency of homozygotes would be of the order of one in one hundred million. Inbreeding might make it a little commoner, but nevertheless it would be excessively rare, and might not, in fact, occur in any one generation. Consequently, we have little idea what the characteristics of individuals homozygous for genes such as those which in heterozygotes result in such conditions as acute intermittent porphyria or pitressin-sensitive diabetes insipidus, are likely to be.

In 'recessive' conditions both the homozygotes and the heterozygotes are available for investigation. While it is true that in most cases the heterozygotes appear to be indistinguishable from the homozygotes for the normal allele, a number of examples are now known where detailed investigation of the heterozygotes has revealed minor peculiarities which are evidently due to the effect of the abnormal gene in single dose. The abnormality in the heterozygote in these cases is usually qualitatively similar to that found in the homozygote, but much less in degree. In consequence, it usually does not lead to any pathological consequences and superficially the heterozygotes appear quite normal. A useful general term to cover such situations is to say that the abnormality is 'incompletely recessive'. However, the important point is that with the progressive development of the subject and the more detailed investigation of heterozygotes in many more different 'recessive' disorders, it seems probable that this will turn out to be the general situation rather than the exceptional one.

The effect of a particular gene may be examined at many levels and by a variety of different techniques. A consideration of the results obtained in those situations where peculiarities in both the heterozygotes and the homozygotes for a particular gene have been clearly characterised suggests that whether a gene is spoken of as completely recessive or not depends largely on what facet of the abnormality produced is being investigated, and what techniques are available for its study. In phenylketonuria, for example, the abnormal homozygotes are usually grossly mentally defective, excrete large amounts of phenylpyruvic acid and other unusual metabolites in their urine and have a very high level of phenylalanine in their blood plasma. These phenomena are probably all consequences of a specific enzyme deficiency. The heterozygote is not mentally defective, and does not show any abnormal excretion of phenylpyruvic acid in his urine. His fasting plasma phenylalanine is, however, on the average slightly higher than that found in normal individuals, and when subjected to a large dose of phenylalanine his plasma phenylalanine level rises to somewhat greater values than do those of normal people under the same conditions. Presumably there is a partial enzyme deficiency in the heterozygotes, but the amount of enzyme still formed is adequate to cope with normal metabolic requirements and no ill-effects ensue. Thus the mental defect and the phenylpyruvic acid excretion could be regarded as 'recessive' characters, and the fasting plasma phenylalanine levels and the response to the phenylalanine tolerance test as 'incompletely recessive' characters. The differences, however, are essentially reflections of the amount of the specific enzyme activity present in the livers of the two kinds of individuals. This in turn depends on whether the abnormal gene is present in single or double dose, or perhaps more correctly in this case on whether the normal allele is present in single dose or not at all. At this level of analysis the terms dominance and recessivity are not very useful.

Another interesting example of the same sort of thing is provided by one of the types of classical cystinuria. The homozygotes excrete grossly abnormal quantities of cystine, lysine, arginine and ornithine in their urine. The heterozygotes excrete moderately increased quantities of cystine and lysine, but the excretion of arginine and probably also of ornithine are not usually elevated. Thus, if one only had available a method for determining arginine in urine, the peculiarity would appear to be completely recessive. If, however, one can estimate cystine or lysine, a different picture emerges. In fact, the abnormal excretion of these four aminoacids appears to depend on a specific defect in renal tubular reabsorption, and the relative quantities excreted in the heterozygotes and the homozygotes on the degree of this abnormality.

The same principle is illustrated by the findings in the sickle-cell trait and in sickle-cell anaemia, which occur respectively in individuals heterozygous and homozygous for a single abnormal gene. The sickling phenomenon, that is the characteristic alteration of shape of the erythrocytes on deoxygenation, is found in both heterozygotes and homozygotes. Anaemia occurs only in the homozygotes. Thus the former might be regarded as a dominant character and the latter as a recessive one. The reason for these differences is that while most of the haemoglobin formed in the homozygote is of the abnormal or sickle-cell type, less than half of the haemoglobin formed in the heterozygotes is of this kind. There is enough sickle-cell haemoglobin synthesised in both heterozygotes and homozygotes to cause the sickling phenomenon, but only in the homozygotes is the disturbance sufficiently great to result in chronic haemolytic anaemia.

In general it appears that, while the terms dominance and recessivity may be useful descriptively, the important problem with respect to any particular gene is the detailed characterisation of the effects produced in the heterozygous and homozygous states.

An interesting point which emerges from the consideration of gene frequencies is that, although a disorder produced by a gene in homozygotes may be relatively rare, nevertheless individuals who are heterozygous for the gene may constitute an appreciable fraction of the population. Thus phenylketonuria occurs with an incidence of about 1 in 40,000 in the United Kingdom. The gene frequency is about 1 in 200, and the incidence of heterozygotes about 1 in 100. Thus approximately 1 per cent of the general population carry an abnormal gene which in double dose results in a severe form of mental defect. There are many similar rare 'recessive' diseases known, and it seems probable therefore that a substantial proportion of the so-called 'normal' members of the population are heterozygous for one or another gene which in homozygotes produces a severe disease. Probably many genes also exist which in homozygotes are lethal in pre- or neonatal life, and whose effects have not in consequence been clearly characterised. Indeed, it has been suggested that most people may be heterozygous for at least one gene which results in severe pathological consequences when it occurs in double dose. Thus the genetical structure of a population, even with respect only to those genes which cause rare 'recessive' abnormalities, is very much more complex than might seem apparent at first sight.

It has already been pointed out that in some cases of apparently 'recessive' abnormalities, the heterozygotes can in fact be shown to exhibit some minor peculiarity. The metabolism of phenylalanine, for example, is slightly different in phenylketonuric heterozygotes from that in other normal people. The effect here can be regarded as constituting one part of the so-called normal individual variation in phenylalanine metabolism. In other words, a gene which in homozygotes produces a major metabolic disorder can also play a part in determining biochemical variation between normal, healthy individuals. This illustrates an interesting facet of the general interrelation between so-called 'normal variation' and so-called 'pathological variation'.

Sex linkage

The application of the Hardy-Weinberg principle to genes which are located on that part of the X chromosome which has no homologue in the Y chromosome, necessitates a consideration of the two sexes separately, because males have only one X chromosome, while females have two. Where there are two allelic genes **A** and **a** with frequencies p and q, there will be three types of females **AA**, **Aa** and **aa** whose relative incidence will be $p^2:2pq:q^2$. There will however be only two types of male **A** and **a**, and the relative incidence here will be the same as the gene frequencies (that is, $p:q$).

A sex-linked 'recessive' abnormality is one which is apparent in all the males carrying the gene, but only in females who are homozygous for it. In consequence, affected males will be commoner than affected females, and when the responsible gene is rare, the condition will be almost entirely confined to males.

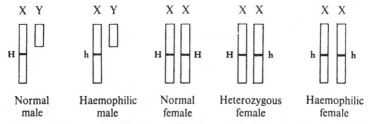

X Y   X Y   X X   X X   X X

H   h   H   H   H   h   h   h

Normal male   Haemophilic male   Normal female   Heterozygous female   Haemophilic female

Fig. 3. Diagramatic representation of the X and Y chromosomes and of different genotypes involving the gene for haemophilia **h**, and its normal allele **H**.

Males transmit their X chromosomes to each of their daughters and their Y chromosomes to each of their sons. Females transmit one or other of their X chromosomes to each of their daughters and also to each of their sons. Consequently, rather characteristic pedigrees occur. The classical example is haemophilia which is thought to be determined by a rare 'recessive' gene on the X chromosome (Fig. 3). Since a male receives his X chromosome from his mother and his Y chromosome from his father, haemophilic males will receive the abnormal gene only from their mothers. They will pass the gene on to all their daughters but not to their sons. A heterozygous (or carrier) female will carry the abnormal gene on one X chromosome and its normal allele on the other. If, as is usually the case, she marries a normal male, half the male offspring will on the average receive the abnormal gene and be affected, and half the female offspring will be heterozygous like their mothers. Thus although the disease is almost entirely peculiar to males, it will appear to be transmitted by females.

Female haemophilics can be produced from a mating between a male haemophilic and a female heterozygote. In these circumstances, half the daughters would on the average be homozygous for the abnormal gene and show the disease. Such matings, however, must be extremely rare. It has been estimated that about 1 in 10,000 of all male children born are haemophilic [6]. This means that the frequency of the haemophilia gene is about 1 in 10,000. It follows that among females about 1 in 5000 are heterozygous for this gene (**h**). Thus a male haemophilic if he survives to adult life is about 5000 times more likely to marry a normal female (**HH**) than a heterozygous one (**Hh**). Inbreeding in the population might make this type of mating a little commoner, but even allowing for this it will still be extremely rare. Nevertheless, what appear to have been authentic examples of such matings giving rise to female haemophilics have been described [7, 8].

Genetical equilibrium

The relative frequencies of the different genotypes in a population as predicted by the Hardy-Weinberg formulae represent a state of equilibrium. Such an equilibrium is said to be neutral in type rather than stable, because any chance fluctuations in gene frequency from one generation to another are perpetuated and there is no tendency for the system to revert to its original state. Fortuitous changes in gene frequency may occur because the relative proportions of different types of mating deviate by chance from those theoretically expected, or because the actual proportions of the different genotypes resulting from some of the matings happen to depart from those theoretically predicted. Such fortuitous changes in gene frequency from one generation to the next are referred to as 'genetic drift'. They are likely to be relatively insignificant where the interbreeding population is large, but may be important in small populations or in subpopulations which have become separated for some social or geographical reason from a larger group. It is possible that some of the diversity in gene frequency which is observed between different human populations in respect to certain genes may have been the consequence of this kind of phenomenon. Theoretically the gene frequency will only be exactly the same in successive generations if the population size is infinitely large.

Another underlying assumption is that the different genotypes present in the population are of equal biological fitness. That is to say, no one genotype has a selective advantage over any other in terms of viability or fertility. This also probably represents an ideal situation. In practice, it is thought likely that virtually all gene differences do result in selective differences of some kind. However, in the case of many common genetically determined polymorphisms which are observed in human populations, any selective differences between the various genotypes are evidently rather small, and the frequencies of the different genotypes which are observed agree remarkably well with those expected from the Hardy-Weinberg formulae. This is so, for example, in the case of most of the genes which determine the various blood group systems. In other instances, however, it is quite apparent that marked differences in fitness do exist between the various genotypes, and the Hardy-Weinberg formulae require appropriate modification to allow for this.

In general, genes which produce deleterious effects in certain genotypes will tend to be eliminated from the population by natural selection. The biological fitness of a particular genotype is a reflection of how far individuals with this genotype contribute offspring to the next generation compared with other people. Their fitness may be reduced because they suffer from some condition which makes them less likely to survive to adult life, or because even if they do survive they are handicapped in some way, so that on the average they have fewer children than other individuals. The pressure of natural selection against a particular gene and hence the rate at which it will tend to be eliminated from the population will depend on the biological fitness of the various genotypes in which it occurs and on their relative frequencies. For example, individuals homozygous for the gene which causes phenylketonuria are usually imbeciles or idiots. They rarely have children and their contribution to the next generation is virtually zero. On the other hand, heterozygotes for this gene appear to be at least as fit as people not carrying it at all. Consequently, only the small proportion of phenylketonuric genes which are present in the homozygotes are being subjected to selection in any one generation. In contrast to this, where an abnormality associated with some loss of fitness occurs in individuals heterozygous for a particular gene, then all the abnormal genes in the population will be exposed to some measure of selection.

However, even when the occurrence of a particular gene in certain genotypes results in an obvious selective disadvantage, an equilibrium may still occur in which the gene is maintained at more or less the same frequency from generation to generation. There are two general types of situation in which such equilibria may be established. The first type involves a balance between mutation and selection, and the second type involves a fitness differential such that heterozygotes are at some advantage compared with homozygotes. The latter situation can be referred to as 'balanced polymorphism'. Both types of situations represent stable equilibria. Provided the conditions remain the same, the system tends to revert to its original state following any disturbances of gene frequency of a chance or fortuitous character. Both of these forms of equilibria are probably important in determining the incidence of different inherited diseases and other inborn peculiarities in human populations.

The occurrence of a mutation of a 'normal' gene to its abnormal allele will tend to offset the loss of the abnormal gene due to natural selection. At a certain point one could expect an equilibrium to be set up in which the loss of the gene, due to the reduced fitness of those genotypes in which it produces deleterious consequences, is balanced by the occurrence of fresh mutations. Once such an equilibrium point has been reached the frequency of the gene, and the incidence of the abnormality which it causes will tend to remain the same in successive generations. The prevalence of the abnormality will be determined by the fitness of the affected individuals, and the mutation rate of the gene in question. For example, in the case of a rare sex-linked recessive condition such as haemophilia an equilibrium would be expected when

$$\mu = \tfrac{1}{3}(1-f)\,q,$$

where μ = the rate of mutation of the normal gene **H** to the haemophilic gene **h**, per chromosome per generation.

q = the gene frequency of **h**. In this case the frequency of haemophilia in all male children at birth.

and f = the fitness of haemophilics. That is the mean number of progeny of all haemophilics born compared with the number of progeny of other members of the population.

The factor $\tfrac{1}{3}$ is introduced because for every haemophilic gene in males there are two in heterozygous females, and selection only acts against the affected individuals.

Haldane [6], using the data obtained in an extensive survey of haemophilia in Denmark by Andreasen, estimated that the frequency of haemophilia in all males at birth was about 13 in every 100,000, and that their biological fitness was about 0·28 of that of normal people. He concluded that if the haemophilic gene was being held in equilibrium in this population by a balance between mutation and selection, then the abnormal gene would occur by fresh mutation in about 1 in 30,000 of all X chromosomes in each generation.

It seems likely that the incidence of many other rare inherited diseases is determined in much the same way. Where this is so in the case of genes which produce abnormality with a marked loss of fitness in the heterozygous state, then a substantial fraction of the affected cases will be found to occur sporadically, that is without any history of the abnormality in any of their antecedents. They will result in fact from spontaneous mutation occurring during gametogenesis in one or other of their parents.

Balanced polymorphism will occur when the loss of a particular 'abnormal' gene from a population, due to a selective disadvantage of individuals homozygous for it, is balanced by a relative superiority in fitness of the heterozygote over the homozygotes for the 'normal' allele. The essential point is that the heterozygotes must be at some advantage compared with either homozygote. However, in the case of a relatively uncommon abnormal gene which produces a severe disorder in homozygotes, the increase in fitness of the heterozygote over the homozygotes for the normal allele need be only very small. Thus in the case of a recessive disease occurring with a frequency of 1 in 10,000 of all births, and which is effectively lethal, a superiority in viability or fertility of the heterozygotes of only one per cent over that of the normal homozygote will result in a balanced system, and the maintenance of the same gene frequency from generation to generation.

An interesting property of such a balanced system is that the frequencies of the various genotypes will be different in the population of children (or more generally of zygotes) from that in the population of parents from which they are derived. The gene frequencies in the two populations, however, will be the same. Typical conditions for such an equilibrium in the case of two allelic genes A and a with frequencies p and q are given in Table 6a[9]. A numerical example in which it is assumed that the abnormal gene a has a gene frequency of 0·1, and the affected homozygotes aa have zero fitness is given in Table 6b.

The difference in fitness between the heterozygote (Aa) and the normal homozygote (AA) is in practice only like to be marked when the abnormal homozygote (aa) has a drastically reduced fitness and also occurs with an appreciable frequency in the population. One example of such a common lethal or sublethal condition is sickle-cell anaemia, which in certain populations in Africa may occur with an incidence approaching 4 per cent of the total population of children. In these populations it seems likely that the high frequency of the abnormal gene (q=approximately 0·2) is maintained by a balanced system in which the heterozygotes have something like 20–30 per cent better chance of surviving to adult life than do the normal homozygotes. The details of this situation will be considered later (p. 166).

Table 6. (*a*) *Frequencies of foetal and parental genotypes in a population at equilibrium. The force of selection is indicated by the constant K.* (*b*) *Numerical example $p = 0.9$, $q = 0.1$, $k = 0.01$. Fitness of genotype* **aa** *is zero.* (*After Penrose*, 1954)

Genotype	Zygote or foetal frequency	Fitness	Parental frequency
(*a*)			
AA	p^2	$1-K/p^2$	$p^2(1-K/p^2)$
Aa	$2pq$	$1+K/pq$	$2pq(1+K/pq)$
aa	q^2	$1-K/q^2$	$q^2(1-K/q^2)$
(*b*)			
AA	0·81	80/81	0·80
Aa	0·18	$1\frac{1}{9}$	0·20
aa	0·01	0	0·00

In other conditions where the abnormal homozygote is less common, or its reduction in fitness less marked, the superiority of the heterozygote over the normal homozygote is likely to be quite small, and in practice extremely difficult to detect. The extent to which this kind of phenomenon occurs in human populations is consequently still largely unexplored. A typical example of a condition where such a situation might plausibly be expected is fibrocystic disease of the pancreas. This has been said to occur with an incidence of about 1 in 500 of all births in certain populations[10]. The affected individuals are homozygous for an abnormal gene, and they rarely survive to adult life. A very slight superiority of the heterozygote over other 'normal' individuals could explain the high incidence of the disease. The only alternative is to postulate a mutation rate of a magnitude much higher than is generally thought to occur.

It is also possible that many common polymorphisms, such as the various blood group systems, may in fact be balanced systems, in which the gene frequencies are maintained in stable equilibrium by a very slight selective advantage of the heterozygotes over the homozygotes. Such balanced polymorphisms may play an important part in maintaining genetical and hence biochemical diversity in human populations. This in itself is likely to be of adaptive significance, because it implies that the population as a whole may respond more flexibly to fluctuations in environmental conditions.

In a balanced polymorphism the selective advantage of a heterozygote is likely to vary in degree from one environment to another, so that the equilibrium frequencies obtained in populations living in diverse environments may well be markedly different. Similarly, changes in environmental conditions in a particular locality will be expected, in so far as they result in changes in the fitness differential between genotypes, to lead to a change in gene frequencies. The genetical structures of different populations may thus be expected to reflect to some extent the character of the environment in which they live.

It appears that even with respect to those genes whose effects have so far been characterised, there are often large divergences in frequency from one human population to another. This has been found to be the case both for genes which result in little or no obvious selection differential, such as many of the blood group genes[11], and also for genes which at least in some combinations produce a drastic effect on fitness such as is found, for example, with the genes causing sickle cell anaemia or thalassaemia major. It is true not only for common peculiarities typified by the blood groups, the haptoglobin types, and the gamma globulin types of Grubb and Laurell each of which occurs with widely divergent frequencies in different areas, but also for relatively rare abnormalities such as xyloketosuria and phenylketonuria. Xyloketosuria has been observed with quite an appreciable frequency in Jews originating in central and eastern Europe, but appears to be extremely rare in other European or American populations. Phenylketonuria is evidently significantly less frequent among Negroes and Jews than in other population groups in the U.S.A.

The pattern of population structures that we observe today, and the differences from one population to another, probably represent a complex product of mutation, differential selection, balanced polymorphism, genetical drift, and population migration and intermixture. The relative significance of each of these will in general vary from one gene difference to another, and from one population to another.

REFERENCES

(1) Hardy, G. H. (1908). *Science*, **28**, 49.
(2) Weinberg, W. (1908). *Jh. Ver. vaterl. Naturk. Wurttemb.* **64**, 369.
(3) Grubb, R. and Laurell, A. B. (1956). *Acta path. microbiol. Scand.* **39**, 390.
(4) Dahlberg, G. (1947). *Mathematical Methods for Population Genetics.* Karger, Basle.
(5) Munro, T. A. (1947). *Ann. Eugen., Lond.* **13**, 282.
(6) Haldane, J. B. S. (1947). *Ann. Eugen., Lond.* **13**, 262.
(7) Merskey, C. (1951). *Quart. J. Med.* **20**, 299.
(8) Israels, M. C. G., Lempert, H. and Gilbertson, P. (1951). *Lancet*, **1**, 1375.
(9) Penrose, L. S. (1954). *J. Gén. Humain.* **3**, 159.
(10) Anderson, D. H. (1953). 'Cystic Fibrosis of the Pancreas', in *Paediatrics*, 12th ed. Appleton-Century Crofts Inc., New York. Edited by L. E. Holt and R. McIntosh.
(11) Mourant, A. E. (1954). *The Distribution of the Human Blood Groups.* Blackwell, Oxford.

CHAPTER 3

AMINOACID METABOLISM: 1

Blocks in the metabolism of phenylalanine and tyrosine

Garrod's idea that the 'inborn errors of metabolism' were, in essence, blocks in metabolism due to the congenital deficiency of specific enzymes was largely derived from his work on alkaptonuria. He suggested that homogentisic acid which occurred in such large amounts in the urine of these patients was an intermediate in the metabolic pathway by which the aminoacids phenylalanine and tyrosine were usually degraded. If so, the abnormal excretion of homogentisic acid in alkaptonuria could be attributed to the congenital deficiency of the enzyme immediately concerned in the further oxidation of this substance. The failure to detect appreciable quantities of homogentisic acid in the tissues and body fluids of normal individuals was presumably due to the fact that under ordinary circumstances it was broken down as rapidly as it was formed.

Albinism was another inherited abnormality which he regarded as due to a defect in the metabolism of the aromatic aminoacids. Here one of the steps in the reaction sequence by which tyrosine was converted to the pigment melanin appeared to be affected. The conspicuous feature of this condition, however, was the failure to form the pigmented derivative, rather than any obvious accumulation of its precursor.

Since then a number of other conditions have been discovered in which similar blocks appear to occur at different points in the metabolism of phenylalanine and tyrosine. These include such disorders as phenylketonuria, tyrosinosis and the various forms of goitrous cretinism. In each case the biochemical findings suggest a deficiency of some particular enzyme, and they each illustrate in various ways different facets of Garrod's general hypothesis.

The main pathways now thought to be involved in the metabolism of phenylalanine and tyrosine are summarised diagrammatically in Fig. 4, and the site of the presumed lesion in the different disorders is indicated.

Phenylketonuria

Phenylketonuria was first recognised by Folling[1] in 1934 when he demonstrated the presence of considerable amounts of phenylpyruvic acid in the urine of several mentally defective patients. Since then a large number of other examples of this metabolic disorder have been identified and extensive investigations have been carried out both from the genetical and biochemical points of view.

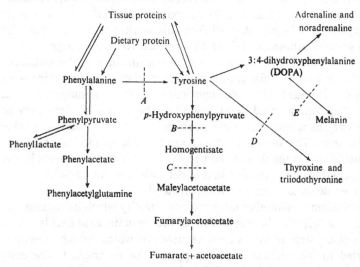

Fig. 4. Possible blocks in the metabolism of phenylalanine and tyrosine. *A*, phenylketonuria; *B*, tyrosinosis; *C*, alkaptonuria; *D*, goitrous cretinism; *E*, albinism.

Nearly all the individuals who have so far been found to excrete phenylpyruvic acid continuously in their urine have exhibited some degree of intellectual impairment. Generally this is severe, amounting to idiocy or imbecility, but occasionally higher grade feeble-minded and border-line cases may be encountered. Jervis[2], reviewing 330 patients with this disorder, found the distribution of intelligence quotients shown in Table 7. Patients of this type account for about $\frac{1}{2}$ to 1 per cent of all cases present in hospitals for the mentally deficient. Munro[3], working in the United Kingdom, estimated the incidence in the general population to be somewhere between 2 and 6 per 100,000, more probably nearer the lower figure.

Neurologically there are no conspicuous findings, though a high proportion of cases show some accentuation of both the superficial and deep reflexes. Epileptic attacks occur in about 25 per cent of the cases, usually in infancy and childhood. They are not very frequent, and severe prolonged epilepsy is exceptional.

Table 7. *Distribution of intelligence quotients in* 330 *phenylketonurics.* (*After Jervis*, 1954)

I.Q.	Number	%
<10	122	37·0
11–20	88	26·7
21–30	41	12·4
31–40	34	10·3
41–50	31	9·4
51–60	7	2·1
61–70	4	1·2
>70	3	0·9
Total	330	—

General physical development is not markedly impaired. The patients are slightly stunted and have somewhat smaller head size when compared with an equivalent normal group, though probably not when compared with an equivalent group of non-phenylketonuric mentally retarded patients.

On the average, phenylketonurics tend to be lighter in hair and skin pigmentation than the population from which they are drawn. Occasionally this dilution of pigmentation may be very striking, as for example in an Italian family reported by Jervis [4] in which both parents had very dark colouring but the affected child was quite fair. Cowie and Penrose [5] used reflectance spectrophotometry to compare the hair colour of a series of phenylketonuric patients with that of their sibs and parents (Fig. 5). They found that while the dilution of hair colour in the phenylketonurics was quite significant, there was nevertheless much overlapping of the distributions. The degree of hair pigmentation appeared to increase with age rather more slowly in the phenylketonurics than in the controls.

Genetics

The familial distribution of phenylketonuria is typical of a Mendelian recessive character. The disease is common among the brothers and sisters of the patients, but rare in their parents, uncles, aunts, cousins and other relatives. Typical findings in three large family surveys are shown in Table 8. Appropriate calculations show that the segregation ratios are in good agreement with those expected theoretically. On the average one in four of the brothers and sisters of affected patients may be expected to be similarly affected. The disease is equally frequent in the two sexes.

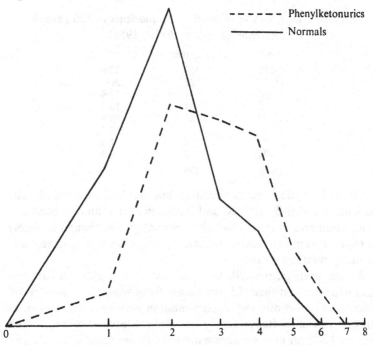

Hair colour. Reflectance % at 700 mμ (corrected for age)

Fig. 5. Distribution of reflectance measurements at 700 mμ from hair from phenylketonuric patients and normal individuals. (After Cowie and Penrose.)

The incidence of first cousin marriage among the parents of phenyl-ketonuric patients varied between 5 per cent and 14 per cent in the different series of cases reported. This, in each instance, is consider-ably in excess of that generally occurring in the populations from which the cases were drawn. Munro has shown that, in his series, the incidence of parental consanguinity agreed fairly well with that expected on theoretical grounds when current estimates of the frequency of first cousin marriages and the incidence of the disease in the general population were used (see p. 22).

Heterozygotes for the abnormal gene are not as a rule noticeably clinically abnormal, though it has been suggested that they might be slightly more prone than other people to develop some form of psychosis in later life[6]. Recently it has been shown that they may be distinguished biochemically (see p. 48).

Table 8. *Familial distribution of phenylketonuria*

	Sibships containing at least one phenylketonuric			Parents		
Source	Number of sibships	Phenyl-ketonuric	Normals	Phenyl-ketonuric	Normals	First cousins
Munro[3]	47	85	141	0	94	10
Jervis[44]	125	197	270	2	248	14
Fölling, *et al.*[45]	22	40	86	0	44	6
Total	194	322	497	2	386	30

Biochemical findings

The urine. Although phenylpyruvic acid was the first metabolite to be found in abnormal quantities in the urine of phenylketonuric patients, it is now known that a number of other substances are also

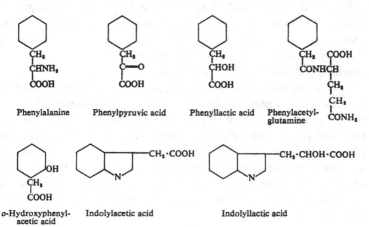

Phenylalanine   Phenylpyruvic acid   Phenyllactic acid   Phenylacetyl-glutamine

o-Hydroxyphenyl-acetic acid   Indolylacetic acid   Indolyllactic acid

Fig. 6. Substances excreted in unusual amounts in phenylketonuria.

regularly present in unusual amounts (Fig. 6). Quantitatively the most important of these are phenylalanine and its derivatives phenyl-lactic acid[7,8,9] and phenylacetylglutamine[10]. The amounts of phenylpyruvic acid excreted and also of these other related substances varies with the diet and the body size of the patient, but they are of the order of ½–2 g. a day.

Besides these o-hydroxyphenylacetic acid has been found in amounts of 0·1–0·4 g. per day, and indolylacetic and indolyllactic acids in quantities of 0·02–0·15 g. daily (11, 12). It has also been reported that the excretion of p-hydroxyphenyllactic and p-hydroxyphenyl-acetic acids may be somewhat increased (13). 5-hydroxyindolylacetic acid may be excreted in somewhat smaller amounts than is normal (14).

The blood plasma. The outstanding abnormal finding here is a grossly elevated concentration of phenylalanine. Values varying from 20 to 60 mg. per cent have been reported (15, 16, 17, 18), while in normal individuals this aminoacid is only present in concentrations of the order of 1 mg. per cent. In contrast, the other aminoacids in the plasma do not occur in unusual concentrations.

Some increase in phenylpyruvic acid concentration has been noted in the plasma (19), but the concentrations are still very small. The other metabolites found in increased quantities in the urine have not been detected in appreciable concentrations in the plasma. It has been claimed that 5-hydroxytryptamine (serotonin) may occur in lower concentrations than is normal (14).

The cerebrospinal fluid. Phenylalanine is present in greatly in-creased amounts, but other aminoacids are not abnormal. The concentration of phenylalanine is of the order of 7 mg. per cent and this represents an increase over normal values of the same order of magnitude as that found in the blood (15, 16).

Thus biochemically the main feature of phenylketonuria is the high concentration of phenylalanine in the blood, cerebrospinal fluid and the urine of the affected individuals. This is associated with the excretion in the urine of phenylpyruvic acid, phenyllactic acid and phenylacetylglutamine in grossly abnormal amounts, and also the abnormal excretion of certain hydroxyphenolic acids and indoles. It is apparent that these findings must reflect a severe disturbance of the metabolism of the aromatic aminoacids in general and of phenyl-alanine in particular.

Feeding experiments

That the abnormal biochemical findings can be attributed to an inability to metabolise phenylalanine efficiently has been clearly shown by the results of a variety of dietary experiments.

Feeding phenylalanine itself, or giving a high protein diet, results

in an increase in the excretion of phenylalanine, phenylpyruvic acid
and its other derivatives in the urine (20,21). Feeding other aminoacids
does not have this effect. If, on the other hand, the protein content
of the diet is diminished or if its phenylalanine content is restricted,
the excretion of the abnormal metabolites is reduced proportionately.

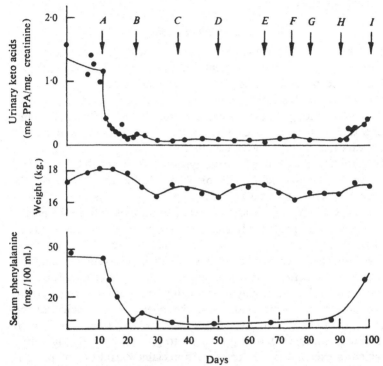

Fig. 7. Effect of dietary restriction of phenylalanine in phenylketonuria. (After
Armstrong *et al.* (22).) *A*, phenylalanine-deficient diet initiated; *B*, 90 mg. L-phenylalanine daily; *C*, 100 mg. L-phenylalanine daily; *D*, 110 mg. L-phenylalanine
daily; *E*, 120 mg. L-phenylalanine daily; *F*, 250 mg. L-phenylalanine daily;
G, 500 mg. L-phenylalanine daily; *H*, 1000 mg. L-phenylalanine daily; *I*, natural
diet.

A number of patients have now been kept on diets which contained
only sufficient phenylalanine to allow of normal protein synthesis and
growth (about 15–20 mg. per kg. body weight in children), but containing normal amounts of all other dietary ingredients (17,22,23).
Under these conditions of severely restricted phenylalanine intake,
it has been found that the phenylalanine concentration in the plasma
falls to normal or near normal levels, and the abnormal excretion of

phenylalanine and also of all the other substances usually found, including the indoles, is abolished (Fig. 7). This correction of the various biochemical abnormalities characteristic of the disease has been maintained for many months and during this period the rate of growth has been satisfactory and the children did not go into negative nitrogen balance.

The metabolic lesion

Rose and his collegues (24) showed that, in man, phenylalanine is an indispensable dietary constituent and that its omission from the diet is followed by pronounced negative nitrogen balance. Thus phenylalanine is an 'essential' aminoacid. Tyrosine, however, is not 'essential', though it may become a limiting factor for growth and nutrition if the diet does not contain enough phenylalanine. It appears that while tyrosine can be formed from phenylalanine, the formation of phenylalanine from tyrosine is not possible.

This irreversible conversion of phenylalanine to tyrosine is now generally believed to be the first step in the oxidation of phenylalanine, derived either from the protein in the diet or from the breakdown of tissue protein. It has a central place in the intermediary metabolism of phenylalanine in the normal subject.

A subsidiary series of reactions in which phenylalanine may be normally concerned involve changes in the side-chain. They are illustrated in Fig. 8. It may be reversibly converted to phenylpyruvic acid and phenyllactic acids, and the phenylpyruvic acid can be irreversibly changed to phenylacetic acid. Phenylacetic acid in man is mainly conjugated with glutamine to give phenylacetylglutamine which is excreted in the urine. Appreciable quantities of phenylacetylglutamine occur in normal urine (25) and this is presumably derived from phenylalanine via phenylpyruvic acid.

The characteristic biochemical findings in the blood, cerebrospinal fluid, and the urine of phenylketonuric patients can for the most part be readily understood on the hypothesis that the enzyme system normally concerned in the conversion of phenylalanine to tyrosine is in some way defective. Under these circumstances one would expect the composition of the body fluids to reflect a block in intermediary metabolism at this point. Phenylalanine derived from protein in the food, or from the breakdown of tissue proteins would tend to accumulate in the blood and cerebrospinal fluid and be excreted in abnormal amounts in the urine. Phenylpyruvic acid, phenyllactic acid, and phenylacetylglutamine would be formed in excess, but since the renal threshold for these substances is very low they would be found in large amounts in the urine but hardly at all in the blood.

Such a block in the intermediary metabolism of phenylalanine was first clearly demonstrated by Jervis[26]. He showed that in normal people the administration of phenylalanine leads to a marked rise in the level of tyrosine in the blood. In phenylketonurics this did not occur (Fig. 9).

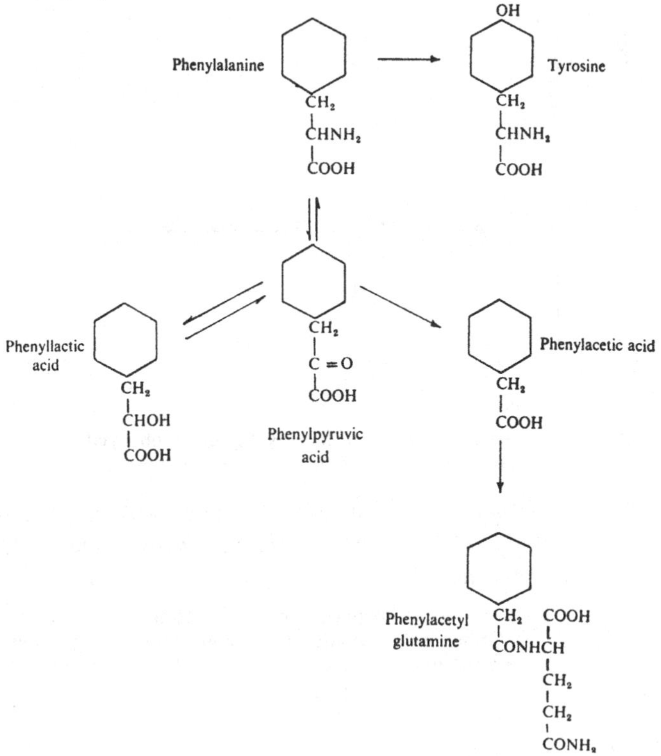

Fig. 8. Pathways in phenylalanine metabolism.

The defect has also been demonstrated by Udenfriend and Bessman using ^{14}C-labelled phenylalanine[27]. The labelled phenylalanine was given by mouth and subsequently tyrosine and phenylalanine were isolated from the plasma proteins and their specific activities determined. The ratio of the activity in tyrosine to that in phenylalanine was taken as an index of the degree of conversion of phenylalanine to tyrosine. Values for this ratio were about ten times as high in the normal subjects as in the phenylketonurics (Table 9). However, some conversion did seem to take place in the phenylketonurics, and this

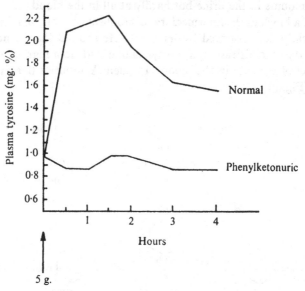

Fig. 9. Effect on plasma tyrosine of feeding 5 g. of DL-phenylalanine to a normal and a phenylketonuric subject. (After Jervis.)

Table 9. *Incorporation of ^{14}C into plasma protein phenylalanine and tyrosine after the administration of 3-^{14}C-DL-phenylalanine. (After Udenfriend and Bessmann, 1953)*

Experiment	Time after administration (hours)	Phenylalanine counts/min./ μM	Tyrosine counts/min./ μM	Ratio tyrosine/ phenylalanine
Control (a)	24	10·4	2·79	0·26
	48	7·84	2·24	0·29
Control (b)	24	24·6	4·90	0·20
	48	21·0	4·70	0·22
Phenylketonuric (c)	24	55·0	0·91	0·016
	48	39·0	0·89	0·023
Phenylketonuric (d)	24	46·0	0·70	0·016
	48	33·0	0·69	0·021

suggested that either the block was not quite complete, or that a small amount of tyrosine was being formed from phenylalanine via some alternative pathway or conceivably by intestinal bacteria prior to absorption.

The enzyme system

The enzyme system concerned with the hydroxylation of phenyl-alanine to tyrosine was described by Udenfriend and Cooper[28]. They found that it is present in water-soluble fractions from liver, but not from other tissues, and it appears to be specific for L-phenyl-alanine. The system is evidently complex and Mitoma[29] has shown that it consists of at least two protein fractions. One of these is very labile and is peculiar to the liver, and the other is more stable and occurs in other tissues as well. The reaction requires both reduced DPN and oxygen. Both protein fractions are necessary for the hydroxylation, and it has not been possible to separate the overall reaction into two steps.

A direct attempt to discover whether any L-phenylalanine hydroxy-lase activity could be detected in the liver of phenylketonuric patients was made by Jervis in 1953[30]. He obtained fragments of liver at autopsy from two phenylketonuric patients and three controls. Crude liver extracts were tested in the system of Udenfriend and Cooper, and it was found that while activity could be demonstrated in the controls, no activity was detectable in the phenylketonurics. This result has since been confirmed by Wallace, Moldave and Meister[31] using fresh biopsy specimens from a living phenylketonuric patient and appropriate controls. These workers and also Mitoma, Auld and Udenfriend[32] have been able to show that the part of the enzyme system which is deficient in these patients is the labile fraction described by Mitoma. This fraction is only found in the liver. The stable fraction also present in other tissues appears to occur in phenylketonuric patients in normal amounts.

Some difficulties

While there seems little doubt that most of the biochemical disturbances occurring in phenylketonuria can be directly referred to a deficiency in one component of the enzyme system normally concerned with the hydroxylation of phenylalanine to tyrosine, there still remain a number of puzzling aspects of the biochemistry of this disorder which require explanation.

The mechanism by which increased quantities of o-hydroxyphenyl-acetic acid and possibly other hydroxyphenolic compounds are formed is still obscure. o-Hydroxyphenylacetic acid is certainly formed from phenylalanine, as has been demonstrated by ^{14}C-labelling experiments (33). The o-hydroxylation cannot be brought about by the para directing phenylalanine hydroxylase. However, it is possible that other hydroxylating mechanisms exist which only become of importance when phenylalanine accumulates in large amounts because its normal mode of conversion to tyrosine is interrupted. Dalgliesh (34) has shown how a non-specific artificial hydroxylating system may bring about similar changes *in vitro* and has plausibly suggested that this might occur *in vivo* and account for the various abnormal hydroxylated products which have been described in phenylketonuria.

The excretion of certain tryptophane derivatives such as indolylacetic and indolyllactic acids in increased quantities also requires explanation. Tied up with this is the finding that 5-hydroxytryptamine may occur in lower than normal concentrations in the blood and 5-hydroxyindole acetic acid in smaller than usual amounts in the urine. It seems possible that the hydroxylation of tryptophane is to some extent defective in these patients. This effect is quantitatively very much smaller than the phenylalanine hydroxylation defect, and it seems likely to be a secondary consequence of it because the abnormal excretion of the tryptophane derivatives disappears when a phenylalanine restricted diet is fed (22). However, the exact explanation of this phenomenon remains uncertain.

The mental defect

It is natural to suppose that the impairment of intellectual capacity characteristically present in this disease is in some way a consequence of the metabolic disorder. The precise cause of the mental defect is, however, not known.

One attractive hypothesis is that it results from the 'toxic' action of one or another of the various metabolites which occur in unusual amounts as a consequence of the block of phenylalanine hydroxylation. Phenylalanine itself which is the most prominent abnormal constituent in the body fluids is the obvious choice as the main potential culprit in this respect, but other substances such as phenylacetic acid have also been proposed as being the responsible ones. It should, however, be pointed out that in general no clear correlation has been found between I.Q. and the blood level of phenylalanine, or the urine excretion of any of the other abnormally increased metabolites (35).

A high concentration of phenylalanine in the body fluids might be thought of as acting by producing a specific inhibition in the reactions of other related metabolites necessary for normal cerebral functioning. Quastel and his colleagues [36], for example, have demonstrated that tyrosine metabolism may be inhibited by high local concentrations of phenylalanine. Alternatively the disturbance might be a consequence of a more general derangement of intracellular aminoacid balance due to excess of phenylalanine in the tissues [35]. Aminoacids are normally concentrated within cells by more or less specific transport systems and not only the absolute amounts present but the relative proportions of one aminoacid to another are likely to be of importance in intracellular functioning. Major dysfunction of a particular tissue could very well be brought about by the intracellular displacement by phenylalanine of other essential aminoacids and a consequent state of aminoacid imbalance. So far, however, no analysis of free intracellular aminoacids in the brain or other tissues has been reported in phenylketonuria.

The possibility that more remote effects of the disorder in phenylalanine metabolism such as a decreased concentration of 5-hydroxytryptamine may be the cause of the mental defect must also not be overlooked in this connection [14].

If indeed the mental disturbance could ultimately be traced back to the abnormal accumulation of phenylalanine or one of its derivatives in the body, it is at least conceivable that an attempt to reduce the phenylalanine concentration by appropriate restriction of dietary phenylalanine might alleviate or perhaps 'cure' the mental retardation. This line of therapy is being actively pursued at a number of centres and a variety of reports on its possible value have already appeared [17, 22, 23, 37, 38, 39]. Since phenylalanine is an essential aminoacid, it is obvious that a little must be present in the diet to allow of normal protein synthesis. The idea is to make sure that no more than this bare essential minimum is present. It is still too early to assess the ultimate value of this therapeutic approach, although it seems that as far as is known all the biochemical abnormalities of the body fluids can be corrected in this way. Improvement in mental capacity is difficult to assess in young children, and although some of the workers in the field are hopeful about the outlook, at least in certain cases, the matter will not become clear until fairly prolonged trials have been undertaken. All the workers stress, however, that it is probably important, if the treatment is going to be of value, to start it at the earliest opportunity in infancy. It is thought that in older

children the long continued interference in cerebral function may
well have produced irreversible damage, or that at any rate the loss
of time available for mental development cannot subsequently be
made up even if no structural damage has occurred.

Melanin formation

The cause of the dilution in hair colour, which though rather variable
in degree, can be regarded as a characteristic feature of phenylketonuria, has not been certainly determined. Broadly speaking three
kinds of hypothesis might be advanced to explain the reduction in
melanin formation which seems to occur; an absence or relative
deficiency of the melanin-forming enzyme system tyrosinase; a
decrease in the amount of tyrosine, the melanin precursor, available
for conversion to the pigment; some inhibition of the tyrosine-
tyrosinase system by phenylalanine or related substances which
accumulate in phenylketonuria.

There is no evidence that the enzyme system itself is deficient, or
that there is any overt deficiency of tyrosine in these patients on
normal diets, though there may be a relative deficiency under certain
circumstances. It has, however, been demonstrated that L-phenylalanine may act as a competitive inhibitor of the tyrosine-tyrosinase
system *in vitro* [40] and it seems likely, therefore, that the high
concentrations known to be present in the body fluids may result in
a similar effect *in vivo*. Some support for this is provided by reports
that noticeable darkening of new-grown hair has occurred in patients
on phenylalanine restricted diets, and also in other patients when
tyrosine intake has been increased by massive doses over a period of
several months [41].

The detection of heterozygotes

Both parents of patients with phenylketonuria must carry the
abnormal gene in single dose, and it has now been shown that they
exhibit a biochemical disturbance qualitatively similar to that encountered in the affected homozygotes, but of course very much less
in degree. On the average the fasting phenylalanine level in the blood
is slightly higher in the heterozygotes than in the controls [42]. Although
the distributions overlap considerably the difference appears to be
quite significant. The discrimination of the heterozygotes can be
further accentuated by means of the phenylalanine tolerance test
(Table 10). If plasma levels of phenylalanine are determined at one-,

two- and four-hourly intervals after feeding a standard dose of
L-phenylalanine the heterozygotes show a phenylalanine level of
about twice that of the controls at each period [43]. The most plausible
interpretation of the results is that the heterozygotes, as a group,
have significantly less than the normal amount of phenylalanine
hydroxylating enzyme activity.

Table 10. *Mean plasma phenylalanine concentration in parents of
phenylketonuric patients and in controls, in the fasting state and after
the administration of a standard dose of phenylalanine.* (*After Hsia,
et al.* 1956)

Plasma phenylalanine conc. μM/ml.

		Controls			Parents of phenylketonuric patients		
		No. tested	Mean	S.D.	No. tested	Mean	S.D.
Fasting		34	0·067	0·032	37	0·103	0·029
Hours after oral	1 hr.	19	0·55	0·186	19	1·14	0·187
administration of	2 hr.	19	0·55	0·168	19	1·03	0·187
L-phenylalanine (0·1 g./kg. body weight)	4 hr.	19	0·30	0·076	19	0·76	0·292

Alkaptonuria

Alkaptonuria is readily recognised by the characteristic changes in
colour which occur in the urine. The urine when freshly passed is
normal in appearance but if left to stand it soon begins to darken.
Alkalinity speeds up the change and the urine passes through a series
of shades of brown and finally may appear quite black. Linen and
woollen fabrics moistened with the urine become darkly stained and
as a result the condition is frequently recognised in early infancy by
the characteristic staining of the napkins. On other occasions the
abnormality is detected for the first time in the course of a life-
insurance examination or a routine medical investigation when the
urine is found to have strongly reducing properties, and then its other
peculiar characteristics are noted.

These curious properties of the urine persist unchanged throughout
life. In other respects the affected individuals appear quite healthy,
except as they grow older their ligaments and cartilages tend to
become darkened and they are particularly prone to develop a form
of osteoarthritis which may be quite severe. These changes are called
ochronosis.

Biochemical findings

The urinary changes in colour are due to the presence of large quantities of homogentisic acid. This, although colourless itself, is readily oxidised to give a black pigment.

Alkaptonurics excrete several grams of homogentisic acid daily. The amount excreted varies somewhat with the diet and is larger as the protein intake is increased. Consequently the output of homogentisic acid in these patients is highly correlated with the total nitrogen output and the ratio of homogentisic acid to total nitrogen excretion has often been used as a convenient index in the study of this condition. Given a constant diet this ratio is probably much the same in all alkaptonuric patients.

Apart from homogentisic acid, no other substance has been reported as occurring in abnormal amounts. In particular, Neuberger and his colleagues[46] in a search for other aromatic compounds, failed to find any abnormal quantities of tyrosine, p-hydroxyphenyllactic acid, p-hydroxyphenylpyruvic acid, or phenylpyruvic acid. The reducing properties of the urine could be attributed entirely to the homogentisic acid present.

In spite of the high concentration of homogentisic acid in the urine, the blood level of homogentisic acid in alkaptonuria appears to be extremely low[46]. The concentrations present are in the range of the lower limits of the applicability of the methods which have been available, and since minute amounts of other reducing substances reacting like homogentisic acid are known to be present in plasma, even from non-alkaptonuric subjects, the precise amount present has not been determined with any accuracy. It is, however, thought to be of the order of 3 mg. per cent. No other abnormal constituents have been reported in the blood of these patients.

Metabolic investigations

Homogentisic acid is believed to be an intermediate in normal metabolism. Normal individuals after taking by mouth amounts of the substance of the order of 5 g. appear to metabolise it completely and no homogentisic acid appears in the urine[47,48]. Embden[49] did in fact succeed in producing a slight transitory alkaptonuria by giving as much as 8 g. of the acid, but he found that smaller doses had no such effect. In sharp contrast with these findings in the normal, homogentisic acid when fed to alkaptonurics is excreted almost quantitatively, in addition to that being put out in any case by these patients. It appears, therefore, that the alkaptonuric is completely incapable of metabolising this substance.

Homogentisic acid is an intermediate on the main, though not the only, metabolic pathway in the degradation of the two aromatic aminoacids phenylalanine and tyrosine. Some 70–90 per cent of these aminoacids present in the diet are converted to homogentisic acid by the alkaptonuric, and a similar conversion rate is obtained when either L-phenylalanine or L-tyrosine are fed alone.

Alkaptonurics also excrete 'extra' homogentisic acid after the administration of phenyllactic acid, and 2·5 dihydroxyphenylpyruvic acid[46]. On the other hand o-tyrosine, m-tyrosine and the corresponding α-keto acids do not produce this effect[50].

The immediate product of the oxidation of homogentisic acid in the liver[51] is now thought to be maleylacetoacetate and it seems that in alkaptonuria the enzyme (homogentisic acid oxidase) which normally catalyses this reaction is either not present at all or is present only in very minute amounts. La Due and his colleagues[52] have demonstrated that in liver material obtained by biopsy from an alkaptonuric patient assays of those enzymes catalysing the conversion of tyrosine to homogentisic acid, and also of those concerned in the catabolism of maleylacetoacetate showed high activity. The enzyme required to convert homogentisic acid to maleylacetoacetate could not, however, be demonstrated, though it was readily detected in control material from non-alkaptonuric individuals (Table 11). Furthermore, there was no evidence for the presence of any inhibitors,

Table 11. *Activity of tyrosine oxidation enzymes in alkaptonuric and non-alkaptonuric liver (activity calculated as μM of substrate oxidised per hour per 0·1 g. wet weight of liver). (After La Due et al. 1958)*

Enzyme	Activity		
	Non-alkaptonuric liver (autopsy)	Non-alkaptonuric liver (biopsy)	Alkaptonuric liver (biopsy)
Tyrosine transaminase	0·67	3·6	3·2
p-Hydroxyphenylpyruvic acid oxidase	4·3	6·7	4·6
Homogentisic acid oxidase	11·8	26·8	< 0·0048
Maleylacetoacetic acid isomerase	14·5	960	780
Fumarylacetoacetic acid hydrolase	14	29	22

so that some defect in the synthesis of this enzyme appears to be the key lesion in this condition.

The renal threshold of homogentisic acid. It is probable that both in normal subjects and in alkaptonurics the renal threshold for homogentisic acid is extremely low, and little if any renal tubular absorption goes on. Leaf and Neuberger (48) were able, by intravenous injection of quantities of the order of 0·3 g., to produce a transient alkaptonuria in normal individuals. On the average about one-third of the dose administered appeared in the urine. The concentration in the plasma was of the order of 1·5 to 3·5 mg. per cent and they concluded that the renal threshold must be well below 4·0 mg. per cent.

In normal subjects alkaptonuria cannot be produced by feeding tyrosine or phenylalanine, and it must be assumed that homogentisic acid, if it is formed as an intermediate, never appears in the blood in appreciable quantities, and it may well be rapidly oxidised in the organ where it is first formed. The alkaptonuric probably has the same low renal threshold for this substance as does the normal and this could account for the high urine concentration and the low concentration in the plasma, which is observed.

However, the values for the renal clearance of homogentisic acid in alkaptonuria actually obtained in one patient (46) were of the order of 400–500 ml. per min. This was much more than could be readily accounted for by filtration alone, as a substance which was filtered by the glomeruli and not at all reabsorbed by the tubules might have been expected to show a clearance of about 100 ml. per min. in this individual. It is possible, therefore, that homogentisic acid when circulating in increased amounts may be actively secreted by the renal tubules at a rate comparable to that shown by certain dyes such as diodrast. However, further work along these lines will be required before this interpretation can be substantiated.

Ochronosis. Apart from the excretion of homogentisic acid in the urine the most notable clinical feature of alkaptonuria is the development of the condition known as ochronosis. This does not generally become apparent till adult life, and is due to the development of a dark pigmentation of the cartilages, tendons and ligaments, and of the sclerotics of the eyes. The earliest signs are bluish discoloration of the ears, and the appearance of triangular brown patches in the sclerotics with their bases towards the corneae. Later owing to the staining of the underlying tendons the nose may appear bluish and a blue tint may appear on the knuckles. The post-mortem appearances are very striking. The cartilages and fibrocartilages are deeply pigmented, the staining of the tracheal rings, and of the interstitial disks being particularly noticeable. Pigmentation in the tendons, sclerotics, and in advanced cases the bones may be observed, and patches of pigment in the endocardium and intima of the arteries have also been described (53, 54).

These patients are particularly prone to develop arthritic changes. The changes are usually most prominent in the spine and may lead to rigidity and kyphosis. Typical X-ray appearances have been described (55), the main features of which are extensive calcification in tendon sheaths, bursal sacs, synovial membranes and in the intervertebral disks.

The black pigment deposited in the ligaments and cartilages is evidently derived from homogentisic acid which is probably circulating in the blood stream in abnormal though still extremely low concentrations. Similar pigmentation may be demonstrated *in vitro* by placing normal cartilage in a solution of homogentisic acid. The mode of formation of the pigment is, however, not understood, nor has it been established in what way its deposition is related to the development of the osteoarthritis.

Genetics. Garrod was the first to point out that alkaptonuria had a characteristic familial distribution. It occurred frequently among the brothers and sisters of affected relatives, but rarely among their parents, children or more distant relatives. Furthermore he drew attention to the unusually high incidence of parental consanguinity. He concluded that this must imply that the condition is genetically determined and that it is in fact inherited in the manner of a typical mendelian recessive character. The affected individuals would thus be homozygous for the rare abnormal gene involved. These conclusions have been largely confirmed by further work (56) and there is little doubt that the majority of cases of alkaptonuria are determined in this way (Table 12).

However, several pedigrees of the condition have been reported which do not fit this interpretation (56, 57). In these pedigrees individuals in a series of successive generations of a family were affected and there was no indication of consanguineous marriage (Fig. 10). In other words the pedigrees were of typical heterozygous or 'dominant' type. The simplest view is that there are in fact two genetically distinct types of alkaptonuria—the usual type determined by a 'recessive' gene,

Table 12. *Incidence of parental consanguinity in 125 cases of alkaptonuria reported in the literature up to 1931. (After Hogben et al. 1932)*

Relationship of parents	Alkaptonurics
First cousins	26
Consanguineous (degree unknown)	1
Unrelated	36
Not ascertained	62
Total	125

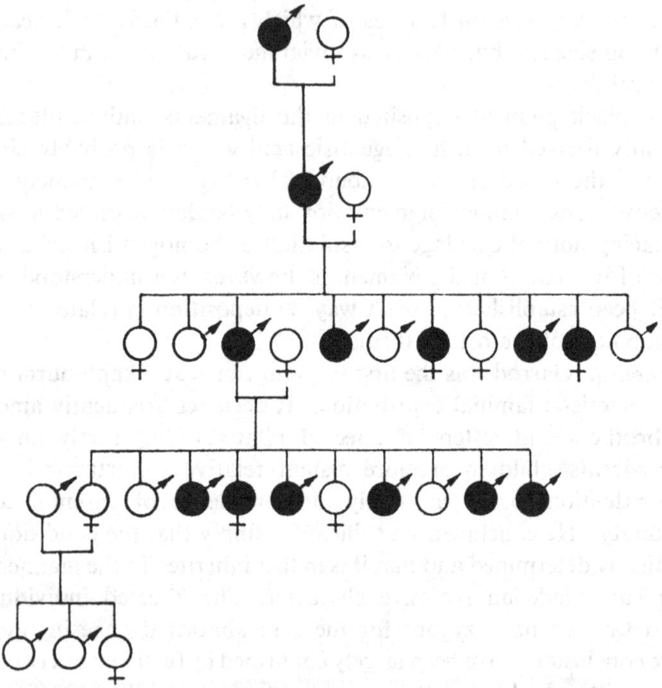

Fig. 10. Pedigree of heterozygous alkaptonuria. (After Pieter.)

and a rare type, perhaps representing only a few per cent of all cases, in which the affected individuals are heterozygous for some other gene. Whether the gene involved in the second type of case is allelic with the first or is at some different chromosomal locus is not known. The existence of such genetical heterogenity in alkaptonuria naturally raises the question as to whether the two types are biochemically distinct. The answer to this is not known. It remains possible that

ALKAPTONURIA 55

the nature of the biochemical disturbance leading to the excretion of homogentisic acid in the rare type of alkaptonuria may be quite different from that found in the common type. All the detailed metabolic studies so far conducted have probably been done on the commoner recessive form of the condition.

Table 13. *Sex ratio in published cases of alkaptonuria.*
(*After Hogben* et al.)

	Males	Females	Total
Isolated cases	28	9	37
Probably recessive (i.e. homozygous) cases			
(a) Derived from consanguineous parents	20	7	27
(b) Derived from non-consanguineous parents	21	15	36
(c) Consanguinity between parents not ascertained	14	6	20
Possibly 'dominant' (i.e. heterozygous) cases	17	9	26
Total	100	46	146

One curious feature of the incidence of alkaptonuria as recorded in the literature is the relatively high proportion of male to female cases. The ratio is about 2:1 and the cause of this is still obscure. Hogben and his colleagues tabulated all the cases reported up to 1931 and divided them into three groups: isolated cases in which no family data were available, cases apparently inherited recessively, and the cases which seemed to fall into the heterozygous class. In all three groups the sex ratio was substantially the same (Table 13) and there was no indication of sex linkage. There is no evidence to suggest that incomplete manifestation in females accounts for the phenomenon. On such a hypothesis one would have to assume that only approximately half the females genetically predisposed to the development of alkaptonuria actually manifest the condition. The clear-cut character of the disorder and the lack of any suggestion that the metabolism of the aromatic aminoacids is sex-influenced make this unlikely, although at present it cannot be rigorously excluded. If we assume some selection in favour of males in the type of case that comes to be recorded in the literature, then we are faced with the problem of how such selection arises. The possibility that the disorder is semi-lethal in the female, so that, on the whole fewer female cases come under observation, is extremely unlikely in view of the generally benign clinical nature of the condition. While occasionally cases are detected at life-insurance examinations and this could lead to a selection in favour of males, this does not seem to be a sufficiently general cause to account for the discrepancy. The occurrence of ochronosis and arthritis in middle and late life often draws attention to the disability, and certainly is a frequent reason for the particular case to become recorded in the literature. It might be, that if such development occurred more frequently in men than in women, the preponderance of the male sex in recorded cases could be accounted for.

Tyrosinosis

Only one authenticated example of tyrosinosis has been described (58). It was, however, studied in considerable detail and there seems little doubt that it represents an error of metabolism analogous to those observed in phenylketonuria and in alkaptonuria. Nothing is known of its possible genetical basis.

In this patient there was a continuous excretion in the urine of large amounts of p-hydroxyphenylpyruvic acid and of tyrosine. If the protein intake was increased or if tyrosine itself was fed, the quantities of these compounds excreted were increased and also some p-hydroxy-phenyllactic acid appeared. When the tyrosine intake was raised further, 3:4-dihydroxyphenylalanine could be demonstrated in the urine. When p-hydroxyphenylpyruvic acid was administered most of it was excreted unchanged, though some p-hydroxyphenyllactic acid also appeared. Feeding phenylalanine led to an increased output of tyrosine and p-hydroxyphenylpyruvic acid.

In contrast to these results, it was found that on administering homogentisic acid, none appeared in the urine, and there was no indication that it influenced the excretion of any other compounds. Presumably it was completely metabolised.

These observations are consistent with a situation in which there is an inability to convert p-hydroxyphenylpyruvic acid to homogentisic acid. In other words the block lies between those located for phenyl-ketonuria and alkaptonuria (see Fig. 4).

The patient concerned also suffered from myasthenia gravis. However, many examples of myasthenia gravis since investigated have failed to show the same biochemical basis, and the association was probably a fortuitous one.

Thyroid hormone formation and goitrous cretinism

The iodination of tyrosine and the formation of the thyroid hormones thyroxine and triidodothyronine is the result of a complex series of reactions, a disturbance of which at several different points can result in gross failure of hormone production. In the last few years it has become possible in the case of several rare genetically determined types of cretinism to identify the site of the lesion in the metabolic sequence and to give a plausible explanation of the pathogenesis of the disease[59]. It is probable in view of the rapid developments in this field that further examples of different inherited disorders in thyroid metabolism will be delineated in the next few years.

Cretinism is a state characterised by a gross retardation in physical and mental development due to a failure in the formation of thyroid hormones either in foetal life or during early postnatal growth. It is found most frequently in areas where goitre is common and here it is believed to be due to iodine deficiency. Where dietary iodine is adequate cretinism may occasionally occur as a result of a failure in development of the thyroid gland, which is either absent or rudimentary. It may also, however, be found in association with large goitres. It is among these so-called goitrous cretins from localities where there is apparently no deficiency of iodine in which the various genetically determined metabolic errors have been identified.

Iodine metabolism

Current views on the pathways involved in the normal formation of the thyroid hormones may be summarised in a somewhat over-simplified way as follows. Detailed reviews are given by Berson[60], and Roche and Michel[61].

Iodine mainly enters the body in the form of inorganic iodide which is absorbed in the gastrointestinal tract and becomes rapidly distributed in the extracellular fluids. The thyroid takes up iodide and concentrates it relative to the plasma so that a considerable concentration gradient is built up. The nature of the process of iodide concentration is not fully understood, but it is inhibited by substances such as thiocyanate and perchlorate. The administration of such compounds after iodide concentration leads to a discharge of inorganic iodide from the gland but not of any organically bound iodide which may have been formed.

5

The iodide concentrated by the gland is then oxidised to free iodine. This process is inhibited by substances of the thiocarbonamide group such as thiouracil. The free iodine reacts immediately with tyrosine residues which are probably in peptide linkage in the intact protein, thyroglobulin. Monoiodotyrosine and diiodotyrosine are believed to be formed sequentially in this way (Fig. 11). They then give rise to

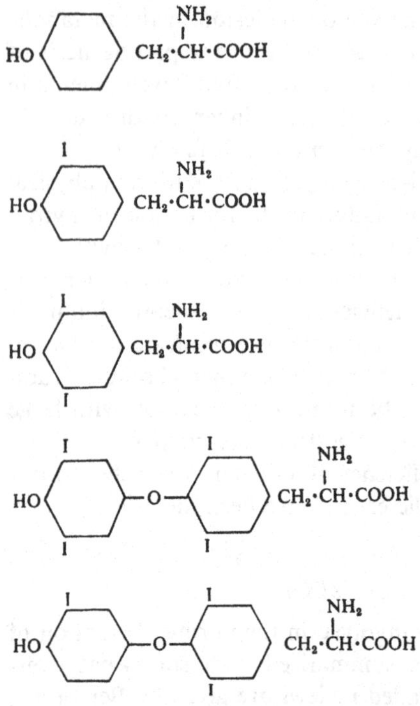

Tyrosine

3-Monoiodotyrosine

3:5-Diiodotyrosine

3:5, 3′:5′-Tetraiodothyronine (thyroxine)

3:5, 3′-Triiodothyronine

Fig. 11. Iodinated derivatives of tyrosine.

the iodinated thyronines of which thyroxine and triiodothyronine are the best known. Thyroxine is thought to result from the conjugation of two diiodotyrosine residues with the elimination of one alanine sidechain. This is believed to occur in the intact protein thyroglobulin, and the proportion of iodinated tyrosine residues which can take part will depend on their spatial relationships within the protein molecule. The formation of triiodothyronine may be a consequence of a condensation of one molecule of monoiodotyrosine with one molecule of diiodotyrosine, or it may result from partial deiodination of thyroxine once this has been formed. The exact mechanisms involved in these processes and the characters of the different enzymes concerned are still uncertain.

The active hormones appear to be stored in the thyroid colloid in the thyroglobulin. This is slowly broken down by proteolytic enzymes and the liberated thyroxine and triiodothyronine are released into the blood stream. In this process of thyroglobulin breakdown mono-iodotyrosine and diiodotyrosine will also be released. However, these substances are rapidly deiodinated, probably by the so-called 'dehalogenating' enzyme described by Roche and his colleagues (62). This enzyme removes the iodine from free monoiodo- or diiodo-tyrosine but not from thyroxine or triiodothyronine or from the tyrosine residues in the intact thyroglobulin. It seems, therefore, that while the hormonally active substances pass into the circulation their inactive precursors are deiodinated. The iodine so liberated can be reutilised in the biosynthetic pathway.

Absence of ' Dehalogenase'

In one group of patients the occurrence of goitrous cretinism can be fairly confidently attributed to a genetically determined failure of 'dehalogenase' activity.

Characteristically, labelled monoiodo- and diiodotyrosine appear in unusual amounts in the blood and in the urine following the administration of radioactively labelled iodine (63). Analysis of the gland removed at thyroidectomy shows that most of the labelled iodine is present as mono- or diiodotyrosine, although small and approximately equal amounts of thyroxine and triiodothyronine are also found.

Following the administration of labelled diiodo- or monoiodo-tyrosine a large proportion of the labelled compound is excreted unchanged in the urine (64). By contrast, in normal subjects, con-siderable deiodination occurs and only a small proportion of the diiodo- and none of the monoiodotyrosine administered is excreted unchanged in the urine. These results indicate that the normal mechanism for removing iodine from mono- and diiodotyrosine is at fault.

This defect has been demonstrated directly using tissue slices of the thyroid gland removed from one of the patients and similar material from patients with ordinary nodular goitre as a control (65). The substrate was DL-diiodotyrosine and deiodination could be readily demonstrated in the control material but was absent when the test tissue was from the cretin.

The findings are consistent with the hypothesis that the basic defect is a failure to form the deiodinating enzyme 'dehalogenase'. Stanbury and McGirr[59] have summarised the probable sequence of events

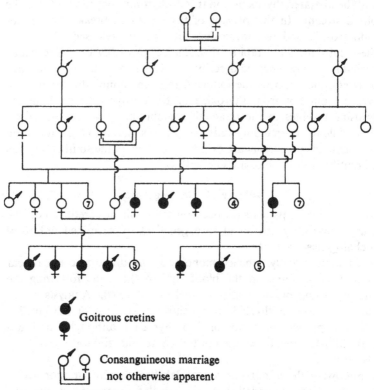

Goitrous cretins

Consanguineous marriage
not otherwise apparent

Fig. 12. Family of Scottish tinkers showing occurrence of goitrous cretinism. (After Hutchison and McGirr.)

which would be expected to result from such a deficiency and account for the pathological findings. The absence of the normal mechanism for removing iodine from mono- and diiodotyrosine as they become freed from thyroglobulin by proteolysis would lead to an abnormal escape of these substances into the circulation, and to their consequent loss in the urine. This could result in a chronic deficiency of iodine, compensatory hyperplasia of the gland, and an inadequate formation of thyroid hormone.

Most of these investigations were carried out in Leiden in a family in which there were two affected brothers and one normal sib. The parents were unrelated. However, a large family in which apparently the same kind of abnormality was segregating has also been investigated in Scotland (66). The members of this family were a group of itinerant tinkers and the pedigree (Fig. 12) is remarkable for the high degree of inbreeding which has occurred. Among thirty-one individuals in four different sibships ten goitrous cretins were identified. There seems little doubt that the affected patients in these families were homozygous for a rare recessive gene.

In another Dutch family (64) it was found that a number of the relatives of the goitrous cretin also showed some evidence of thyroid disease. These included the mother, the sister, an aunt and a cousin of the patient, all of whom had nodular goitres. None of them, however, showed any signs of hypothyroidism. When labelled diiodo-tyrosine was given intravenously, it was found that while all gave clear evidence of deiodination, nevertheless the rate of deiodination was significantly less rapid than in a control group of patients. It seems possible that these relatives with a detectable, but much less obtrusive biochemical abnormality, and with no clinical symptoms apart from the goitre, were heterozygous for the abnormal gene.

Failure to form organically bound iodine

Another form of goitrous cretinism due to a quite different defect in thyroid metabolism has been described by Stanbury and Hedge (67). There were four typical goitrous cretins in a group of seven brothers and sisters. The parents were first cousins and this defect also was presumably due to a rare 'recessive' gene.

When labelled iodine was given by mouth to the patients a large proportion of it accumulated extremely rapidly in the thyroid. Maximal values were observed within 2 hr. If, when this accumulation of labelled iodine had reached a plateau, an oral dose of potassium thiocyanate was given, there immediately occurred a striking and rapid release of iodine from the gland (Fig. 13). In normal individuals the labelled iodine accumulates in the gland at a much slower rate and it is not discharged in such large amount by the administration of thiocyanate.

The metabolism of iodine in this group of patients appeared to be identical with that occurring in patients on full doses of anti-thyroid drugs of the thiouracil type. These drugs are thought to exert their effect by inhibiting the transfer of iodide to tyrosyl residues by blocking in some way the enzymically controlled oxidation of iodide to iodine. It seems likely that this is the point at which iodide metabolism is blocked in the thyroid glands of this group of goitrous cretins.

Direct analysis of thyroid gland material from these patients failed to reveal any iodinated compounds, though these could readily be demonstrated in normal or hyperplastic glands using the same

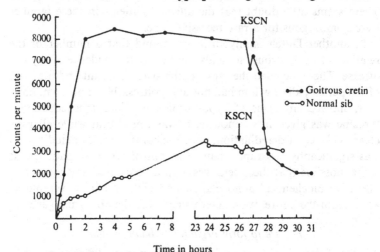

Time in hours

Fig. 13. Uptake of radioactive iodine by the thyroid in a goitrous cretin and his normal sib. At zero time a tracer dose of 100 microcuries of radioactive iodine was given by mouth. Potassium thiocyanate was administered a day later. (After Stanbury and Hedge[67]).

method. Thus the glands may contain iodide and even show excessive avidity for iodide but no incorporation into the organic form occurs. In effect there appears to be a complete block in hormone formation at a very early stage, and the large goitres and intense cellular hypertrophy and hyperplasia can be regarded as compensatory phenomena.

Other types of defect

It seems likely that several other types of condition also exist, each of which is probably genetically distinct and represents a failure at some specific point in normal thyroid metabolism. For example, Stanbury, Ohela and Pitt-Rivers [68] have described a condition in two sisters where the essential defect appeared to be a failure in the ability to couple iodotyrosines to form active hormones. In another group of cases there appears to be an inability to deiodinate diiodotyrosine, while deiodination of monoiodotyrosine goes on satisfactorily [59]. The nature of the enzyme defect here is obscure. Still other types of goitrous cretins are known which do not fit readily into any of these categories.

Melanin formation and albinism

The term melanin is used to refer to a series of insoluble brown and black pigments of high molecular weight which result from the polymerisation of dihydroxyphenolic compounds. It appears probable that in man, their main precursor is 3:4-dihydroxyphenylalanine which is derived from tyrosine. Melanin is formed predominantly in specialised pigment cells in the skin and uveal tract. In these cells it seems to be firmly bound to protein.

The processes concerned in the conversion of tyrosine to melanin are evidently complex and are not completely understood [69, 70]. The sequence of reactions which is believed to occur is shown in Fig. 14. It used to be thought that the first step, the conversion of tyrosine to dihydroxyphenylalanine, was mediated by a different enzyme from that concerned in the subsequent oxidation of dihydroxyphenylalanine. It is now considered more likely that the same enzyme or enzyme system is involved in both cases, but that the initial reaction involving tyrosine requires a certain amount of dihydroxyphenylalanine to be present for it to take place [71]. The enzyme system is referred to as 'tyrosinase'. It requires copper for its activity, and it is inhibited by compounds with $-SH$ groups.

The degree to which normal melanin formation may occur in different individuals varies considerably and it seems to be to a large extent genetically determined. Little, however, is known about the manner in which the genetical determinants influence the process. Melanin formation is also influenced by a variety of other factors such as exposure to sunlight, local inflammation, and so on. Again the processes involved are obscure. It has, however, been suggested that in the normal pigment-forming cell the tyrosine-tyrosinase system is to a greater or lesser extent inhibited by the presence of $-SH$ groups, and that the action of such agents as for example ultraviolet light might be to result in oxidation of $-SH$ groups, and so release the inhibited enzyme system [72].

Albinism is an inherited condition in which there appears to be a complete or nearly complete failure to form melanin. In its most extreme form (total albinism) the skin appears pinkish white, the hair is white or pale yellow, and the eyes show a similar absence of pigment. The iris is pink and translucent, the pupils red, and there is usually marked photophobia nystagmus and defective vision. Less extreme forms are also seen in which melanin may be formed but only in very restricted amounts.

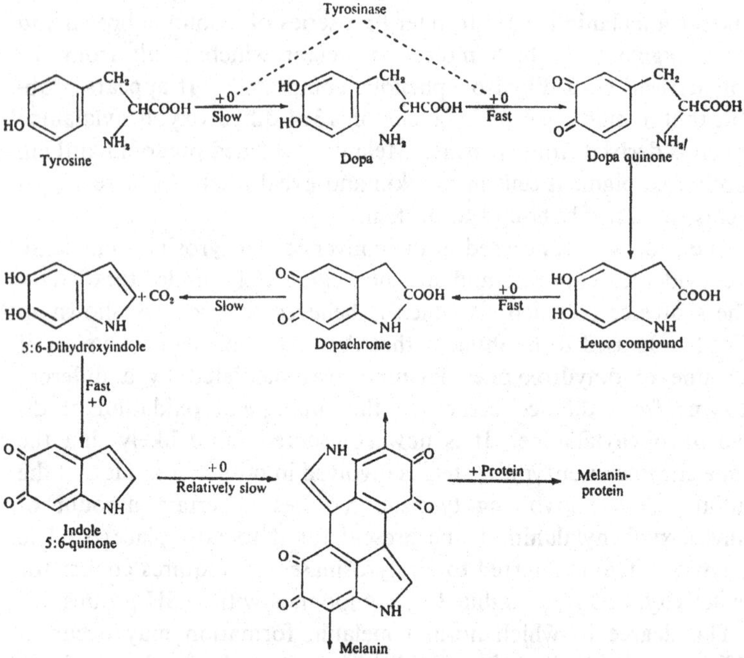

Fig. 14. The formation of melanin from tyrosine. (After Fitzpatrick and Lerner [70].)

The particular cells which normally form pigment (the melanocytes) have been demonstrated in their normal numbers in albino skin [73]. They lack, however, the capacity to form melanin, and it has been suggested that this is due to a deficiency of the enzyme 'tyrosinase'. Histochemical studies of albino skin have failed to reveal any evidence of 'tyrosinase' activity under conditions in which it could be readily demonstrated in normal skin.

The familial distribution of severe albinism suggests that in most cases it is inherited as a mendelian 'recessive' character [74]. There is a strikingly high incidence of parental consanguinity (about 20–30 per cent), and this is in fact rather higher than estimates of the incidence of the condition (about 1 in 20,000 in Great Britain) would lead one to anticipate[75]. A plausible explanation of the discrepancy is that several gene mutations at different loci may each lead to a similar defect in pigment formation. Further support for this idea of such genetical heterogeneity in this condition has been provided by the description of a family in which both parents were albinos but the children were quite normal[76]. Presumably here the parents were homozygous for different abnormal genes, probably at separate chromosomal loci.

Localised forms of albinism also occur. One example of this is 'ocular albinism' where the defect in pigmentation is peculiar to the globe of the eye, and there are no obvious albinotic changes elsewhere. This is inherited as a sex-linked character. Nothing is known about its possible biochemical basis.

REFERENCES

(1) Fölling, A. (1934). *Hoppe-Seyl. Z.* **227**, 169.
(2) Jervis, G. A. (1954). *Res. Publ. Ass. Nerv. Ment. Dis.* **33**, 259.
(3) Munro, T. A. (1947). *Ann. Eugen., Lond.* **14**, 60.
(4) Jervis, G. A. (1937). *Arch. Neurol. Psychiat.* **38**, 944.
(5) Cowie, V. and Penrose, L. S. (1951). *Ann. Eugen., Lond.* **15**, 297.
(6) Penrose, L. S. (1935). *Lancet*, **2**, 192.
(7) Zeller, E. A. (1943). *Helv. Chim. Acta*, **26**, 1614.
(8) Dann, M., Marples, E. and Levine, S. Z. (1943). *J. Clin. Invest.* **22**, 87.
(9) Jervis, G. A. (1950). *Proc. Soc. Exp. Biol. N.Y.* **75**, 83.
(10) Woolf, L. I. (1951). *Biochem. J.* **49**, 9.
(11) Armstrong, M. D. and Robinson, K. S. (1954). *Arch. Biochem. Biophys.* **52**, 287.
(12) Armstrong, M. D., Shaw, K. N. F. and Robinson, K. S. (1955). *J. Biol. Chem.* **213**, 797.
(13) Boscott, R. J. and Bickel, H. (1935). *Scand. J. Clin. Lab. Invest.* **5**, 380.
(14) Pare, C. M. B., Sandler, M. and Stacey, R. S. (1957). *Lancet*, **1**, 551.
(15) Borek, E., Brecher, A., Jervis, G. A. and Waelsch, H. (1950). *Proc. Soc. Exp. Biol. N.Y.* **75**, 86.
(16) Jervis, G. A., Block, R. J., Bolling, D. and Kanze, E. (1940). *J. Biol. Chem.* **134**, 105.
(17) Bickel, H., Gerrard, J. and Hickmans, E. M. (1954). *Acta Paed.* **43**, 64.
(18) Armstrong, M. D. and Low, N. L. (1957). *Proc. Soc. Exp. Biol. N.Y.* **94**, 142.

(19) Jervis, G. A. (1952). *Proc. Soc. Exp. Biol. N.Y.* **81**, 715.
(20) Jervis, G. A. (1938). *J. Biol. Chem.* **126**, 305.
(21) Penrose, L. S. and Quastel, J. H. (1937). *Biochem. J.* **31**, 266.
(22) Armstrong, M. D. and Tyler, F. H. (1955). *J. Clin. Invest.* **34**, 565.
(23) Woolf, L. I., Griffiths, R. and Moncrieff, A. (1955). *B.M.J.* **1**, 57.
(24) Rose, W. C., Haines, W. J., Johnson, J. E. and Warner, D. T. (1943). *J. Biol. Chem.* **148**, 457.
(25) Stein, W. H., Paladini, A. C., Hirs, C. H. W. and Moore, S. (1954). *J.A.C.S.* **76**, 2848.
(26) Jervis, G. A. (1947). *J. Biol. Chem.* **169**, 651.
(27) Udenfriend, S. and Bessman, S. P. (1953). *J. Biol. Chem.* **203**, 961.
(28) Udenfriend, S. and Cooper, J. R. (1952). *J. Biol. Chem.* **194**, 503.
(29) Mitoma, C. (1956). *Arch. Biochem. Biophys.* **60**, 476.
(30) Jervis, G. A. (1953). *Proc. Soc. Exp. Biol. N.Y.* **82**, 514.
(31) Wallace, H. W., Moldave, K. and Meister, A. (1957). *Proc. Soc. Exp. Biol. N.Y.* **94**, 632.
(32) Mitoma, C., Auld, R. M., Udenfriend, S. (1957). *Proc. Soc. Exp. Biol. N.Y.* **94**, 634.
(33) Udenfriend, S. and Mitoma, C. (1955). In *Symposium on Aminoacid Metabolism*, ed. by W. D. McElroy and B. Glass, Baltimore.
(34) Dalgliesh, C. E. (1955). *Arch. Biochem. Biophys.* **58**, 214.
(35) Knox, W. E. and Hsia, D. Y. Y. (1957). *Amer. J. Med.* **22**, 687.
(36) Bickis, I. J., Kennedy, J. P. and Quastel, J. H. (1957). *Nature, Lond.* **179**, 1124.
(37) Armstrong, M. D., Low, N. L. and Bosma, J. F. (1957). *Amer. J. Clin. Nutrit.* **5**, 543.
(38) Blainey, J. D. and Gulliford, R. (1956). *Arch. Dis. Child.* **31**, 452.
(39) Woolf, L. I., Griffiffs, R., Moncrieff, A., Coates, S. and Dillistone, F. (1958). *Arch. Dis. Child.* **33**, 31.
(40) Miyamoto, M. and Fitzpatrick, T. B. (1957). *Nature, Lond.* **179**, 199.
(41) Snyderman, S. E., Norton, P. and Holt, L. E. (1955). *Amer. J. Dis. Child.* **90**, 616.
(42) Hsia, D. Y. Y., Paine, R. S. and Driscoll, K. W. (1957). *J. Ment. Def. Res.* **1**, 53.
(43) Hsia, D. Y. Y., Driscoll, K. W., Troll, W. and Knox, W. E. (1956). *Nature, Lond.* **178**, 1239.
(44) Jervis, G. A. (1939). *J. Ment. Sci.* **85**, 719.
(45) Fölling, A., Mohr, O. L. and Ruud, L. (1945). *Norske Videnskaps-Akad. i Oslo Mat.-Naturv. Klasse,* **13**.
(46) Neuberger, A., Rimington, C. and Wilson, J. M. G. (1947). *Biochem. J.* **41**, 438.
(47) Falta, W. (1904). *Dtsch. Arch. Klin. Med.* **81**, 231.
(48) Leaf, G. and Neuberger, A. (1948). *Biochem. J.* **43**, 606.
(49) Embden, H. (1893). *Z. Phys. Chem.* **17**, 182.
(50) Blum, L. (1908). *Arch. exp. Path. Pharmak.* **59**, 268.
(51) Knox, W. E. and Edwards, S. W. (1955). *J. Biol. Chem.* **216**, 489.
(52) La Due, B. N., Zannoni, V. G., Laster, L. and Seegmiller, J. E. (1958). *J. Biol. Chem.* **230**, 251.

(53) Garrod, A. E. (1923). *Inborn Errors of Metabolism*, 2nd ed. Oxford University Press.
(54) Lichtenstein, L. and Kaplan, L. (1954). *Amer. J. Path.* **30**, 99.
(55) Pomeranz, M. M., Friedman, L. J. and Tunick, I. S. (1941). *Radiology*, **37**, 295.
(56) Hogben, L. T., Worrall, R. L. and Zieve, I. (1932). *Proc. Roy. Soc. Edinb.* **52**, 264.
(57) Pieter, H. (1925). *Pr. Méd.* **33**, 1310.
(58) Medes, G. (1932). *Biochem. J.* **26**, 917.
(59) Stanbury, J. B. and McGirr, E. M. (1957). *Amer. J. Med.* **22**, 712.
(60) Berson, S. A. (1956). *Amer. J. Med.* **20**, 653.
(61) Roche, J. and Michel, R. (1955). *Physiol. Rev.* **35**, 583.
(62) Roche, J., Michel, O., Michel, R., Gorbman, A. and Lissitzky, K. (1953). *Biochim. Biophys Acta*, **12**, 570.
(63) Stanbury, J. B., Kassenaar, A. A. H., Meijer, J. W. A. and Terpstra, J. (1955). *J. Clin. Endocrin.* **15**, 1216.
(64) Stanbury, J. B., Meijer, J. W. A. and Kassenaar, A. A. H. (1956). *J. Clin. Endocrin.* **16**, 848.
(65) Querido, A., Stanbury, J. B., Kassenaar, A. A. H. and Meijer, J. W. A. (1956). *J. Clin. Endoc.* **16**, 1096.
(66) Hutchison, J. H. and McGirr, E. M. (1956). *Lancet*, **1**, 1035.
(67) Stanbury, J. B. and Hedge, A. N. (1950). *J. Clin. Endocrin.* **10**, 1471.
(68) Stanbury, J. B., Ohela, K. and Pitt-Rivers, R. (1955). *J. Clin. Endocrin.* **15**, 54.
(69) Lerner, A. B. and Fitzpatrick, T. B. (1950). *Physiol. Rev.* **30**, 91.
(70) Fitzpatrick, T. B. and Lerner, A. B. (1954). *A.M.A. Arch. Derm. Syph.*, *N.Y.* **69**, 133.
(71) Fitzpatrick, T. B., Becker, S. W., Lerner, A. B. and Montgomery, H. (1950). *Science*, **112**, 223.
(72) Flesch, P. and Rothman, S. (1948). *Science*, **108**, 505.
(73) Becker, S. W., Fitzpatrick, T. B. and Montgomery, H. (1952). *A.M.A. Arch. Derm. Syph.*, *N.Y.* **65**, 511.
(74) Pearson, K., Nettleship, E. and Usher, C. H. (1913). *Monograph on Albinism in Man.* Cambridge University Press.
(75) Hogben, L. (1939). *Nature and Nurture.* Allen and Unwin, London.
(76) Trevor-Roper, P. D. (1952). *Brit. J. Ophthal.* **36**, 107.

CHAPTER 4

AMINOACID METABOLISM: 2

The significance of aminoaciduria

The excretion of aminoacids in unusual amounts in urine occurs in a variety of different inherited biochemical disorders [1] and very often the detection of the aminoaciduria has represented the starting-point in the investigation of such conditions. The abnormal excretion of aminoacids can result from diverse causes and frequently shows characteristic and highly specific features. Some general questions concerning the mechanism by which aminoaciduria may arise are therefore worth considering before discussing in more detail certain of the syndromes in which it has been observed.

In practice [2] it is useful to classify aminoacidurias into two main groups; the 'overflow' aminoacidurias, and the 'renal' aminoacidurias. The 'overflow' aminoacidurias arise because there is some defect in intermediary metabolism leading to an increase in plasma level of one or more aminoacids to such a degree that the normal renal tubular reabsorptive mechanism is unable to deal with them adequately and they therefore pass in increased quantities into the urine. The 'renal' aminoacidurias are due to some defect in the processes of renal tubular reabsorption so that even at normal plasma concentrations, and hence normal concentrations in the glomerular filtrate, inefficient reabsorption of one or more aminoacids takes place, and so abnormal amounts are found in the urine. The particular aminoacids occurring in excess in the urine will depend in the 'overflow' type on the specific character of the disturbances in intermediary metabolism, and in the 'renal' type on the particular way in which the renal tubules are defective. It is possible of course that in certain circumstances both types of cause may operate, but in most cases the aminoaciduria appears to fall quite clearly into one or other of these two classes. Theoretically renal aminoaciduria might also be caused by active tubular secretion but so far no definite example of this has been discovered.

Differentiation between the two general causes of aminoaciduria can usually be made from a consideration of the plasma concentrations of the aminoacids excreted in increased quantities. Characteristically in 'overflow' aminoaciduria the plasma levels of the relevant aminoacids will be appreciably in excess of those normally found. A typical example is phenylketonuria where the abnormal urinary concentration of phenylalanine is associated with plasma concentrations of this aminoacid which are some thirty times greater than those which normally occur. In 'renal' aminoaciduria on the other hand the plasma aminoacid concentrations will not be elevated and may indeed be lower than those usually encountered. An example of this is classical cystinuria in which although there is a grossly abnormal urinary excretion of the four aminoacids cystine, lysine, arginine, and ornithine, the plasma concentrations of these substances are certainly not elevated, and in fact appear to be on the average slightly lower than the equivalent normal values.

More precise clarification of the situation requires renal clearance studies of the particular aminoacids concerned, preferably at several different plasma concentrations [3]. In practice this type of investigation is often difficult to carry out. It is, however, essential in situations where it may be thought that there is both a 'metabolic' and a 'renal' component of the abnormal aminoacid excretion. It is also necessary in evaluating quantitatively the degree of impairment of tubular reabsorptive capacity in typical 'renal' aminoaciduria, and also in assessing the possibility of active tubular secretion.

Most of the common aminoacids are constituents of proteins and are also found in appreciable amounts in the circulating fluids. They are in general very efficiently reabsorbed by the renal tubules in the normal subject. Usually more than 99 per cent of the amounts present in the gomerular filtrates are removed from this fluid during its passage down the tubules and only small quantities appear in the urine. The renal clearances are mostly of the order of 1–2 ml. per min., though in the cases of glycine and histidine somewhat higher values (approximately 5–15 ml.) are observed [4, 5]. Such figures contrast with inulin clearances of the order of 120–130 ml. per min. which indicate the expected value when no tubular reabsorption is occurring.

Not all metabolites, however, are reabsorbed by the renal tubules with such a high degree of efficiency, and some may not be reabsorbed at all. Substances which are not reabsorbed can be referred to conveniently as 'no-threshold' substances, and it seems possible that certain aminoacids and closely related substances which are not protein constituents and which do not usually occur in appreciable quantities in the circulating fluids belong to this class. Dent and his colleagues[6] have suggested the term 'no-threshold' aminoaciduria to cover the situation where these substances are excreted in abnormal quantities in the urine. Argininosuccinicaciduria in the syndrome described by Allan, Cusworth, Dent and Wilson[6] probably represents an example of just such a situation and it is possible that β-aminoisobutyricaciduria and cystathioninuria are other examples. If so, such conditions could be regarded as essentially 'overflow' aminoacidurias in which the plasma concentrations of the relevant substance are maintained at low levels because of the absence of appreciable tubular reabsorption. The substances involved may be essentially intracellular metabolites whose circulation in the plasma could have no functional significance. The important practical point about such conditions is that it may sometimes be difficult, using available methods, to demonstrate that the plasma concentration of the relevant substances is appreciably different from that in normal people, simply because the amounts present are very small. Thus the distinction from a renal type of aminoaciduria may not be very obvious at first sight.

These general considerations are of course not peculiar to variations in aminoacid excretion, though it so happens that they have been most prominently discussed in this connection. They obviously apply to other substances as well. Thus the glycosuria of diabetes mellitus and the fructosuria of essential fructosuria are typically 'overflow' phenomena, while the glycosuria of renal glycosuria as the name implies is 'renal' in origin. Similarly the abnormal urinary concentrations of ethanolamine phosphate in hypophosphatasia, of porphobilinogen in acute porphyria, of L-xyloketose in essential pentosuria, and of homogentisic acid in alkaptonuria, probably represent the increased excretion of 'no-threshold' substances. Sometimes more than one different metabolite may be excreted in unusual quantities and the cause of this can be complex. Thus in galactosaemia the massive excretion of galactose is usually associated with a moderate to marked aminoaciduria. The galactosaemia is certainly an 'overflow' type of phenomenon, while the aminoaciduria is renal in origin.

A number of inherited conditions are now known in which some degree of renal aminoaciduria has been found. These include diseases as diverse as cystinuria, galactosaemia, and Wilson's disease. While each of them will be considered in more detail elsewhere, certain general points arise about the significance of the aminoaciduria in relation to pathogenesis in the various conditions(7). In classical cystinuria, for example, there occurs a grossly abnormal excretion of four aminoacids, cystine, lysine, arginine and ornithine. This can be attributed to a specific defect in renal tubular reabsorption which appears to be constant and lifelong. The various clinical features of the condition can all be satisfactorily explained in terms of the high urinary concentration of the relatively insoluble aminoacid cystine and the consequent propensity to renal calculus formation. There is no evidence that any other metabolic abnormality exists, or that the transport of these four aminoacids across other cell membranes in the body is disturbed in the same way as is their transport across the renal tubules. While it is true that the latter possibility is difficult to exclude, all the known facts about the condition can be explained in terms of a primary abnormality of a specific aspect of renal tubular function, and one may speculate that this is due to a failure in the formation of some enzyme or transport substance necessary for the efficient reabsorption of these particular aminoacids.

In contrast to this the renal aminoaciduria observed in conditions such as galactosaemia and Wilson's disease almost certainly represent secondary disturbances of renal tubular function due to a more generalised metabolic disorder not primarily concerned with aminoacid metabolism. In galactosaemia the tubular disturbance is probably a consequence of the intracellular accumulation of galactose-1-phosphate. This defect is not peculiar to the kidney. It occurs in other sites in the body such as the liver and the erythrocytes and it is probably the cause of all the diverse clinical and biochemical features of this disease of which the aminoaciduria is but one relatively unimportant facet. Similarly in Wilson's disease the aminoaciduria is probably a consequence of renal tubule damage secondary to excessive copper deposition, a process occurring throughout the body and having manifold consequences. In both cases the aminoaciduria is rather variable and not particularly specific in character.

Thus it is clear that the occurrence of aminoaciduria in a particular syndrome does not necessarily mean that one is dealing primarily with a defect in aminoacid metabolism. Similarly the demonstration of a renal tubular disturbance does not imply necessarily that this has a central place in the pathogenesis of the particular disease.

Cystinuria

In 1810 Wollaston [8] described a 'new species of urinary calculus'. During the following hundred years many further examples of the same kind of stone were identified and it was shown that they were composed almost entirely of the aminoacid, cystine. Furthermore, patients who formed such stones were found to be excreting continuously in their urine large amounts of cystine. The disorder was frequently familial and it was recognised to be in some way genetically determined.

It is now known that cystine is not the only aminoacid excreted in unusual quantities by those patients who form cystine calculi. The basic aminoacids, lysine, arginine and ornithine, are also regularly present in the urine in grossly abnormal amounts [9,10,11] and the quantities involved are remarkable. Stein [10], for example, in five cases found that an average of 0·73 g. of cystine, 1·8 g. of lysine, 0·83 g. of arginine and 0·37 g. of ornithine were excreted per day. This massive aminoaciduria is continuous and probably persists with little change throughout life. Furthermore, the abnormality appears to be highly specific for these four substances.

Earlier reports that the diamines, cadaverine and putrescine, sometimes occurred in large amounts in cystinuric urines have not been confirmed when modern analytical methods have been applied to fresh urine samples. It is possible that they represented artefacts due to infection or that the substances were misidentified.

Cystine may also be excreted in unusual amounts in a number of other genetically determined conditions. Among these may be mentioned cystinosis and the different variants of the Fanconi, De-Toni, Debré syndrome, and Wilson's disease or hepato-lenticular degeneration. In the past, cystinosis has certainly been confused with the type of cystinuria described above. It is now clear, however, that these disorders may be sharply differentiated on clinical, biochemical and genetical grounds [12]. In particular, the aminoaciduria found in such conditions is of a much more generalised type involving some ten or more aminoacids and cystine stone formation rarely if ever occurs. It is convenient, therefore, to reserve the term 'cystinuria' for the classical condition involving recurrent cystine calculus formation, described by Wollaston, and now known to be characterised by the abnormal excretion of cystine, lysine, arginine and ornithine.

The term 'cystine-lysinuria' has also occasionally been used in recent years to designate the condition. This, however, is unsatisfactory because, as will be seen later, true cystine-lysinuria when it occurs without concomitant arginine and ornithinuria is only rarely associated with stone formation. The incorporation of all four aminoacids in the name for the disease is, however, somewhat cumbersome, and now the situation has been clarified it seems simplest to retain the classical term 'cystinuria' for the disease.

The loss of the four aminoacids, even in these considerable amounts, does not lead to any obvious nutritional disturbances in the patients, providing that they are on a normal diet with an adequate protein content. All the clinical features of the condition can be attributed simply to the complication of recurrent formation of stones in the renal tract. Apart from the tendency to calculus formation and consequent obstruction in the renal tract, these patients may remain remarkably well. Surprisingly enough, chronic renal infection does not usually occur. The prime cause of the stone formation is undoubtedly the high urinary concentration of cystine. Cystine is one of the least soluble of aminoacids and in urine between pH 5 and 7 it can be kept in solution only to the extent of 300–400 mg. per litre [13] (Fig. 15). In patients excreting between $\frac{1}{2}$ g. and 1 g. of cystine per day the concentration of this substance may frequently reach saturation level, particularly at night time when the urine passed is most concentrated. Consequently, the cystine will tend to come out of solution and this will lead to calculus formation. Lysine, arginine and ornithine, on the other hand, are freely soluble and therefore do not become incorporated in the stones.

The nature of the lesion

Until quite recently it had been assumed that cystinuria represented a disorder in the intermediary metabolism either of cystine itself or of the other sulphur containing aminoacids, cysteine and methionine. (For full reviews see [14, 15].) The exact nature of the postulated 'block' in the metabolism of these substances had, however, always remained obscure. The demonstration that lysine, arginine and ornithine were equally involved introduced further complications because of the absence of any obvious specific interrelation between the intermediary metabolism of these aminoacids and the sulphur-containing ones.

An alternative hypothesis was put forward by Dent in 1949, when he suggested that the abnormality in cystinuria was essentially renal in character. If the renal tubule cells were unable to reabsorb the cystine, lysine, arginine and ornithine normally present in the glomerular filtrate, then these substances would appear in large amounts in the urine, and the various features of the disease could be readily explained. A considerable body of evidence has now accumulated in favour of this hypothesis.

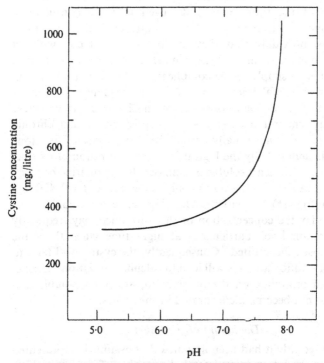

Fig. 15. The solubility of cystine in urine at different pHs.
(After Dent and Senior.)

If cystinuria arises from some kind of block in the intermediary metabolism of cystine, one would expect cystine to accumulate in the body fluids and the plasma level should be considerably higher than in normal people. If, however, cystinuria were a purely renal abnormality, no such rise in plasma cystine would be expected. Similar arguments also hold for the other aminoacids excreted in abnormal amounts. The plasma cystine level has now been measured in a number of cystinuric patients by a variety of different methods (16,17,18,19). It is, in fact, not elevated as would have been expected on the metabolic block hypothesis but is if anything slightly less than normal, as may be anticipated on the renal hypothesis. The same seems to be true for lysine, arginine and ornithine (19,20,21).

Estimates of the renal clearances of cystine and of lysine, arginine and ornithine have shown that they are all grossly elevated compared with the normal (18, 20,21). In the case of cystine, the clearance values in several instances were of the same order of magnitude as the expected rate of glomerular filtration and in one subject where the inulin and cystine clearances were measured simultaneously close agreement was obtained. The clearances for lysine, arginine and ornithine were however somewhat less than the rate of glomerular filtration and this suggests that the reabsorption defect, though gross, is not complete. Doolan and his colleagues (21), for example, measured inulin and lysine clearances simultaneously in four different cystinuric subjects. They found that the average endogenous lysine clearance was 55 ml. per min. compared with normal values of rather less than 1 ml. per min. About 45 per cent of the filtered load appeared to be reabsorbed under these conditions compared with normal reabsorption of more than 99 per cent. When the filtered load was increased by infusing lysine, no significant increase in the quantity of lysine reabsorbed occurred. Thus the residual reabsorption presumably represents an active process and not simply passive diffusion.

The renal hypothesis implies that in normal individuals the tubular reabsorption of cystine, lysine, arginine and ornithine involves at least one step which is common to and specific for these four aminoacids, and that in cystinuria this process is in some way defective. If this is so, one may expect that if one artificially elevated the plasma concentration of one of these aminoacids to very high levels in a normal person, then, as a result of overloading the reabsorptive mechanism, an increased excretion of the other three aminoacids should occur. This phenomenon has recently been demonstrated by Robson and Rose (22). They infused 5 g. lysine intravenously into normal subjects and found that an increased excretion of cystine, arginine and ornithine as well as of lysine resulted. Little change in the excretion of other aminoacids occurred. Similar experiments carried out on cystinuric patients caused little or no increase in the already grossly elevated excretion of cystine, arginine and ornithine. This, of course, would be expected on the renal hypothesis.

The results of experiments which have been carried out at different times involving the feeding of cystine, cysteine and methionine to cystinuric subjects have rarely been clear cut and have been variously interpreted. They can, however, probably be most comprehensively understood on the renal hypothesis.

If cystine itself is fed to cystinuric patients, there is little or no rise in the plasma cystine level and no appreciable increase in the urinary cystine. It appears, however, to be absorbed and metabolised because an appropriate increase in the urinary sulphate can be demonstrated. Feeding cystine to normal individuals gives substantially the same results, so that there appears to be no peculiarity in the cystinuric with respect to his ability to deal with dietary cystine.

Ingestion of cysteine by cystinurics leads to quite different phenomena; their interpretation is, however, made somewhat difficult by the absence of any satisfactory methods for differentiating plasma cystine from cysteine. In general, there occurs a rapid rise in the plasma level of cystine (or cysteine) and a very marked increase of cystine in the urine[17,18,23,24]. In all these experiments the urinary cystine output varied with the plasma levels. However, for equivalent plasma levels the cystine excretion was much greater in the cystinurics than in the normal subjects. Since the plasma tolerance curves after feeding cysteine to normal and cystinuric subjects were substantially the same, these findings are consistent with the idea that it is the renal tubular reabsorption mechanism that is at fault. Estimates of the renal clearances at different plasma levels following the feeding of cysteine further support this concept. In the cystinuric subjects the clearances did not change significantly with increasing plasma levels but remained virtually constant at a value of the same order of magnitude as the glomerular filtration rate. In normal subjects the clearances were very much lower but did rise significantly with increasing plasma levels.

The reason why both in normal and in cystinuric subjects cystine ingestion fails to lead to any marked change in plasma level, whereas cysteine leads to a rapid elevation in plasma level, remains uncertain. Dent and his colleagues[18] suggest that this is due to different rates of absorption probably depending on the relative solubilities of the two substances. Cysteine, being readily soluble, is likely to be rapidly absorbed through the intestinal mucosa and so reach the portal blood in high enough concentrations to temporarily saturate the mechanisms for maintaining a constant blood level. A large dose of cystine, however, will at first remain largely undissolved in the intestinal fluids and so be taken up into the portal blood only slowly and consequently be adequately dealt with by the liver. Earlier workers (23), however, had postulated that there existed entirely different metabolic pathways for cystine and cysteine.

Various results have been reported after feeding methionine. Earlier workers did find an increase in cystine excretion after feeding methionine to cystinurics, while Dent and his colleagues failed to find this. Such minor discrepancies may be a result of different time scales of the experiments.

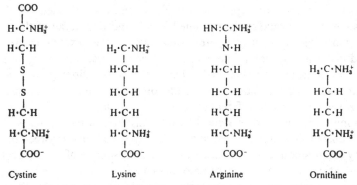

Fig. 16. Formulae of cystine, lysine, arginine and ornithine.

In general, none of these feeding experiments suggest that cystinurics differ in any material respect from normal subjects in their intermediary metabolism of the sulphur-containing aminoacids. The results, on the other hand, are all consistent with the renal hypothesis.

If it is true that in normal individuals there is a pathway in tubular reabsorption common to and specific for cystine, lysine, arginine and ornithine, and that in cystinuric patients this is defective, then one is confronted with the problem as to what property peculiar to these four aminoacids leads to their being handled by renal tubules differently from other amino acids. Some evidence for a common reabsorptive mechanism for lysine and arginine has been obtained experimentally in dogs (25). These particular substances resemble each other and also ornithine sufficiently closely in structure and chemical properties to make this association not very surprising. The specific association of cystine with the basic aminoacids is, however, rather unexpected. Dent and Rose suggested on the basis of the structural formulae (Fig. 16) that the important similarity might be the occurrence of two positively charged amino-groups separated by a chain of four to six atoms. The transport mechanism, for example, might involve the combination of these positively charged amino-groups with similarly spaced negatively charged carboxyl groups projecting from alternate glutamate or aspartate residues on a protein surface. So far, however, there is no direct evidence bearing on this problem, nor has any more plausible explanation been put forward.

Family studies

When the urine from apparently healthy relatives of patients with cystine stone formation is examined it is found that some of them, though clinically in no way abnormal, nevertheless excrete cystine and lysine in unusual amounts in their urine. Occasionally arginine and ornithine are found as well. Quantitative estimations of cystine, lysine and arginine have been made on a large number of such relatives from many different families (11,26,27) and it is evident that among them there exists a considerable variation in the amounts of the substances excreted. Indeed all values may be found between the very small amounts encountered in a random sample of the general population and the very large amounts encountered in patients with cystine stone formation. Determinations of several samples from particular individuals over periods of two or three years showed that each person had a fairly characteristic level of excretion of these substances.

Among these relatives of cystinuric patients there is a good correlation between the output of cystine and the output of lysine (Fig. 17). Differences between individuals with regard to their cystine excretions are more or less paralleled by equivalent differences in the lysine excretion. On the other hand, abnormal arginine excretion in such individuals is only consistently found when the cystine and lysine outputs are relatively high (Fig. 18). Below these levels, even though the cystine and lysine outputs may be well above the values found in normal individuals the arginine output is either within normal limits or is at most only slightly elevated. Apparently, the cystine and lysine excretion must be above a certain threshold before arginine is excreted in excess. The same may be true in the case of ornithine, but detailed quantitative results have not as yet been obtained.

Thus healthy individuals occur in some of these families with a moderately increased but quite definitely abnormal excretion of cystine and lysine and with normal arginine and perhaps ornithine outputs. Such individuals only very occasionally form stones, presumably because the urinary cystine concentration will only rarely rise to saturation levels.

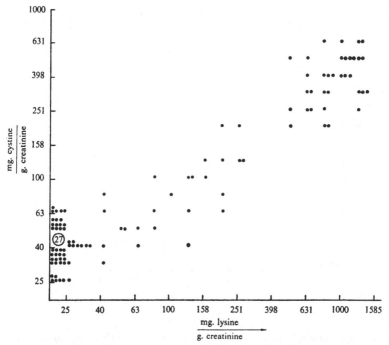

Fig. 17. Cystine and lysine contents of urine from a series of cystinuric patients and their relatives. Each point represents one person. The concentration of cystine and of lysine has been related to the creatinine concentration in each sample in order to minimise variations due to different rates of urine formation.

Now, if it is the case that in cystinuric patients with stone formation the essential defect lies in a gross failure to reabsorb in the renal tubules cystine, lysine, arginine and ornithine, then the fact that all degrees of cystine and lysine excretion may be found among their apparently healthy relatives suggests that considerable variation in the degree of failure of tubular reabsorption may occur. Furthermore, the results on arginine excretion among the relatives indicate that when the reabsorptive capacity for these four aminoacids is only partially limited, then arginine is reabsorbed preferentially to cystine and lysine. Qualitative results suggest that ornithine may in this respect resemble arginine.

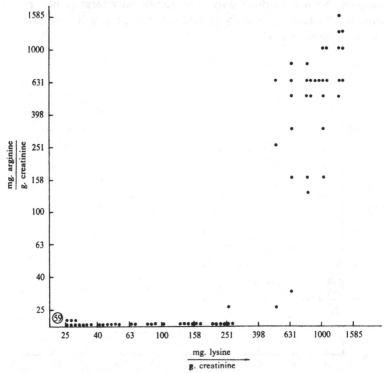

Fig. 18. Arginine and lysine contents of urine from a series of cystinuric patients and their relatives. Each point represents one person. The concentration of arginine and lysine has been related to the creatinine concentration in each sample in order to minimise variations due to different rates of urine formation.

Genetical analysis

Genetical analysis has revealed a rather complex situation. If a series of families each containing at least one member with cystine stone formation and a massive excretion of cystine, lysine, arginine and ornithine is studied, it can be shown that they are heterogenous [26, 27]. Those individuals who are clinically unaffected but have a moderately abnormal excretion of cystine and lysine with little or no detectable abnormality in arginine and ornithine excretion are not found in some families, while in others they occur quite frequently. It is possible to divide the families into two groups on this basis.

In the first group of families the intermediate phenotype does not occur, and only two classes of individual can be identified: those with a grossly abnormal excretion of cystine, lysine, arginine and ornithine, and those with excretions of these substances within the normal range. The segregation is sharp and without any overlap. The familial distribution here is typical of a Mendelian recessive character (Fig. 19).

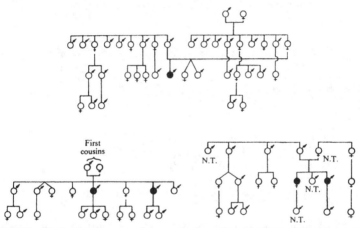

Fig. 19. Typical pedigrees of 'recessive' cystinuria. ●, grossly abnormal excretion of cystine, lysine, arginine and ornithine; ○, normal aminoacid excretion; N.T. not tested.

Abnormal individuals occur usually in only a single sibship in each individual family; the parents, children and other relatives are normal, and there is an increased incidence of parental consanguinity. Appropriate calculations indicate that the observed segregation ratios are consistent with those theoretically expected. One can conclude that here one is dealing with a rare abnormal gene whose effects are only manifest in homozygous individuals. The heterozygotes, that is to say both parents, all the children and a proportion of the other relatives have no detectable abnormality. The individuals who carry the abnormal gene in double dose appear to have a severe defect in the tubular reabsorption of the four aminoacids concerned, while individuals carrying the gene only in single dose can reabsorb these substances as efficiently as other people, at least at normal loads.

The type of condition found in this group of families has been called 'recessive cystinuria'.

In the second group of families, which is somewhat less common than the first group, the position is rather more complex. Three types of individual may be identified; those with grossly abnormal excretion of the four aminoacids; those with a moderate excretion of cystine and lysine, but a normal or only slightly elevated excretion of arginine and ornithine; and those with normal excretion. The intermediate phenotype is rather variable and some overlap in the

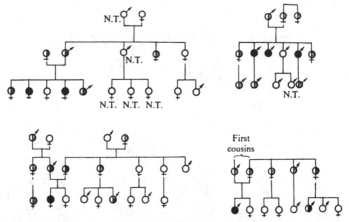

Fig. 20. Typical pedigrees of 'incompletely recessive' cystinuria. ●, grossly abnormal excretion of cystine, lysine, arginine and ornithine; ◑, abnormal excretion of cystine and lysine, arginine and ornithine excretion normal or only slightly elevated; ○, normal aminoacid excretion; N.T. not tested.

three distributions occurs. This is particularly noticeable in the lower ranges of the intermediate class which overlaps with the upper range of the distribution of normals, and some difficulty in unequivocal classification occurs. However, there seems little doubt about the reality of these three phenotypes and most individuals in such families can be fairly readily assigned to one or the other on the basis of the quantities of the individual aminoacids found in the urine. The distribution of these three phenotypes in these families fits well with the idea that the most extreme phenotype where there is presumably a gross failure in tubular reabsorption of all four aminoacids occurs in individuals homozygous for the abnormal gene; and the inter-mediate phenotype with only a moderate defective tubular dysfunc-tion represents the heterozygous individuals (Fig. 20). Such a hypothesis implies that both parents and all the children of the most severely affected individuals would be heterozygotes and thus belong to the intermediate phenotype. Similarly, half the uncles and aunts, one of each pair of grandparents and an appropriate proportion of the cousins and other relatives, both on the maternal and paternal sides of the family, would also belong to the intermediate phenotype. These expectations are in good agreement with the observed findings in these families, providing appropriate allowance is made for some overlapping of the distributions. The fact that there is an increased incidence of parental consanguinity among the parents of the affected patients in these families gives further support to the hypothesis. For this and other reasons the type of condition found in this group of families has been called 'incompletely recessive cystinuria'.

Individuals with this abnormal gene in double dose show a gross defect in the renal tubular handling of the four characteristic aminoacids. In this respect it resembles the gene responsible for the so-called 'recessive cystinuria'. On the average the rate of excretion of the four aminoacids is much the same in the two sorts of homozygote. The important difference appears to be that while in the one case the gene even in single dose results in a detectable though minor abnormality of tubular function, in the other case the heterozygote is by available methods indistinguishable from the normal. The relative amounts of cystine, lysine and arginine excreted in individuals of different genotypes are indicated in Table 14.

Table 14. *Average cystine, lysine and arginine concentrations (mg./g. creatinine) in urine from individuals of different cystinuria genotypes. (After Harris et al. 1955)*

Genotype		Cystine*	Lysine†	Arginine†
'Recessive' cystinuria	Homozygotes	456	1074	769
	Heterozygotes	40	<25	<25
'Incompletely recessive' cystinuria	Homozygotes	453	1025	689
	Heterozygotes	124	194	<25
Normal homozygotes		40	<25	<25

* Estimated polarographically.
† Estimated microbiologically.

Thus it has become possible to differentiate on genetical grounds two main forms of classical cystinuria: the 'recessive' and the 'incompletely recessive'. In both forms the abnormal homozygotes excrete large quantities of the four characteristic aminoacids. However, even among such homozygotes considerable variation in the relative proportions of the different aminoacids excreted from case to case may be found, and analysis of this variation has revealed further complexities in the genetical situation (28).

A convenient index of this variation in pattern of excretion is the ratio of the quantity of lysine to the quantity of arginine in urine samples from different homozygous individuals. Values for this ratio as high as 4·2 and as low as 0·8 may occur in different homozygotes and these differences are larger than can be reasonable attributed to experimental error. Furthermore, the variation in the lysine/arginine ratios are very much greater among the recessive homozygotes than among the incompletely recessives. This difference in variance is highly significant. On the other hand, the mean value for the ratio among the recessive homozygotes is not significantly different from that for the incompletely recessive ones. In the recessive group of homozygotes affected pairs of sibs closely resemble one another in the lysine/arginine excretion ratio, a sib-sib correlation coefficient of the order of 0·90 being found. In the incompletely recessive homozygotes, on the other hand, no sib-sib correlation is demonstrable. All this suggests that the large variation in the pattern of excretion of the recessive group of homozygotes is to a great extent genetical in origin. It seems probable that this group is heterogenous and consists of several distinct conditions caused by separate recessive genes. The affected individuals would either be homozygous for one of these genes or heterozygous for two of them. Whether or not the several genes causing 'recessive cystinuria' and the gene causing the 'incompletely recessive' condition are alleles or at different chromosomal loci remains to be discovered.

Calculus formation

Stone formation is a fairly frequent occurrence among individuals homozygous for one or other of the genes causing cystinuria. Probably more than 65 per cent of such individuals develop calculi at some time in their lives and in such people stone formation is very often recurrent. The majority of them form their first stone before the age of thirty and an appreciable fraction of these do so in infancy and childhood. Thus, although cystine calculi may account for no more than 1 per cent of all renal calculi encountered, they probably form a very much larger proportion of all calculi occurring in childhood. The exact proportion has, however, not yet been estimated.

Stone formation has also occasionally occurred in heterozygotes of the incompletely recessive type who happen to have rather a high level of cystine excretion. This, however, is rather unusual and the vast majority of heterozygotes remain symptom-free and quite healthy.

Stone formation is, in the main, undoubtedly a function of the cystine concentration attained in the urine. If this should frequently reach saturation level, then the patient is at risk. The concentration attained at any time will depend on the rate of excretion of cystine and the volume of urine being formed. Differences in stone formation between homozygotes may, therefore, depend not only on differences in the absolute rates of cystine excretion, but also on individual variations in rates of urine formation. This latter is likely to be of considerable importance in view of the known variations from one person to another in habits of fluid intake. No doubt other factors such as malformations in the structure of the renal tract, infection, transfer to tropical climates with inadequate adjustment of fluid intake to maintain urine volume, and so on, may also play a part in deciding why one homozygote is more prone to form stones than another.

What may, however, be of particular significance in stone formation is the diurnal rhythm in urine flow. Most people pass very much more concentrated urine at night time than in the daytime and it may well be that most of the stone formation occurs in the night. This possibility is emphasised by the results of an experiment carried out by Dent and Senior[13] on a cystinuric patient. Urine collections were made in two periods each day; a day-time period from 6 a.m. to 10 p.m. and a night-time period of 10 p.m. to 6 a.m. During this time the patient was allowed to follow her normal habits of food and fluid intake. The volumes of urine passed and their cystine content were measured in each period (see Table 15). The average day-time excretion of cystine was 538μg. per min. and the night excretion average was 492μg. per min. There was thus little difference in the rate of cystine excretion in the two periods. On the other hand, the urine output fell from an average day-time level of 2·1 ml. per min. to an average night-time one of 0·67 ml. per min. In consequence, the concentration of cystine in the night urine was very much more than in the corresponding day urine. During part of this experiment solubility studies were also carried out. The addition of solid cystine to the day urines caused an increased concentration in the urine

Table 15. *Day and night excretion of cystine in the urine of a cystinuric patient.* (*After Dent and Senior*, 1955)

Day	Period	Urine output (ml./min.)	Cystine concentration(μg./ml.)	Cystine excretion (μg./min.)	pH	Cystine in solution after equilibration with added cystine (μg./ml.)
First	Day	2·2	275	602	6·2	380
	Night	0·78	690	540	6·1	340
Second	Day	2·2	225	504	6·1	450
	Night	0·49	890	435	6·5	440
Third	Day	1·8	290	530	7·2	500
	Night	0·5	975	486	5·9	310
Fourth	Day	2·4	225	540	—	—
	Night	0·92	575	536	—	—
Fifth	Day	1·7	250	425	—	—
	Night	0·65	610	420	—	—
Sixth	Day	1·8	375	695	—	—
	Night	0·75	745	557	—	—
Seventh	Day	1·9	250	468	—	—
	Night	0·67	700	466	—	—

filtrate, while in the case of the night urines the concentration decreased. Thus, the day-time urines were undersaturated with cystine and the night-time urines were super-saturated.

The Fanconi syndrome

The Fanconi syndrome is a complex syndrome or group of syndromes which has been described from different points of view under a variety of different names (for example, Syndrome of de Toni, Fanconi, and Debré; Lignac-Fanconi disease; cystine rickets; aminoacid diabetes, etc.). Characteristically there is a marked aminoaciduria involving many aminoacids, renal glycosuria, and low plasma inorganic phosphate. This is associated with Vitamin D resistant rickets in childhood or osteomalacia in adult life. Other common features are chronic acidosis, proteinuria, polyuria and electrolyte disturbances which may result in potassium depletion. There are probably several genetically distinct types of condition which have these features in varying degree and which have tended, therefore, to be classified together.

In what is probably the commonest group of cases sharing these features there is one additional important biochemical finding. This is a widespread deposition of cystine crystals throughout the tissues [29].

It is often referred to as cystinosis. Although this was first recognised in post-mortem examinations, it was later found that it could be detected during life by the demonstration of cystine crystals in aspirated bone marrow and lymph nodes removed by biopsy, or by slit lamp examination of the cornea. Affected children usually do quite well for the first few months of life and then may present because of vomiting failure to thrive, or polyuria. In other cases the first indication of the disease is a severe resistant type of rickets with dwarfing and concomitant deformities. The prognosis is poor and death usually occurs before puberty.

The amounts of cystine deposited in the tissues in such cases may be very considerable. Dent and Fowler(30), for example, found quantities of the order of 300 and 900 mg. of cystine per g. tissue total nitrogen in liver and spleen respectively as compared with control values of the order of 2 or 3 mg. per g. nitrogen. There is obviously a very gross disorder in the handling of cystine and possibly of other more soluble aminoacids by the tissues, but the nature of this is at present quite obscure.

Despite the profound disturbance in aminoacid metabolism implied by this widespread deposition of cystine in the tissues, the aminoaciduria which includes an increased cystine output as one of its components appears to be essentially renal in origin. The aminonitrogen level in the plasma is usually within normal limits and the amino-nitrogen clearance is significantly raised(31). It has indeed been plausibly argued that many of the features of the disorder can be attributed to a gross defect in the proximal convoluted tubules of the kidney resulting in imperfect reabsorption of many aminoacids, glucose, phosphate, bicarbonate, and perhaps potassium from the glomerular filtrate. A low renal threshold for phosphate, for example, could account for the hypophosphataemia, and this could be regarded as determining the peculiarities in bone formation which are similar in type to those found in other forms of Vitamin D resistant rickets and osteomalacia, where inadequate tubular reabsorption of phosphate seems to occur without any associated renal aminoaciduria.

Support for this concept of a defect in tubular function has been provided by the elegant microdissections of nephrons from kidneys of such patients carried out by Darmady and his colleagues(32). They have found a peculiar and characteristic morphological abnormality of the proximal tubule. This is shorter than normal and is joined to the glomerulus by a narrow swan-like neck. It is present in all or nearly all the nephrons.

It is not, however, possible to account for the cystinosis in terms of the renal peculiarity, and as yet no simple unifying hypothesis which adequately explains the manifold features of the disease has been forthcoming.

The disorder is not infrequently found among sibs of affected patients, the parents are occasionally consanguineous, and the data as a whole are consistent with the hypothesis that the affected individuals are homozygous for a rare abnormal gene(29, 33). No peculiarity has been detected so far in the presumed heterozygotes.

A similar kind of condition but presenting for the first time in adolescence or adult life as a severe osteomalacia has also been recognised. This is usually referred to as the 'adult Fanconi syndrome' (34). These patients resemble the infantile group of cases in that there is a marked generalised aminoaciduria, glycosuria, hypophosphataemia, and a mild degree of chronic acidosis. They differ in that there is no cystinosis. The pattern of abnormal aminoacid excretion is similar to that found in the cystinosis cases and it is certainly renal in character. The plasma aminoacids are within normal limits and the clearances of these aminoacids excreted in excess have been shown to be greatly elevated (3, 4). The glycosuria and low plasma phosphate levels can likewise be attributed to defective function of the proximal renal tubules. Here again Darmady and his colleagues have been able to observe the peculiar 'swan neck' deformity in microdissections of the nephrons, and in this respect the adult cases without cystinosis resemble the infantile cases with cystinosis.

The renal tubular dysfunction precedes the development of the osteomalacia, and so individuals may occur who show the typical biochemical findings but who appear to be quite well. This was strikingly illustrated in the family shown in Fig. 21. Here the initial case was a housewife(12) aged 41 who had for the previous seven years suffered severe 'rheumatic' pains in various parts of the body. The pains had gradually restricted her movements until she became completely bedridden. Investigation revealed all the typical biochemical features of the adult Fanconi syndrome with well advanced osteomalacia and multiple 'pseudofractures'. Examination of the urines of some forty of her relatives revealed that two of her brothers and one sister though at that time quite well showed an aminoaciduria and glycosuria identical in every respect with that of the affected patient. They also had a somewhat reduced level of plasma inorganic phosphate and a mild acidosis. These sibs were followed for several years and the early signs of bone diseases detected as they developed. Since the bone changes which are the most disabling feature of the disease in the adult respond very well to large doses of vitamin D, the recognition of the condition in its preclinical state is of great therapeutic significance because treatment can commence before disablement develops.

While it seems highly probable that in this family and in most other cases of the adult Fanconi syndrome, the disorder is genetically

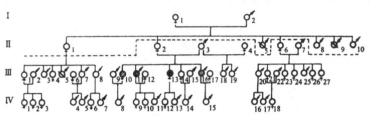

Fig. 21. Pedigree showing the segregation of the 'adult' Fanconi syndrome. Urines from all the individuals below the dotted line with the exception of III_5 were examined. III_{13} was the patient with the full clinical manifestations of the disease, through which the family was identified. III_{10}, III_{11}, and III_{16} were found to have the typical biochemical features of the syndrome, but were at that time clinically unaffected. (After Dent and Harris.)

determined (probably by a rare 'recessive' gene), it is possible that occasionally a similar symptom complex with the associated characteristic urinary findings may result as a secondary consequence of renal tubular damage from other causes. Such an effect has been plausibly attributed to multiple myelomatosis in at least two instances [35].

Hypophosphataemia, generalised renal aminoaciduria, and renal glycosuria, combined with marked vitamin D resistant rickets in infancy has also been found in association with severe and progressive cirrhosis of the liver [36]. The aminoaciduria is peculiar in that tyrosine excretion is a particularly prominent feature [37]. In these cases cystinosis is not observed. At least one family has been studied in which two sibs were affected in this way, and the condition is probably a distinct genetically determined disease entity. A similar syndrome but presenting later in life with cirrhosis and osteomalacia has also been encountered [38]. This may represent a

milder version of the same kind of disease process. It is almost
certainly a different condition from the other type of adult Fanconi
syndrome without liver damage.

Hartnup disease

This condition was described in 1956 under the title 'hereditary
pellagra-like skin rash with temporary cerebellar ataxia, constant
renal aminoaciduria and other bizarre biochemical features'[39].

The pedigree of the family in which the condition was first
recognised is shown in Fig. 22. Case II_1 had been seen originally
nearly twenty years previously when at the age of six she had a

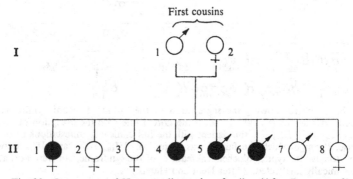

Fig. 22. Occurrence of Hartnup disease in a family. (After Baron *et al.*)

peculiar neurological episode characterised by ataxia, nystagmus,
incontinence, and mental confusion. She also had a skin rash
localised to exposed areas and apparently due to photosensitivity.
The clinical appearances closely resembled pellagra and she was
treated with the appropriate vitamin preparations, making what
appeared to be a more or less complete recovery. Subsequently,
however, she had periodic attacks of the dermatitis despite the
absence of any obvious vitamin deficiency in her diet. Some fourteen
years later her brother II_4, then aged twelve, developed a similar kind
of neurological disturbance with marked cerebellar features. He also
had an extensive dry scaly rash on his face, neck, arms and legs.

At this point it was discovered that both these patients had a gross
and remarkable aminoaciduria. Furthermore investigation of the
rest of the family revealed that two younger brothers, then aged eight
years and six years respectively, both shared the same type of

abnormal aminoacid excretion, identical in all its details to that present in the older children. II$_5$ had some degree of dermatitis, but II$_6$ appeared at that time to be clinically normal. The urinary aminoacids in the other sibs and also in both parents were normal.

The pattern of abnormal aminoacid excretion in the four affected sibs was rather different in detail from that which had been previously encountered in other types of generalised aminoaciduria. Alanine, serine, asparagine, glutamine, valine, leucine, isoleucine, phenylalanine, tyrosine, tryptophan and histidine were present in much greater quantities than is normally found; cystine, lysine and glycine were moderately elevated compared with the normal; taurine was present in normal amounts; and proline methionine and arginine were not detected. The relative proportions of the different aminoacids seemed to be much the same in all four sibs. Since the recognition of the syndrome in this family, a number of further cases have been identified in which the same symptom complex, often originally diagnosed as pellagra, has been found to be associated with precisely the same pattern of aminoacid excretion, so that this seems to be characteristic and diagnostic.

The aminoaciduria is evidently mainly, if not entirely, renal in origin. No abnormality has been detected in the plasma aminoacid concentrations, and where it has been possible to estimate the renal clearances of those aminoacids excreted in excess, they have been found to be grossly elevated. There is, however, some uncertainty as to whether in the particular case of tryptophan, the increased excretion is entirely renal in origin. This is because the plasma concentrations of this aminoacid could not be estimated satisfactorily with the methods available, and because the abnormal indole excretion mentioned below suggests that some defect in the intermediary metabolism of tryptophan may exist. However, in general there is little doubt that in each of these individuals there exists a highly specific disturbance in the renal tubular reabsorption of many different aminoacids. This appears to be continuous and unvarying and evidently precedes the development of the clinical disturbances.

The other outstanding biochemical finding in these patients is an abnormal excretion of indolylacetic acid (50–200 mg. a day), and also indolylacetyl glutamine [40]. Indican may also be excreted in markedly increased amounts, but this seems to be more variable than the other urinary abnormalities, and may in fact be completely abolished by the administration of aureomycin, a fact which suggests that it is formed by bacterial action in the gut. Unusual amounts of other tryptophan derivatives such as serotonin or indolyllactic acid were not observed.

So far no adequate unifying hypothesis has been found which will relate the gross and characteristic renal aminoaciduria and the unusual excretion of tryptophan derivatives to the peculiar pellagra-like symptom complex which develops in these individuals. Evidently true vitamin deficiency pellagra does not result in similar abnormalities in aminoacid or indole excretion. Furthermore, while the urine findings seem to be relatively constant, the clinical manifestations are variable and episodic. It has been suggested that the condition may represent some primary disorder of tryptophan metabolism. In this case the specific renal tubular dysfunction would have to be regarded as in some way secondary to this. Another possibility is that there is some primary disorder of aminoacid transport systems of which the renal tubular disorder is but one facet, and the other findings are secondary consequences.

The segregation pattern in the original family and the fact that the parents were first cousins made it seem likely that the affected individuals are homozygous for a rare abnormal gene. This hypothesis has been supported by the family studies in a few of the other examples of what appear to be the same disorder. No peculiarity has as yet been reported in the presumed heterozygotes.

β-Aminoisobutyric acid excretion

β-Aminoisobutyric acid was discovered as a biologically significant substance when the technique of paper chromatography began to be applied in a routine way to the study of the free aminoacids in urine [41,42]. It was observed that urine samples obtained from some 5–10 per cent of normal people consistently showed the presence of an unknown ninhydrin-reacting material which was one of the most prominent spots on the chromatogram. This material was subsequently isolated and identified as β-aminoisobutyric acid (Fig. 23).

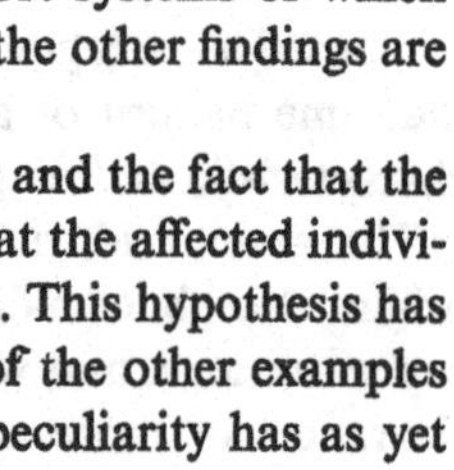

$$CH_3 \underrel{\displaystyle C}{\overset{\displaystyle CH_2NH_2}{\rule{0pt}{1em}}} H$$

Fig. 23.
β-Aminoisobutyric acid.

The rate of excretion of this substance varies greatly from individual to individual. In some people quantities of the order of

50–200 mg. are put out daily, and this represents a significant fraction of the total free aminoacid excretion. In most people, however, much smaller quantities are excreted though it is probably almost always present in the urine in at least trace amounts [4]. The distribution of individual excretion rates appears to be continuous and there is still doubt whether it is bimodal or not. This uncertainty is partly due to the technical difficulties involved in estimating concentrations of this substance in the lower excretion ranges with sufficient accuracy. The most satisfactory methods of estimation (for example, Moore and Stein column chromatography) are too laborious and time consuming for extensive survey work. Thus although it has often proved convenient to classify individuals into high and low excretors of β-aminoisobutyric acid, this dichotomy is still essentially arbitrary and does not necessarily signify that there are two biologically distinct groups in the population.

The quantity of β-aminoisobutyric acid excreted daily by any one person appears in normal circumstances to remain relatively constant. It is hardly at all influenced by ordinary dietary variation, and can reasonably be regarded as an individual characteristic. There is little doubt in fact that it is genetically determined [43, 44, 45, 46]. The incidence of 'high excretors' among the offspring of matings where one parent is a 'high excretor' is significantly greater than among the offspring of parents neither of whom would be classified in this way. Similarly twin studies have shown that uniovular twins resemble each other more closely in their β-aminoisobutyric acid excretion than do binovular twins [47]. The precise mode of inheritance, however, remains uncertain. Some of the published data is consistent with the hypothesis that a large part of the variation in individual rates of excretion can be explained in terms of a single gene substitution, the so-called 'high excretors' being homozygous for one of these genes. However, more complex hypotheses involving a multiplicity of genetical factors influencing the excretion of this substance in normal individuals cannot be excluded. Whatever the nature of the genetical determinants turns out to be, however, there seems little doubt that they occur with varying incidence in different populations. Appreciably higher frequencies of 'high excretors' than are found in European populations have been encountered in studies of Apache Indians, British Honduras Carib Negroes [48] and certain Chinese and Japanese populations [44, 49].

It was originally thought likely [41] that the variation in excretion rates of β-aminoisobutyric acid was due to differences between people in the capacities of their renal tubules to reabsorb this substance from the glomerular filtrate. This idea was based on the fact that in people excreting relatively large quantities (100–200 mg. per day), the substance was either not detectable or only just detectable in the blood plasma. Rough estimates of the maximal possible plasma concentrations indicated that these must be very small, and that therefore the renal clearance of β-aminoisobutyric acid in these subjects was high. However, there is as yet little direct evidence that in normal subjects

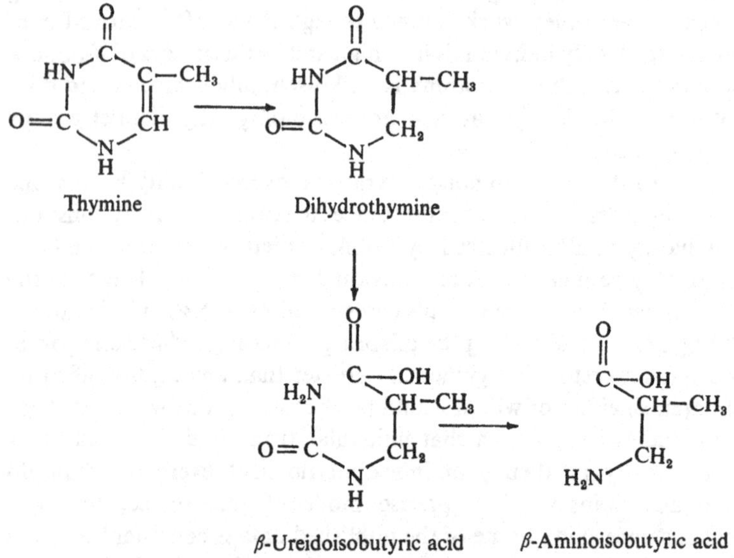

Fig. 24. Possible pathway for the formation of β-aminoisobutyric acid from thymine. (After Fink *et al.*)

who excrete only small quantities of this substance any appreciable degree of tubular reabsorption takes place and it may well be that the renal clearance is very high here as well. If this were so, the variations in excretion could be a reflection of variations in intermediary metabolism, and a search for a metabolic difference of some sort between individuals at the extremes of the excretion range might be rewarding. So far no such studies have been reported.

The metabolic origin of β-aminoisobutyric has been studied experimentally in the rat by Fink and her colleagues [50,51,52]. They found that the administration of thymine led to increased excretion of β-aminoisobutyric acid by these animals and the effect was even more pronounced following the administration of dihydrothymine. The conversion of these substances to β-aminoisobutyric acid was also demonstrated *in vitro* using liver slices. This was confirmed with radioactively-labelled thymine. These workers suggest the pathway for the formation of β-aminoisobutyric acid from thymine shown in Fig. 24.

How far such a reaction sequence represents the mode of origin of urinary β-aminoisobutyric acid in man remains to be seen. It is of interest that a relatively increased incidence of high β-aminoisobutyric acid excretion has been noted in leukaemia, and other neoplastic conditions[48]. This may well be a consequence of increased nucleic acid catabolism. Increased β-aminoisobutyric acid output has also been observed in individuals who have been completely starved for several days[53], and also in lead poisoning[54].

Other aminoacidurias

A number of other specific kinds of aminoaciduria which are most probably genetically determined have also been reported.

Allan, Cusworth, Dent and Wilson[6] described two sibs who were mentally defective and who were found by chromatography to be excreting large amounts of a substance which gave reactions typical of an aminoacid or closely related type of compound. The quantities excreted were of the order of 1–2 g. per day. Two other sibs, both parents and a number of other relatives were examined and found to be apparently quite normal. In the affected children the unusual substance was also found in appreciable amounts in the blood plasma and the cerebrospinal fluid. Its concentration in the cerebrospinal fluid was, however, two and a half to three times that in the plasma and this led to the suggestion that the substance was being formed in the brain possibly as a result of a block in cerebral metabolism. An alternative hypothesis would be that the material was formed elsewhere but specifically concentrated in the cerebrospinal fluid. Estimates of the renal clearance of this substance were of the same order of magnitude as the rate of glomerular filtration, and this implies that little or no renal tubular reabsorption was going on.

The substance has now been isolated and identified by Westall[55] as argininosuccinic acid. This is thought to be an intermediate in the urea-cycle, but whether it is the sequence of reactions involved in urea synthesis or some other metabolic process in which argininosuccinic acid may be concerned which is defective in this disease remains to be elucidated. It is of interest that the blood urea was within normal limits in the affected patients.

Another unusual form of aminoaciduria has recently been studied in the author's own laboratory. Large amounts of cystathionine were found in the urine of an elderly imbecile in the course of a survey of urines from patients in a mental deficiency institution. The cystathionine excretion amounted to about 500 mg. per day. It was markedly increased following the administration of methionine. No cystathionine could be detected in the blood plasma by paper

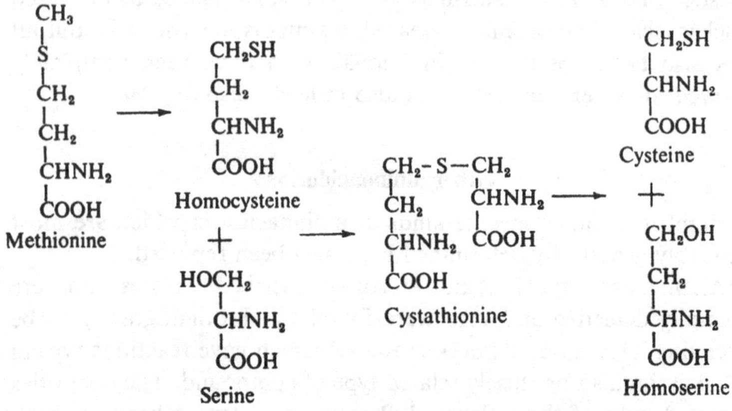

Fig. 25. Formation and cleavage of cystathionine.

chromatography, so that the renal clearance of this substance was presumably very high. Preliminary studies of extracts prepared from tissues obtained at post-mortem indicate that there was a significantly greater amount of cystathionine in the liver and kidney compared with appropriate controls.

Cystathionine is believed to be an intermediate in the formation of cysteine from methionine (Fig. 25), and the findings in this patient could be interpreted as due to an enzymic block at the point where normally cystathionine is cleaved to give cysteine and homoserine. Such a block has been produced experimentally in rats rendered deficient in vitamin B_6. However, there was no evidence to suggest that this patient's diet was vitamin deficient. Furthermore, investigation of a number of the relatives of the patient revealed that a clinically normal brother and also a nephew of the patient, both of whom had lived separately, and under quite different conditions from the patient all their lives, also excreted significant though smaller amounts of cystathionine.

Westall, Dancis, Miller and Lepitz[56] have discovered another peculiar form of aminoaciduria in an infant suffering from the so-called 'maple syrup urine' syndrome. This is a severe neurological disturbance occurring in young infants and usually fatal in a few weeks or months. It was originally described by Menkes and his colleagues[57] in a family where four out of six children were affected. The outstanding feature to which they drew attention was the peculiar smell of the urine which closely resembled that of maple syrup. Westall and his colleagues showed that the urine contained abnormal amounts of the branched chain aminoacids valine, leucine and isoleucine, and that the plasma concentrations of these particular aminoacids were also markedly elevated. The nature of the defect in the metabolism of these substances remains to be elucidated. It is also still not known what material is responsible for the curious smell of the urine.

REFERENCES

(1) Harris, H. (1956). *Proc. 3rd Int. Congr. Biochem.* p. 467. Academic Press Inc., New York.
(2) Dent, C. E. (1950). *Schweiz. med. Wschr.* **80**, 752.
(3) Dent, C. E. (1954). *Exp. Med. Surg.* **12**, 229.
(4) Evered, D. F. (1956). *Biochem. J.* **62**, 416.
(5) Doolan, P. D., Harper, H. A., Hutchin, M. E. and Shreeve, W. W. (1955). *J. Clin. Invest.* **34**, 1247.
(6) Allan, J. D., Cusworth, D. C., Dent, C. E. and Wilson, V. K. (1958). *Lancet*, **1**, 182.
(7) Harris, H. (1956). In *Modern Views on the Secretion of Urine*, ed. F. R. Winton, p. 186. Churchill, London.
(8) Wollaston, W. H. (1810). *Phil. Trans. Roy. Soc.* p. 223.
(9) Dent, C. E. and Rose, G. A. (1951). *Quart. J. Med.* N.S. **20**, 205.
(10) Stein, W. H. (1951). *Proc. Soc. Exp. Biol.*, N.Y. **78**, 705.
(11) Harris, H., Mittwoch, U., Robson, E. B. and Warren, F. L. (1955). *Ann. Hum. Genet.* **19**, 196.
(12) Dent, C. E. and Harris, H. (1951). *Ann. Eugen.*, *Lond.* **16**, 60
(13) Dent, C. E. and Senior, B. (1955). *Brit. J. Urol.* **27**, 317.
(14) Bach, S. J. (1952). *The Metabolism of the Protein Constituents in the Mammalian Body.* The Clarendon Press, Oxford.
(15) Garrod, A. E. (1923). *Inborn Errors of Metabolism*, 2nd ed. Oxford University Press.
(16) Fowler, D. I., Harris, H. and Warren, F. L. (1952). *Lancet*, **1**, 544.

(17) Dent, C. E., Heathcote, J. G. and Joron, G. E. (1954). *J. Clin. Invest.* **33**, 1210.

(18) Dent, C. E., Senior, B., Walshe, J. M. (1954). *J. Clin. Invest.* **33**, 1216.

(19) Stein, W. H. and Moore, S. (1954). *J. Biol. Chem.* **211**, 915.

(20) Arrow, V. and Westall, R. G. (1958). *J. Physiol.* **142**, 14.

(21) Doolan, P. D., Harper, H. A., Hutchin, M. E. and Alpin, E. L. (1957). *Amer. J. Med.* **23**, 416,

(22) Robson, E. B. and Rose, G. A. (1957). *Clin. Sci.* **16**, 75.

(23) Brand, E., Cahill, G. F. and Harris, M. M. (1933). *Proc. Soc. Exp. Biol., N.Y.* **31**, 348.

(24) Brand, E., Cahill, G. F. and Harris, M. M. (1935). *J. Biol. Chem.* **109**, 69.

(25) Beyer, K. H., Wright, L. D., Skeggs, H. R., Russo, H. F. and Shaner, G. A. (1947). *Amer. J. Phys.* **151**, 202.

(26) Harris, H. and Warren, F. L. (1953). *Ann. Eugen., Lond.* **18**, 125.

(27) Harris, H., Mittwoch, U., Robson, E. B. and Warren, F. L. (1955). *Ann. Hum. Genet.* **20**, 57.

(28) Harris, H. and Robson, E. B. (1955). *Acta Genet.* **5**, 381.

(29) Bickel, H. Smallwood, W. C., Smellie, J. M., Baar, H. S. and Hickmans, E. M. (1952). 'Cystine storage disease with aminoaciduria and dwarfism.' *Acta Paed.* **42**, Suppl. 90.

(30) Dent, C. E. and Fowler, D. I. (Personal communication.)

(31) Dent, C. E. (Personal communication.)

(32) Clay, R. D., Darmady, E. M. and Hawkins, M. (1953). *J. Path. Bact.* **65**, 551.

(33) Dent, C. E. and Harris, H. (1956). *J. Bone Jt. Surg.* **38B**, 204.

(34) Wallis, L. A. and Engle, R. L. (1957). *Amer. J. Med.* **22**, 13.

(35) Engle, R. L. and Wallis, L. A. (1957). *Amer. J. Med.* **22**, 5.

(36) Baber, M. D. (1956). *Arch. Dis. Child.* **31**, 335.

(37) Dent, C. E. (Personal communication.)

(38) Stowers, J. M. and Dent, C. E. (1947). *Quart. J. Med.* N.S. **16**, 275.

(39) Baron, D. N., Dent, C. E., Harris, H., Hart, E. W. and Jepson, J. B. (1956). *Lancet*, **2**, 421.

(40) Jepson, J. B. (1956). *Biochem. J.* **64**, 14P.

(41) Crumpler, H. R., Dent, C. E., Harris, H. and Westall, R. G. (1951). *Nature, Lond.* **167**, 302.

(42) Fink, K., Henderson, K. B. and Fink, R. M. (1951). *Proc. Soc. Exp. Biol., N.Y.* **78**, 135.

(43) Gartler, S. M. (1956). *Amer. J. Hum. Genet.* **8**, 120.

(44) de Grouchy, J. and Sutton, H. E. (1957). *Amer. J. Hum. Genet.* **9**, 76.

(45) Harris, H. (1953). *Ann. Eugen., Lond.*, **18**, 43.

(46) Calchi-Novati, C., Ceppellini, R., Biancho, I., Silvestroni, E. and Harris, H. (1954). *Ann Eugen., Lond.* **18**, 335.

(47) Gartler, S. M., Dobzhansky, T. and Berry, H. K. (1955). *Amer. J. Hum. Genet.* **7**, 108.

(48) Gartler, S. M., Firschein, I. L. and Gidaspon, T. (1956). *Acta Genet.* **6**, 435.

(49) Sutton, H. E. and Clark, P. J. (1955). *Amer. J. Phys. Anthrop.* N.S. **13**, 53.

(50) Fink, R. M., McGaughy, C., Cline, R. E. and Fink, K. (1956). *J. Biol. Chem.* **218**, 1.

(51) Fink, K. (1956). *J. Biol. Chem.* **218**, 9.

(52) Fink, K., Cline, R. E., Henderson, R. B. and Fink, R. M. (1956). *J. Biol. Chem.* **221**, 425.

(53) Sandler, M. and Pare, C. M. B. (1954). *Lancet*, **1**, 494.

(54) Wilson, V. K., Thomson, M. L. and Dent, C. E. (1953). *Lancet*, **2**, 66.

(55) Westall, R. G. (1958). *Proc. IV Int. Congr. Biochem.* Pergamon Press, Lond. (in press).

(56) Westall, R. G., Dancis, J., Miller, S. and Lepitz M. (1958). *Fed. Proc.* **17**, 334.

(57) Menkes, J. H., Hurst, P. L. and Craig, J. M. (1954). *Paediatrics*, **14**, 462.

CHAPTER 5

VARIATIONS IN CARBOHYDRATE METABOLISM

The glycogen storage diseases

In 1929 Von Giercke[1] described a disorder characterised by a gross enlargement of the liver and kidneys, due to an extensive and quite abnormal deposition of glycogen in these organs. Schönheimer[2] isolated glycogen from the liver of Von Giercke's original case and found that it had the same specific rotation as did normal glycogen, that it was exclusively composed of glucose residues, and that while it appeared to be extremely stable in the diseased liver, it was readily degraded when mixed with minced normal human liver. He therefore concluded that the glycogen was normal in character, but that one or other of the enzymes normally concerned with the degradation of glycogen to glucose was absent in Von Giercke's disease.

Since then, many further examples of the same kind of disorder have been studied[3] and it has also emerged that a number of other forms of abnormal glycogen storage exist which differ in various respects from the kind originally described by Von Giercke[4,5]. For example, the abnormal deposition of glycogen may not occur predominantly in the liver and kidney, but may be generalised throughout the body and be particularly prominent in other sites such as the heart or the skeletal muscles. Another peculiar feature of certain of the cases is that a severe degree of hepatic cirrhosis develops in association with the glycogenosis.

Abnormal glycogen storage has not infrequently been found to be familial, and while extensive family studies have not been reported, most of the data is consistent with the idea that the affected individuals are homozygous for a rare abnormal 'recessive' gene. For some years it was thought that the rather variable features which were encountered in different cases were due to a variation in expression of the same underlying pathological process. It is now clear, however, that this is not the case. Modern enzymatic studies, notably by Gerty Cori[6], have shown that in fact there exist a whole series of distinct congenital disorders in which abnormal deposition of glycogen may occur. Each probably represents a specific enzymic deficiency, determined by a distinct abnormal gene. So far at least four different varieties of glycogen storage disease have been characterised, and possibly more exist.

The formation of glycogen

Carbohydrate is stored in the form of glycogen largely in the liver and muscles, although smaller amounts may be found in most other tissues. Glycogen is a polysaccharide composed entirely of glucose

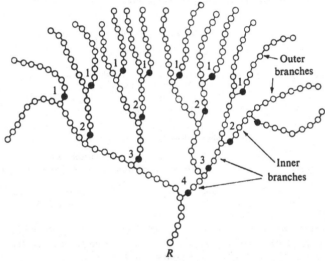

Fig. 26. Model of a segment of a glycogen molecule (after Cori [6]). There are 209 glucose residues, mol. wt. 33,858. Open circles, glucose residues in α-1:4-linkage; black circles, residues in α-1:6-linkage. $R =$ reducing end-group. There are four tiers of branch points (glycogen has at least seven). Inner branches are terminated by branch points in adjacent tiers, outer branches by a branch point and by the non-reducing terminal glucose residue (end-group).

units, and has a molecular weight of the order of one to four million. Its general structure as revealed by modern enzyme analysis is illustrated in Fig. 26. There is a multi-branched tree-like arrangement, the glucose units being joined in chains by α-1:4-glycosidic linkages, except at the branch points where α-1:6-linkages occur.

The sequence of reactions by which glucose units are built up to form glycogen, and glycogen broken down to give glucose is shown in Fig. 27. Four enzymes are involved in both directions, but only two, phosphoglucomutase and phosphorylase, act effectively on both routes. The first step is the formation of glucose-6-phosphate from glucose and ATP with hexokinase as the enzyme. The conversion of glucose-6-phosphate to glucose-1-phosphate with phosphogluco-mutase as the enzyme can then take place. However, glucose-6-phosphate may be a substrate for several other enzymes as well. These include glucose-6-phosphatase, glucose-6-phosphate dehydrogenase, and phosphohexoseisomerase. The regulatory mechanisms which allow one or another of these various enzymes to act on the same substrate are complex and are not clearly understood. They are no doubt closely geared to the general metabolic requirements of the body.

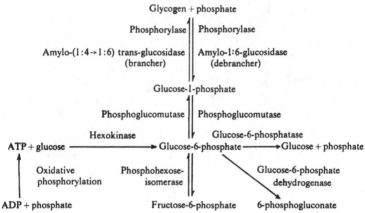

Fig. 27. Pathways in the synthesis of glycogen from glucose, and the breakdown of glycogen to glucose.

Following the formation of glucose-1-phosphate, glycogen formation requires both phosphorylase and the so-called 'brancher' enzyme acting in conjunction. Some glycogen itself is a necessary substrate. Phosphorylase action leads to the removal of the phosphate group from glucose-1-phosphate and the attachment of the glucose residue to the glycogen nidus. In this way successive glucose units joined by 1:4-linkages can be attached in a chain. The reaction is reversible and its direction (that is glycogen synthesis as opposed to glycogen breakdown) depends on the ratio of inorganic phosphate to glucose-1-phosphate present. Oxidative phosphorylation, keeping the inorganic phosphate down, will favour synthesis.

As phosphorylase action successively lengthens the outer chains they reach a critical level of about eight residues when they become a suitable substrate for the 'brancher' enzyme. This establishes the 1:6-linkage by a process of transglycosidation and is correctly described as amylo (1:4 → 1:6) transglycosidase. By repeated action of phosphorylase and 'brancher' enzyme successive new tiers in the glycogen molecule may be formed.

The breakdown of glycogen requires a further enzyme amylo-1:6-glucosidase (debrancher). It is specific for the 1:6 linkages and acts hydrolytically, liberating free glucose. It can, however, only act after phosphorylase in the presence of inorganic phosphate has systematically removed the 1:4-linked glucose residues from the outermost branches. Phosphorolysis stops as the outermost tier of branch points is approached since phosphorylase can neither split nor by-pass the 1:6 linkages. When phosphorylase action comes to a standstill a polysaccharide is left behind with an average molecular size some 25–40 per cent smaller than that of the parent molecule. This polysaccharide is called phosphorylase limit dextrin. The 1:6 linkages are now exposed to the action of the 'debrancher' enzyme. They are split hydrolytically to give free glucose and to leave a new polysaccharide in which the original penultimate tier of branches has now become the outermost tier. Phosphorylase may now act again and in this manner the two enzymes acting successively can degrade the glycogen molecule.

Glucose and glucose-1-phosphate are the final products following the complete degradation of glycogen in this way, and their ratio gives a measure of the proportion of branch points in the whole molecule. About 8 per cent of the whole glycogen molecule emerges directly as free glucose. The remaining 92 per cent is in the form of glucose-1-phosphate and in order to liberate free glucose this must first be converted to glucose-6-phosphate with phosphoglucomutase, and the glucose-6-phosphate hydrolysed by glucose-6-phosphatase. Since glucose-6-phosphatase occurs in the liver and kidney but not in muscle, it is only in the former organs that most of the glycogen present can be converted to free glucose. In muscle the glucose-6-phosphate must be either converted to lactic acid or completely oxidised.

Glucose-6-phosphatase deficiency

The type of glycogen storage disease in which the liver and kidney are predominantly affected is the least uncommon of this rather rare group of disorders. Von Giercke's original descriptions correspond to this form of disease. There appears to be rather a wide range in severity of the condition. In its most severe form the disease presents in infancy with a very gross enlargement of the liver, failure to thrive, and a general retardation in growth. The fasting blood-sugar levels are low and ketosis and ketonuria not uncommon. Characteristically there is little or no elevation of the blood sugar following parenteral administration of adrenaline. Death in infancy or early childhood is not infrequent and at post-mortem the liver cells and the cells of the convoluted renal tubules are found to be heavily loaded with glycogen.

These findings have from the beginning been interpreted as due to a failure of the liver to mobilise glycogen for the formation of blood sugar. Modern enzymic analysis has fully confirmed this interpretation. Studies of specimens of glycogen obtained by biopsy have shown that they are in no way structurally abnormal. The glycogen can be readily degraded if mixed with normal liver mash, and its apparent stability in the affected patients can best be explained as being due to a specific deficiency of the enzyme glucose-6-phosphatase [7]. Direct assay of this enzyme in both liver and kidney specimens from a series of severe cases of the disease has shown that the activity was extremely low. Furthermore, no evidence for the presence of significant inhibitiof of this enzyme by material from the affected patients could be found.

That glucose-6-phosphatase deficiency might be the underlying lesion here was suggested by the characteristic involvement of the liver and kidney, with apparently no abnormal glycogen accumulation in the muscles. Glucose-6-phosphatase is known to occur in liver and kidney, but is not found in muscle. The absence or relative deficiency of this enzyme, while limiting the conversion of glucose-6-phosphate to glucose in these organs, would not be expected to interfere directly with glycogen synthesis. Thus an abnormal accumulation of glycogen might reasonably be expected. A deficiency of glucose-6-phosphatase could also account for the fasting hypoglycaemia not only because it would restrict the formation of glucose from glycogen, but also because the formation of glucose from other sources such as lactic acid, pyruvic acid, aminoacids and glycerol largely goes by way of glucose-6-phosphate. The tendency to ketosis can be explained as a secondary consequence of this general failure in carbohydrate metabolism.

A milder form of what appears at first sight to be essentially the same kind of disorder has also been recognised. Such patients, although they exhibit a considerable enlargement of the liver with marked glycogen accumulation in infancy and childhood may nevertheless survive to adolescence and adult life. Their rate of growth is much retarded at first, but as they grow older they appear to catch up quite successfully and may eventually reach adult life with little or no obvious physical disability. Two such patients have been followed over a period of some twenty-five years by Van Creveld [8]. The liver enlargement became much less prominent after puberty and by adult life was only barely detectable. Similarly the fasting blood-sugar levels which were low in childhood tended to approach normal values later on, and the tendency to ketosis became much less marked. That the original metabolic disturbance still persisted to some degree, however, was shown by the continued absence of a normal response to adrenaline injection.

Cori and her colleagues have assayed glucose-6-phosphatase activity in biopsy specimens of liver from a group of five individuals with what appears to be this milder form of the condition [9]. The enzyme activities were appreciably lower than the activity found in most control subjects. However, the deficiency was certainly very much less profound than that encountered in the group of cases in infancy and early childhood with the severe manifestation of the disease.

The relationship between the milder and the more severe forms of the syndrome has not yet been sorted out. There are several possibilities. It may be that they represent two distinct disorders caused by different genes, possibly alleles, one resulting in almost complete defect in glucose-6-phosphatase synthesis and the other in only a moderate deficiency. The apparent clinical amelioration of the milder type of syndrome as adult life is reached might imply that the partial enzyme deficiency while leading to a fairly marked degree of inbalance of carbohydrate metabolism in infancy, becomes less critical later on. Another possibility is that the disorder reflects a situation in which there is a delay in the development of the process necessary to form the enzyme, so that the disturbance is maximal in early infancy when virtually no enzyme is present and becomes much less marked as the child grows up and the enzyme begins to be formed. A further possibility is that moderate glucose-6-phosphatase deficiency in the milder cases is not the specific cause of the metabolic disturbance here, but is simply a secondary consequence of some other as yet obscure defect in carbohydrate metabolism.

Of some interest in this connection is the curious situation which has been encountered in the foetal guinea-pig (9). Here no liver glycogen is demonstrable before the 57th day of the 66-day gestation period. At this point glycogen begins to accumulate rapidly until term, when the liver glycogen reaches two or three times the concentration found in the maternal liver. After birth the foetal liver glycogen is rapidly depleted. Now glucose-6-phosphatase activity was shown to be absent until term, but appears after birth. Thus the glycogen accumulation in the later stages of the development of the guinea-pig foetus has the same kind of metabolic basis as the kind of glycogen storage disease in man which we have been discussing. That is to say, during this period all the enzymes necessary for glycogen formation are present, but there is a relative deficiency of glucose-6-phosphatase which is necessary for its breakdown to glucose.

Amylo-1:6-glucosidase deficiency

In the course of their survey of the structures of specimens of glycogen from patients with glycogenosis, Illingworth and Cori (10) encountered a case in which the glycogen present approached phosphorylase limit dextrin in structure. That is to say, the glycogen appeared to be highly branched but the chains of glucose units at the periphery of the molecule were abnormally short. The degree of degradation produced by phosphorylase acting alone in the absence of 'debrancher' was much less than normal, and the proportion of branch points appeared to be excessively high.

Unlike the cases with glucose-6-phosphatase deficiency the glycogenosis was generalised, the skeletal and heart muscles being as extensively affected as the liver. Furthermore, the glucose-6-phosphatase activity of the liver was found to be normal. Evidently then this represented a distinct disease entity.

The abnormal glycogen structure was of the sort that might be expected if there were a relative deficiency of the 'debrancher' enzyme (amylo-1:6-glucosidase), and indeed direct assay of this enzyme in skeletal and heart muscle from two of these patients revealed virtually no activity (11). The specific deficiency of this enzyme presumably means that only the glucose residues in the outermost branches of the glycogen molecule could be readily released from the molecule. The inner core would be largely unavailable for rapid glycogenolysis. This could account both for the accumulation of glycogen which is found, and for the rather slight and incomplete blood-sugar response to adrenaline which has been noted in these patients.

Clinically the main features are a marked enlargement of the liver and a fasting hypoglycaemia. The ultimate outlook is still uncertain because so far too few of these patients have been observed for long enough, but in one patient of this type followed over a period of ten years[5] development seemed normal and apart from the hepatomegaly the child was reasonably well.

Glycogenosis with hepatic cirrhosis

Generalised glycogen deposition, particularly marked in the liver where it is associated with a severe degree of cirrhosis, represents another distinct type of glycogen storage disease, in which the glycogen formed has a grossly abnormal structure. Here the glycogen is found to have much longer outer and inner chains than is usual, and the number of branch points is very much reduced[6,10]. Structurally it resembles amylopectin, the branched polysaccharide of starch, much more than it does normal glycogen.

Its physical properties are found to be correspondingly abnormal. It is much less soluble in water at body temperature than is normal glycogen. The X-ray powder diagram resembles that of amylopectins rather than of glycogen, and is of the form that is thought to be produced when the branches of the polysaccharide are long enough to align with neighbouring branches in an orderly array. The molecular weight is rather smaller than that found with typical glycogens, and the polysaccharide gives a purplish colour with iodine rather than the reddish brown colour usually given by glycogen.

The deposition of an abnormal glycogen of this kind could be readily explained on the hypothesis that there is a specific deficiency of the 'brancher' enzyme (amylo-1:4 → 1:6-transglucosidase). As yet, however, direct assays for this enzyme in material from such patients have not been reported.

Symptoms of the disease appear in infancy or early childhood. They are mainly referable to the severe and progressive cirrhosis of the liver which develops and is usually fatal[12]. The blood-sugar is generally within normal limits and there is no acidosis. The occurrence of the hepatic cirrhosis and also the glycogen accumulation can probably be attributed to the peculiar physical properties of the glycogen which is being formed. Although this amylopectin-like polysaccharide can be completely degraded by phosphorylase and amylo-1:6-glucosidase *in vitro*, it is very much less soluble than is normal glycogen and it seems likely that *in vivo* it tends to come out of solution and become relatively unavailable to the action of the degrading enzyme. The fibrosis of the liver which develops can be plausibly interpreted as due to a tissue reaction to the abnormal glycogen similar to that precipitated by an irritating foreign substance (12). It is possible that a number of cases described under the general heading of 'familial hepatic cirrhosis' may in reality be examples of this condition.

Glycogen disease of the heart

An enormous enlargement of the heart due to an excessive deposition of glycogen is the characteristic feature of yet another rare form of generalised glycogenosis (4). On X-ray the heart has a typical globular appearance, and at post-mortem is found to be five or six times the normal size for the age of the patient. It is heavily infiltrated with glycogen. Unusual amounts of glycogen are also found in the rest of the musculature and curiously enough can be particularly prominent in the tongue which may be noticeably enlarged.

The disease becomes obvious in early infancy, cardiac failure and a generalised muscular weakness being the most noticeable features. The course is short and death generally occurs from heart failure or intercurrent infection in the first year of life. The condition is familial and shows the same typical features in affected members of the same family.

Enzyme studies have so far failed to reveal the nature of the underlying abnormality (6). The structure of the glycogen formed is normal in character, and glucose-6-phosphatase activity is within normal limits. Studies of the behaviour of the blood-sugar under a variety of conditions have failed to reveal any characteristic deviations from the normal.

Galactosaemia

Galactosaemia is a genetically determined condition in which there exists a specific inability to metabolise galactose in the normal manner. If galactose is given by mouth there occurs a marked elevation of the galactose level in the blood and a consequent excretion of galactose in the urine. The main dietary source of galactose is milk which contains lactose as its principal carbohydrate component. This is a disaccharide composed of glucose and galactose.

It follows that infants with this disorder who are fed on milk in the ordinary way show a persistently high level of galactose in the blood and a more or less continuous galactosuria. The clinical consequences are somewhat variable but in most cases they tend to be rather severe (13). Characteristically the liver becomes grossly enlarged, and cataracts develop. The infants fail to thrive, growth is slow, and mental development is retarded. Death in infancy is not uncommon.

If such an infant is placed on a diet completely free from galactose, the blood galactose level rapidly falls, and in most cases a remarkable and dramatic improvement in the physical condition takes place. It seems probable that if such treatment is started early enough, and great care is taken to exclude rigorously all traces of galactose from the diet, then growth and development may take place quite normally. If, however, the commencement of the treatment is delayed, some degree of liver damage, cataract, and mental backwardness is likely to persist presumably because of irreversible changes that have already taken place.

Proteinuria and marked aminoaciduria occur when galactose is fed to such patients. These abnormalities, however, disappear within a week or so, once the galactose has been excluded from the diet.

Pathways in galactose metabolism

Galactose is believed to enter the main stream of carbohydrate metabolism via a series of reactions which result in its conversion to glucose-1-phosphate. Several distinct steps are involved (14). They are illustrated in Fig. 28. The first of these is catalysed by galacto-kinase and results in the formation of galactose-1-phosphate. The galactose-1-phosphate then reacts with the nucleotide uridine di-phosphoglucose to give glucose-1-phosphate and uridine diphospho-galactose. The enzyme involved in this reaction has been called galactose-1-phosphate uridyl transferase. The uridine diphospho-galactose so formed can then be converted to uridine diphospho-glucose. The enzyme concerned with this was originally called galacto-'waldenase' but is perhaps more precisely referred to as uridine diphospho galactose-4-epimerase. DPN acts as coenzyme.

Some uridine diphosphoglucose is necessary for these reactions to take place and this may be formed from glucose-1-phosphate via reaction 4.

Reaction 1 is effectively irreversible, but the direction of the other reactions will depend on the nature of the particular situation present at any one time. In this way glucose-1-phosphate may be formed from galactose, and galactose-1-phosphate or uridine diphospho-galactose may be formed from glucose. Thus galactose-containing compounds such as the galactosides of brain may be synthesised in the body from glucose in the absence of galactose in the diet.

$$\text{Gal} + \text{ATP} \xrightarrow{\quad \text{Galactokinase} \quad} \text{Gal-1-P} + \text{ADP} \qquad (1)$$

$$\text{Gal-1-P} + \text{UDPG} \underset{\longleftarrow}{\overset{\text{Gal-1-P uridyl}}{\underset{\text{transferase}}{\rightleftharpoons}}} \text{UDPGal} + \text{G-1-P} \qquad (2)$$

$$\text{UDPGal} \xrightarrow{\quad \text{UDPGal-4-epimerase} \quad} \text{UDPG} \qquad (3)$$

$$\text{UTP} + \text{G-1-P} \underset{\longleftarrow}{\overset{\text{UDPG}}{\underset{\text{pyrophosphorylase}}{\rightleftharpoons}}} \text{UDPG} + \text{PP} \qquad (4)$$

N.B. The sum of reactions (1), (2) and (3) is

$$\text{Gal} + \text{ATP} \longrightarrow \text{G-1-P} + \text{ADP}$$

Fig. 28. Reactions in the formation of glucose-1-phosphate from galactose. (After Kalckar.)

The metabolic lesion

In patients with galactosaemia the metabolism of glucose is apparently unimpaired and trouble only arises when galactose is present in the diet. It follows therefore that the basic metabolic lesion lies at some point in the sequence of reactions between galactose and glucose-1-phosphate.

Although galactose is probably metabolised predominantly in the liver, it is also handled by other tissues as well. Among these are the red blood cells, and because blood is very much more readily obtained for study than is liver material, most of the work on the nature of the metabolic error in this disease has been carried out by comparing the metabolism of erythrocytes from galactosaemic patients with those from normal individuals. Schwartz, Golberg, Komrower and Holzel[15] were the first to demonstrate that in contrast to normal erythrocytes galactosaemic erythrocytes accumulated large amounts of galactose-1-phosphate in the presence of galactose. They concluded that a metabolic block existed between galactose-1-phosphate and glucose-1-phosphate. Direct assay of the different enzymes involved in these reactions was then carried out by Kalcker and his colleagues (16). They showed that reaction 2 in the sequence described above was defective. The transferase concerned in the reaction of galactose-1-phosphate with uridinediphosphoglucose to give uridine-diphosphogalactose was virtually absent in the erythrocytes of the galactosaemic subjects. All the other necessary enzymes, however, were present in normal amounts (Table 16).

Table 16. *Enzymes of galactose metabolism in R.B.C. haemolysates from normal and galactosaemic subjects (activity is given in μM of reactant converted per ml. of lysed erythrocytes per hour). (After Isselbacher et al. 1956)*

Enzyme	Normal		Galactosaemic	
	No. tested	Mean activity	No. tested	Mean activity
Galactokinase	3	0·10	3	0·08
Gal-1-*P*-uridyl transferase	15	0·82	10	0·02
UDP gal-4-epimerase	3	0·32	3	0·35
UDP glucose pyrophosphorylase	9	1·20	8	1·85

Table 17. *Uridyl transferase activity in human liver homogenates (values in μM incorporated into nucleotide/g. liver/hr.). (After Anderson et al. 1957)*

Subject	^{14}C-labelled Gal-1-*P*
Non-galactosaemic adult (autopsy)	>15·0
Non-galactosaemic infant (autopsy)	>25·0
Galactosaemic adult (biopsy)	1·2
Galactosaemic infant (biopsy)	< 0·3

The absence or at least gross deficiency of this enzyme has also been demonstrated in liver biopsy material (Table 17) from such patients (17) and it seems highly probable that this specific enzyme deficiency is common to all the tissues where galactose is normally metabolised. The grossly abnormal galactose tolerance curve, and the intracellular accumulation of galactose-1-phosphate are obvious consequences of such a metabolic block. However, a lesion of this sort would not be expected necessarily to interfere with the synthesis of galactosides and other galactose-containing materials because uridinediphosphogalactose could be formed from glucose.

It has frequently been reported that when galactose is fed to galactosaemic subjects not all the administered galactose can be accounted for by the galactose appearing in the urine. A proportion of this deficiency can probably be explained by the intracellular accumulation of galactose-1-phosphate, but the question still remains as to whether some galactose metabolism does go on, either because the metabolic block is not complete or because alternative metabolic pathways come into operation. Eisenberg, Isselbacher, and Kalckar[18] have examined this question in a detailed study of the metabolism of ^{14}C-labelled galactose administered to an adult galactosaemic patient. They have been able to show that in fact some galactose metabolism does take place, though quantitatively it is only a small fraction (about one per cent) of that possible in normal subjects. In this patient it was also found that liver biopsy material showed some slight capacity to form uridine diphosphogalactose from galactose, though no such activity was found in the red blood cells. It is still uncertain whether this was due to some transferase activity catalysing reaction 2 above being retained and the metabolic block therefore being incomplete or whether an alternative pathway may exist. It seems possible that the variations in the severity of the condition observed clinically may be a reflection of different degrees of this remaining capacity to form uridinediphosphogalactose from galactose by one route or another.

Thus the main metabolic lesion in galactosaemia can be confidently located in a specific deficiency in the activity of the enzyme galactose-1-phosphate uridyl transferase. There is no evidence that any inhibitors are present and it seems likely, therefore, that the genetical factors responsible for the disease result more or less directly in a defect in the synthesis of this enzyme. The question then arises as to exactly how this lesion gives rise to the diverse and rather characteristic signs and symptoms of the clinical condition. These include severe liver dysfunction and enlargement, cataract formation, generalised retardation of growth and of mental development and disturbances in renal function resulting in proteinuria and amino-aciduria. Evidently these disturbances only occur if galactose is being administered to the affected individual, and at first sight these pathological consequences might be attributed to the 'toxic' effects of either the high concentration of galactose in the body fluids, or to the high intracellular concentration of galactose-1-phosphate. Both these phenomena have been shown to be the direct result of the administration of galactose to these patients.

Schwartz and his colleagues compared the respiratory activity of erythrocytes from galactosaemic infants before and after a period of galactose feeding[15]. They found that after exposure of the cells to circulating galactose their oxygen uptake was significantly depressed. Concomitant with this reduction of respiratory activity there was a general fall in ester phosphate in spite of the accumulation of galactose-1-phosphate. Similar observations were made when galactosaemia erythrocytes were incubated with galactose *in vitro*. However, when normal erythrocytes were incubated with similar concentrations of galactose their respiratory activity was if anything enhanced and their ester phosphate increased. It was therefore concluded that galactose *per se* was not 'toxic', but that the 'toxic' effects arose because of the high intracellular concentration of galactose-1-phosphate or one of its derivatives.

One way in which it has been suggested that increased intracellular concentrations of galactose-1-phosphate could lead to disturbances in intracellular metabolism is by the inhibition of the interconversion of glucose-1-phosphate and glucose-6-phosphate by the enzyme phosphoglucomutase[15,19]. It has been suggested that this interconversion takes place by the transfer of phosphate from the phosphorylated enzyme to the 6 position of glucose-1-phosphate to give glucose-1:6-diphosphate and the dephosphoenzyme. The glucose-1:6-diphosphate then reacts with the dephosphoenzyme to give glucose-6-phosphate and regenerated phosphoglucomutase. Now galactose-1-phosphate will also react with phosphoglucomutase. This reaction is very much slower than the corresponding one with glucose-1-phosphate, but in the presence of high concentrations of galactose-1-phosphate could become quantitatively important. Each molecule of galactose-1-phosphate which reacts with phosphoglucomutase consumes one transferable phosphate group and produces galactose-1:6-diphosphate and the dephosphoenzyme. The dephosphoenzyme, however, tends to accumulate because its reaction with the galactose-1:6-diphosphate is excessively slow. The dephosphoenzyme so produced could react with any glucose-1:6-diphosphate present but this will soon become depleted. Thus the overall effect of an increased concentration of galactose-1-phosphate would be to inhibit the interconversion of glucose-1-phosphate and glucose-6-

phosphate, because it would lead to an accumulation of the dephospho form of phosphoglucomutase and this is not reactive with either glucose-1-phosphate or glucose-6-phosphate. Such an effect could have extensive repercussions in carbohydrate metabolism. Similar inhibitions of other enzymes may also be produced. It seems plausible that this is the kind of way the diverse pathological consequences of galactosaemia are brought about.

In this connection it is of interest that cataract, one of the characteristic features of galactosaemia, has been produced experimentally in rats by feeding a diet extremely rich in galactose. The cataractous lenses of animals so treated have been shown to contain high concentrations of galactose-1-phosphate [20]. Since glucose is the main source of energy for the lens and the inhibition of glucose metabolism tends to cataract formation, it seems possible that the development of the cataracts can be attributed to the inhibition of glucose metabolism by galactose-1-phosphate.

Another intriguing facet of the impaired cellular function in galactosaemia is illustrated by the behaviour of the renal tubule cells. When a galactosaemic patient is being fed galactose these cells become relatively inefficient in the reabsorption of certain aminoacids from the glomerular filtrate [21,22]. In consequence a generalised type of aminoaciduria is found. When galactose is removed from the diet the aminoaciduria eventually disappears, but this takes some days. If galactose feeding is reintroduced, the aminoaciduria develops again, but several days elapse before it becomes clearly apparent and the clearance of amino-N is definitely raised. Thus the functional disturbance of the renal tubule is reversible. It is, however, evidently not an immediate effect of the high galactose concentration in the glomerular filtrate because while the galactosuria starts more or less immediately galactose feeding commences, and ceases equally abruptly when it is stopped, there is a marked time lag both in the development and the subsequent disappearance of the aminoaciduria. It appears as if some kind of slow build-up of a 'toxic' substance with a progressive disturbance in cellular function is occurring when galactose is fed, and this in turn results in impairment of aminoacid transport.

Genetics of galactosaemia

Galactosaemia has frequently been found to be familial, and there seems little doubt that it is genetically determined.

The most detailed family investigations are those carried out by Holzel and Komrower [23, 24]. They studied five families in which the disease was segregating and they carried out galactose tolerance tests on many of the apparently normal relatives. Their findings are summarised in Fig. 29.

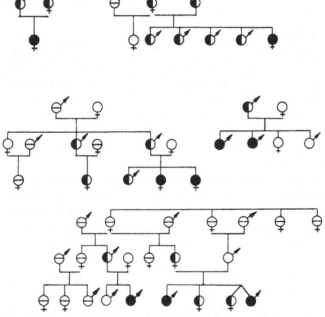

Fig. 29. Pedigrees of galactosaemia. (After Holzel *et al.*) ⊖, not tested; ○, normal galactose tolerance; ●, clinical galactosaemia; ◐, abnormal galactose tolerance.

The definition of an abnormal response in a galactose tolerance test is of necessity somewhat arbitrary because of the considerable variation in response to galactose feeding among random normal individuals, and the general difficulty of finding a suitable single quantitative index for assessing the results of the test. However, even though a fairly conservative criterion of abnormal galactose tolerance was chosen in these studies, it was nevertheless quite clear that a significant proportion of the apparently healthy relatives of galacto-saemic patients showed some defect in handling a standard test dose of galactose. For example, out of twelve parents of galactosaemic patients who were examined, eight showed significant deviations in galactose tolerance. In two families both parents were affected in this way. Among ten sibs of the affected patients, seven had abnormal galactose tolerances. Of the six sibships containing affected patients which were examined by Holzel and Komrower, one was the result of a cousin marriage.

Although the data are still too scanty to draw firm conclusions it is a reasonable hypothesis that the galactosaemic patients are homo-zygous for a rare abnormal gene, and that their relatives who show impaired galactose tolerance are heterozygotes. Using the standard galactose tolerance test it is clear that the variation in response among both the presumed heterozygotes and the normals is so great that only a proportion (about 70 per cent) of the heterozygotes in these families might be expected to be detected in this way. It must also be remembered of course that the galactose tolerance test is not very specific and has indeed been used as a general test for defective liver function, so that abnormalities may be expected for a variety of different reasons.

It remains to be seen whether refinement of the assay of galactose-1-phosphate uridyl transferase in red cells so as to detect a partial and possibly very slight deficiency of the enzyme will help to dif-ferentiate these presumed heterozygotes more precisely.

L-xyloketosuria

This condition, often referred to as 'essential pentosuria', is charac-terised by the excretion in the urine of unusual quantities of the ketopentose, L-xyloketose (xylulose). It may be readily distinguished from the transient pentosuria which may follow the ingestion of large amounts of fruit by the characteristic and very unusual sugar which is found. Affected individuals excrete some 1–4 g. of L-xyloketose daily, and this seems to be continuous and persists unchanged throughout life. In other respects they appear to be quite normal. They seem to suffer no ill-effects in consequence of this curious metabolic anomaly and no other peculiarities in their metabolism of carbohydrates have been detected.

The amount of L-xyloketose excreted daily appears to be fairly constant in any one individual (25,26). It is not markedly influenced by ordinary variations in diet. The quantity excreted can, however, be increased by the administration of a variety of drugs which are themselves excreted as glucuronates. D-Glucuronolactone (26,27) itself produces an even more pronounced effect (Fig. 30). Thus feeding 5 g. of D-glucuronolactone may lead to an increased output of L-xyloketose varying from 0·8 to 1·4 g. In normal people the admini-

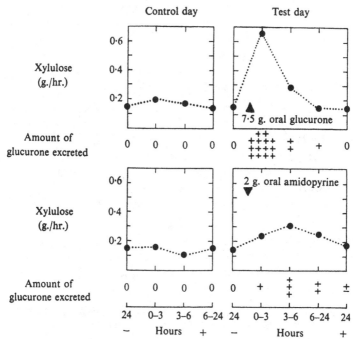

Fig. 30. Excretion of L-xyloketose (xylulose) in a xyloketosuric patient after the administration of glucuronolactone and amidopyrine. (After Flynn (27).)

stration of D-glucuronolactone has also been shown to lead to some L-xyloketose excretion. Here, however, after feeding as much as 17 g. of the lactone, only some 70–90 mg. of L-xyloketose was excreted (28).

These results suggest that L-xyloketose is formed more or less directly from glucuronolactone or glucuronic acid and it may indeed be an intermediate in the normal pathway in the metabolism of this substance. Touster and his colleagues (28) have suggested that the reaction sequences shown in Fig. 31 may be involved.

Further evidence on this matter has been obtained by studies involving the administration of labelled glucuronolactone to a pentosuric individual(29). When 6-^{13}C-D-glucuronolactone was used no excess ^{13}C was found in the xyloketose isolated from the urine. When, however, 1-^{13}C-D-glucuronolactone was administered a significant excess of ^{13}C was found in the isolated xyloketose. The experiments indicated that D-glucuronolactone is a direct precursor of L-xylo-

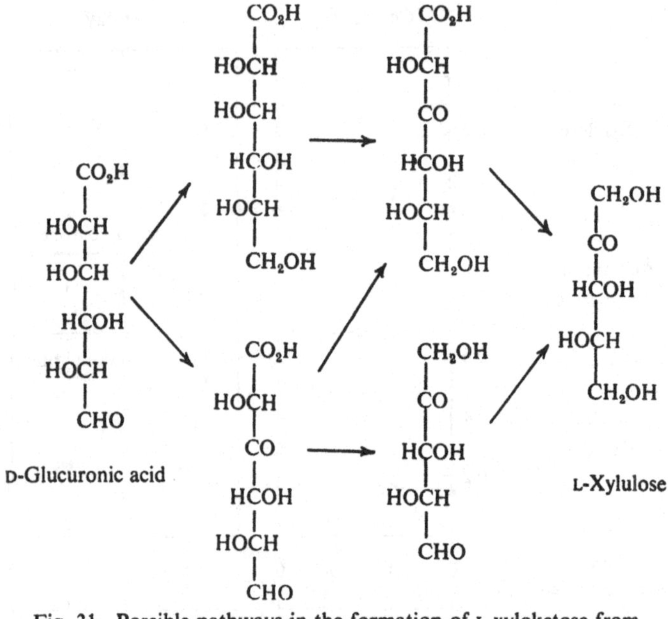

Fig. 31. Possible pathways in the formation of L-xyloketose from glucuronic acid. (After Touster et al.)

ketose, the carboxyl C being lost in the conversion and the aldehydic C becoming C5 of the xyloketose.

Only traces of xyloketose can be demonstrated in the blood plasma of these patients(27). Evidently the renal clearance of L-xyloketose is very high and probably little or no renal tubular reabsorption occurs at all.

Most of the cases of this condition which have been reported appear to have occurred in Jewish people derived from populations in Central Europe. The disorder is evidently extremely rare in other populations. An extensive survey by Lasker, Enklewitz and Lasker of some twenty different families in which the condition was found to be segregating leaves little doubt that the disorder is inherited in the manner of a Mendelian recessive character [30]. So far no peculiarity has been detected in the heterozygotes, but it would be of interest to know whether such individuals would give an abnormal response when fed large doses of D-glucuronolactone.

Fructosuria

Fructosuria probably represents a condition in which only one of several possible pathways in the metabolism of fructose is blocked. As a result the organism is able to metabolise satisfactorily most of the fructose with which it has to deal and only a certain proportion of this substance fails to be utilized.

Table 18. *Percentage of ingested fructose excreted in urine by a fructosuric patient.* (*After Silver and Reiner* [32], *1934*)

Fructose ingested (g.)	Percentage fructose excreted in urine
1	traces
5	16
25	11
50	12
75	14
100	14

In this condition, some 10–20 per cent of the fructose taken in food is excreted in the urine. The proportion appears to be relatively constant and independent of the total amount of fructose taken. This was first noted by Schlesinger [31] and has been found in all subsequent studies where the appropriate investigations were made (Table 18). If the individual is on a diet free from fructose, or if he is fasting, no sugar appears in the urine, and no sugar appears after the ingestion of glucose or glucose-forming polysaccharides. The results of fructose tolerance tests indicate that there is some failure in the intermediary metabolism of fructose in such individuals and the fructosuria is not a renal threshold effect. After 50 g. of fructose, the blood fructose rises to much higher levels in fructosuria than in normal individuals and it disappears from the body more slowly (Fig. 32).

It is known that in normal subjects the ingestion of fructose leads to a rise in respiratory quotient which occurs more quickly and reaches a higher level than when glucose is ingested [33, 34]. This rise in

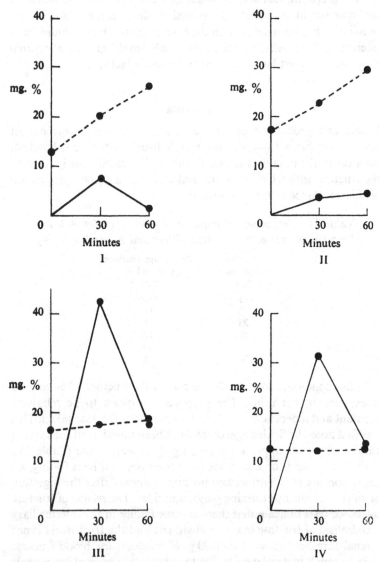

Fig. 32. Effect of feeding 50 g. of fructose to two normal controls, I and II, and to two fructosurics, III and IV, on blood fructose and lactic acid. (After Sachs *et al.*) —— fructose; - - - - - lactic acid.

respiratory quotient is associated with a marked elevation in the level of blood lactic acid, which occurs after the ingestion of fructose but not of glucose. Both these phenomena have been studied in fructo-surics. It was found that the respiratory quotient was only slightly raised, in a manner similar to that observed after glucose had been fed to normal subjects (35). Similarly little or no increase was observed in the level of blood lactic acid (35,36,37) (Fig. 32).

Sachs and his colleagues (37) have explained these findings by postulating that in normal individuals about 80 per cent of the fructose ingested is converted to glycogen, the remainder being broken down to lactic acid. Fructosurics are unable to deal with the part of the ingested fructose which normally goes to lactic acid, and so 10–20 per cent of it is excreted in the urine. Clearly, however, detailed enzyme studies will be necessary before any precise idea of what is going on can be obtained.

Fructosuria is evidently extremely rare. In a series of five sibships containing nine fructosuric individuals collected by Lasker (38), three sibships were derived from consanguineous unions. No peculiarity was found in the parents of the patients. Presumably the affected individuals are homozygous for a rare mutant gene. The peculiarity is evidently quite harmless, and is usually identified because the individual is found at an insurance examination or other routine medical investigation to be excreting a reducing substance in the urine which is not glucose.

Renal glycosuria

Glucose is present only in traces in normal human urine. In certain diseases, such as diabetes mellitus, where there is a gross disorder of carbohydrate metabolism, the level of glucose in the blood may be greatly increased, and consequently large quantities of glucose appear in the urine. Some individuals, however, who in other respects seem to be quite healthy, and who show no obvious abnormality in carbohydrate metabolism or undue elevation of blood-sugar levels, excrete glucose in their urine in quite large amounts. They are said to have 'renal glucosuria' and the peculiarity is generally attributed to an impairment of the capacity of the renal tubules to reabsorb glucose from the glomerular filtrate.

In this condition the blood-sugar, after the administration of a standard dose of glucose by mouth, rises no higher than in normal subjects, and falls to fasting levels in the usual time. This normal glucose tolerance curve indicates that the utilisation of glucose by the tissues is unimpaired. Glycosuria, however, which is usually only encountered in normal individuals if the blood sugar is raised above 160–180 mg. per cent appears in these people at much lower levels. In some cases, the glycosuria occurs even at fasting levels of blood sugar (80 to 100 mg. per cent). In others it is found only if the blood sugar is rather higher than this. Consequently all gradations of this condition occur between individuals where the glycosuria is continuous and is found even when the affected individual is fasting, and those where it is intermittent and only occurs after a carbohydrate meal.

The renal 'threshold'

It is usually said that in renal glycosuria the 'renal threshold' for glucose is lower than in normal people. Detailed physiological analysis of the so-called 'renal threshold' has, however, now made it clear that renal glycosuria may occur as a result of two quite different kinds of renal peculiarity. Both of these types of renal glycosuria are probably genetically determined, although it is also likely that on occasion either may result as a secondary consequence of other kinds of renal damage (39, 40, 41).

In its simplest form the concept of a renal threshold for glucose implies that when the concentration of glucose in the plasma and hence in the glomerular filtrate becomes higher than a definite level, glucose appears in the urine. The relationship between the amount of glucose excreted and the plasma concentration of glucose would appear (Fig. 33) as a straight line (*SE*) starting from the threshold value (*S*). This line would be parallel to the line (*OE*) which measures the amount of glucose filtered through the glomeruli at varying plasma concentrations. The amount of glucose filtered at the plasma level (*S*) corresponding to the threshold would be a measure of the maximum tubular reabsorptive capacity for glucose (the TmG).

In practice, however, the situation is rather more complex. The relation between amount of glucose excreted and the plasma glucose level is found to be a straight line only at plasma levels appreciably greater than the presumed threshold. In the region of the threshold the line is curved (Fig. 34). This is presumably because functional capacity varies somewhat from nephron to nephron, and some nephrons become saturated before others. The blood glucose level at

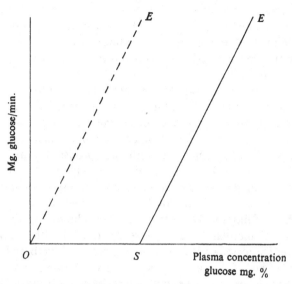

Fig. 33. Theoretical relation between plasma level and glucose excretion, if the capacity of all nephrons is equal. (After Lambert.) - - - - glucose filtered mg./min.; —— glucose excreted mg./min.

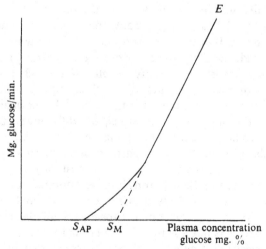

Fig. 34. Relation between plasma level and glucose excretion if the capacities of the nephrons are not equal. (After Lambert.) —— glucose excreted mg./min.; S_M = mean threshold; S_{AP} = apparent or minimal threshold.

which glycosuria first appears has been called the 'appearance threshold or minimal threshold'. The blood glucose level obtained by extrapolating back to the base line the linear part of the curve has been called the 'mean threshold'. This represents an average value for all the nephrons.

To determine these thresholds it is necessary to infuse glucose under carefully controlled conditions, and measure the rate of glucose excretion at blood levels considerably in excess of those normally occurring physiologically. In practice the minimal threshold is extremely difficult to measure with any precision. The mean threshold can, however, be obtained fairly precisely by extrapolation of the line relating glucose excretion to blood glucose concentration obtained in the region of high blood glucose values. It may also be estimated by dividing the TmG determined at a high blood glucose value by the glomerular filtration rate determined with inulin or thiosulphate. The average value of the mean threshold has been found by Lambert to be 246 mg. per cent [40]. It varies, however, considerably from one person to another and in a series of some sixty normal individuals studied values ranging from 180 to 320 mg. per cent were observed. The average value of the minimal threshold is probably of the order of 170 mg. per cent.

Studies of this sort in patients with renal glycosuria have shown that two distinct kinds of abnormality may exist. In one kind (Table 19, numbers 1–6) the mean threshold is distinctly lower than in normal individuals. This can be attributed to a general diminution in the tubular reabsorptive capacity for glucose throughout all the nephrons [41]. In the other kind of renal glycosuria (Table 19, numbers 7–9) the mean threshold is found to be within normal limits. The minimal threshold is, however, significantly lower than in normals. This could occur if the functional capacity of the nephrons is more variable from nephron to nephron than it is normally. Either the glomerular load or the tubular capacity must vary very widely. In consequence some of the nephrons become saturated at quite low levels of blood glucose and glycosuria occurs. This could happen even though the average functional capacity of all the nephrons considered together is not less than in the normal subject.

The exact mechanism by which glucose is transported across the renal tubular cells is not understood. It is certainly an active process, and it has been suggested that it involves phosphorylated intermediates though there is little definite evidence for this. It can be

Table 19. *Mean threshold for glucose in nine patients with renal glycosuria.* (*After Reubi*, 1954)

	Glomerular filtration rate (ml./min.)	Maximal rate of glucose reabsorption (TmG) (mg./min.)	Mean threshold mg. % (normal 241 ± 35)
1	111	204	174
2	152	220	131
3	134	219	150
4	126	144	122
5	116	153	140
6	99	151	155
7	108	275	230
8	109	304	268
9	84	253	255

temporarily inhibited by phloridzin. Shannon [42] has postulated that during tubular reabsorption glucose enters into a reversible combination with some substance present in the tubule cells in constant but limited amounts. Subsequent breakdown of this complex allows transfer of the glucose to the blood to take place (Fig. 35). It is

Glomerular filtrate	Tubular fluid		Tubule cells		Interstitial fluid		Blood
G	→	G	+A → GA → A+		G	→	G

G = glucose; A = substance in tubular cells with which glucose combines.

Fig. 35. Diagrammatic representation of transfer of glucose across renal tubule cells.

suggested that the second reaction (GA → G+A) proceeds rather slowly relative to the attainment of equilibrium in the first reaction (G+A → GA). If the amount of glucose in the glomerular filtrate is increased sufficiently, a point will occur when the glucose is proferred to the tubule cell more rapidly than it can be dealt with. As a result some glucose is not reabsorbed and glycosuria results. This model would describe the situation in an individual nephron. Nephrons evidently vary, however, in the balance between their reabsorptive capacity and the amount of glomerular filtrate formed.

In the first kind of renal glycosuria where the mean threshold is lower than normal, there is presumably a diminished capacity for tubular reabsorption throughout all the nephrons. This could arise either because smaller quantities of the postulated transporting substance are formed, or because one or other of the enzymes mediating the reabsorptive processes is deficient. It is unlikely to be due to some anatomical peculiarity of the nephrons because the defect is in general specific for glucose, and other metabolites are reabsorbed normally.

The second type of renal glycosuria where the abnormality appears to be essentially one of greater variation between the nephrons could perhaps arise because of an uneven distribution of the carrier substance or transport enzymes between the nephrons (41). An alternative possibility is that it is due to some kind of increased morphological variability, resulting for example in an excessive proportion of large glomeruli attached to short tubules, and small glomeruli to long tubules.

Genetics of renal glycosuria

Renal glycosuria has frequently been reported in several members of the same family and a number of pedigrees illustrating the pattern of segregation of the abnormality have been published (43,44,45). In general it seems to turn up in several generations of the same family and to be transmitted directly from an affected parent to a proportion of his or her offspring. The affected individuals are probably heterozygous for a gene causing the condition.

In these family studies the affected individuals have been identified because of the finding of glycosuria in association with a normal glucose tolerance test. This would not enable a distinction between the two physiologically distinct forms of renal glycosuria to be made. While there is some evidence that both types of condition may be genetically determined, no studies in which several affected members of the same family have been subjected to detailed analysis of their renal thresholds have as yet been reported.

Other forms of renal glycosuria

While in most examples of renal glycosuria glucose has been the only metabolite found in the urine in unusual quantities, a number of genetically determined disorders are known in which a defective tubular reabsorption of glucose may occur as part of a more widespread type of renal tubule defect. For example, defective tubular reabsorption of glucose, aminoacids and phosphate and possibly other substances occur in the Fanconi syndrome. Here an anatomical lesion of the proximal convoluted tubule has been demonstrated. In Wilson's disease renal glycosuria may be found in association with defective reabsorption of aminoacids, phosphate and urate. In this case the tubular disorder has been attributed to an excessive deposition of copper. Finally deficient reabsorption of glucose and phosphate but not of aminoacids or other materials has been observed in one kind of vitamin D resistant rickets (46).

Primaquine sensitivity

In 1952 Hockwald and his colleagues (47) observed that the administration of the antimalarial drug primaquine resulted in an acute haemolytic anaemia in some 10 per cent of American negroes to whom it was given. 'Sensitivity' to this drug, however, was apparently rather rare among 'white' Americans. It has since emerged that the sensitive individuals possess an intrinsic red cell defect which probably has as

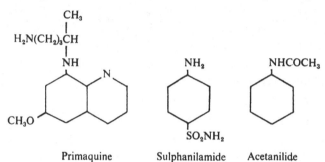

Primaquine   Sulphanilamide   Acetanilide
Fig. 36. Formulae of primaquine, sulphanilamide, and acetanilide.

its basis a genetically determined deficiency of one of the enzymes normally concerned in red cell glucose metabolism, namely glucose-6-phosphate dehydrogenase.

Besides primaquine a number of other drugs such as sulphanilamide and acetanilide (Fig. 36) induce a similar haemolytic crisis in sensitive individuals (48). It also appears probable that favism, the characteristic acute haemolytic reaction occurring in certain individuals after eating fava beans, is due to the same or a very similar type of red cell peculiarity (49).

In the course of their investigations into the nature of this peculiarity, Beutler and his colleagues (50) discovered that the concentration of reduced glutathione in the red cells was on the average lower in 'sensitive' individuals than in other people. Furthermore, an abrupt and profound fall in the reduced glutathione content of the red cells could be observed when primaquine was administered to 'sensitive' individuals, while there was little or no change in 'normals' [51]. It was also found that a similar fall in reduced glutathione concentration could be demonstrated *in vitro* by incubating 'sensitive cells' with acetylphenylhydrazine [52]. The reduced glutathione in normal cells appeared to be quite stable under these conditions. This *in vitro* test of reduced glutathione stability in the presence of acetylphenylhydrazine has been found to be a reliable diagnostic method for identifying the drug-sensitive individuals.

The formation of reduced glutathione (GSH) from oxidised glutathione (GSSG) is thought to occur through the action of reduced

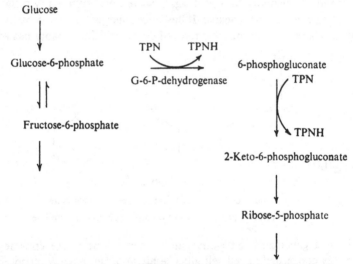

Fig. 37. Pathways in the oxidation of glucose involving TPN reduction. (After Beutler *et al.*[54].)

triphosphopyridine nucleotide (TPNH) and the enzyme glutathione reductase [53]. Triphosphopyridine nucleotide (TPN) may be reduced at at least two different points in red cell metabolism. One of these is the oxidation of glucose-6-phosphate to 6-phosphogluconate, and the other is the oxidation of 6-phosphogluconate to 2-keto-6-phosphogluconate (Fig. 37). Carson and his colleagues [55] were able to show that dialysed haemolysates from primaquine-sensitive individuals differ from those of normal individuals in their inability to reduce oxidised glutathione when supplied with glucose-6-phosphate. If, however, 6-phosphogluconate or TPNH were supplied in appropriate amounts the haemolysates were as effective in reducing GSSG as were those from normals. Thus it appeared that while the enzymes glutathione reductase, and 6-phosphogluconic acid dehydrogenase are present in normal amounts in 'sensitive' cells, glucose-6-phosphate dehydrogenase is deficient. Previous investigations (50) had already shown that there was no apparent peculiarity with respect to other red cell enzymes such as catalase, carbonic anhydrase, cholinesterase, or the various enzymes involved in glycolysis.

The deficiency of glucose-6-phosphate dehydrogenase in these erythrocytes is evidently not complete and probably only becomes of critical significance as the red cells age. Thus if primaquine is administered continuously to a sensitive individual the haemolysis stops after the acute haemolytic crisis, and the blood counts return to normal (56). The abrupt fall in average GSH concentration precedes the major portion of the haemolytic episode, but subsequently returns to pretreatment levels (51). By labelling red cells with a limited age span with ^{59}Fe it was possible to demonstrate that in fact only the older members of the red-cell population were being destroyed through the action of the drug (57).

The precise mechanism by which the different drugs induce the sudden fall in GSH concentration, and the exact relationship of this to the haemolysis is still not clearly understood. Beutler and his colleagues (54) have however suggested that the fall in GSH sensitive cells incubated with acetylphenylhydrazine, and the relative stability of GSH in non-sensitive cells under these conditions may be explained in the following way. On incubation with acetylphenylhydrazine the oxyhaemoglobin of the red cells is altered to a product which in turn oxidises GSH. In normal cells the GSSG so formed is reduced rapidly to GSH through the action of TPNH, which is formed from TPN when glucose-6-phosphate and 6-phosphogluconate are oxidised. In sensitive cells, a defect in glucose-6-phosphate oxidation due to the deficiency of the appropriate dehydrogenase, limits TPN reduction, both directly and indirectly by restricting the amount of 6-phosphogluconate available for further oxidation. The GSSG is therefore not reduced effectively and some of it is broken down by other pathways.

Childs and his colleagues (58) have investigated the incidence of the peculiarity in an American negro population by measuring the level of GSH after incubating red cells with acetylphenylhydrazine under standard conditions. They found that the distributions of GSH values so obtained were sharply bimodal (Fig. 38). However, the incidence of 'sensitive' individuals was much higher in males than in females. About 14 per cent of males but only 2 per cent of females showed GSH values of less than 21 mg. per 100 ml. of packed red cells under these conditions. On the other hand, an appreciably higher proportion of females than males showed low 'normal' values.

The study of the distributions among families each of which contained at least one member giving low values on the acetylphenyl-

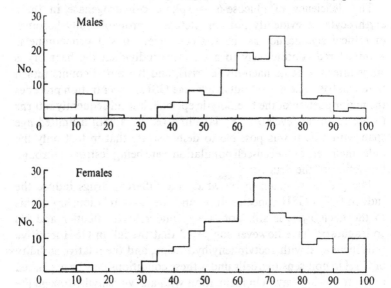

Fig. 38. Distribution of red cell GSH concentrations (after incubation with acetylphenylhydrazine) in a random series of American negroes. (After Childs *et al.*)

hydrazine GSH stability test further emphasized this sex difference (Table 20). About half the males in these families had GSH values below 20 mg. per cent, while only about 16 per cent of the females did so. On the other hand, a high proportion of the females showed intermediate values (21–40 mg. per cent) while such values were not encountered in the males.

Childs and his co-workers suggest, on the basis of their analysis of the manner in which individuals with different GSH values are related to one another, that the curious sex distribution that they had observed could be most plausibly explained on the hypothesis that the peculiarity is determined by an 'incompletely dominant' sex-

Table 20. *Distribution of concentrations of reduced glutathione in red cells among members of sixteen families in which at least one individual had a low value. The measurements were made after the red cells had been incubated with acetylphenylhydrazine.* (*After* Childs et al. 1958)

Reduced glutathione (mg. %)	Males	Females
0–20	30	12
21–40	—	22
41–100	29	43
Totals	59	77

linked gene. They suggest that males carrying the gene, and females homozygous for it, show the abnormality in its most profound form, and usually give values in the GSH stability test of less than 21 mg. per cent. Females heterozygous for the gene have a less pronounced defect and it is rather variable in manifestation. While some of them give GSH values within the normal range, others give intermediate results (21–40 mg. per cent). Thus the females carrying the gene in single dose are on the average less severely affected than are homozygous females, and in fact only a proportion of the heterozygotes can be detected confidently using this test. In essence the hypothesis requires that males should only inherit the peculiarity from their mothers and never from their fathers, and in general this interpretation is consistent with the observed familial distribution. The gene frequency on this hypothesis would be the same as the frequency of affected males (in this population about $0 \cdot 14$). The expected incidence of homozygous females in the population would then be $(0 \cdot 14)^2$ or about 2 per cent, which is what is observed.

REFERENCES

(1) von Giercke, E. (1929). *Beitr. path. Anat.* **82**, 497.
(2) Schönheimer, R. (1929). *Z. physiol. Chem.* **182**, 148.
(3) van Creveld, S. (1939). *Medicine, Baltimore,* **18**, 1.
(4) di Sant'Agnese, P. A., Anderson, D. H., Mason, H. H. and Bauman, W. A. (1950). *Paediatrics,* **6**, 607.
(5) Forbes, G. B. (1953). *J. Paediat.* **42**, 645.
(6) Cori, G. T. (1954). *Harvey Society Lectures,* **48**, 145. Academic Press, N.Y.
(7) Cori, G. T. and Cori, C. F. (1952). *J. Biol. Chem.* **199**, 661.
(8) van Creveld, S. (1952). *Arch. Dis. Child.* **27**, 113.
(9) Nemeth, A. M. (1954). *J. Biol. Chem.* **208**, 773.

(10) Illingworth, B. and Cori, G. T. (1952). *J. Biol. Chem.* **199**, 653.
(11) Illingworth, B., Cori, G. T. and Cori, C. F. (1956). *J. Biol. Chem.* **218**, 123.
(12) Anderson, D. H. (1952). In *A symposium on the clinical and biochemical aspects of carbohydrate utilisation in health and disease.* Najjar, V. A., ed. Johns Hopkins Press, Baltimore.
(13) Holzel, A., Komrower, G. M. and Schwartz, V. (1957). *Amer. J. Med.* **22**, 703.
(14) Kalckar, H. M. (1957). *Science*, **125**, 105.
(15) Schwartz, V., Golberg, L., Komrower, G. M. and Holzel, A. (1956). *Biochem. J.* **62**, 34.
(16) Isselbacher, K. J., Anderson, E. P., Karahashi, K. and Kalckar, H. M. (1956). *Science*, **123**, 635.
(17) Anderson, E. P., Kalckar, H. M. and Isselbacher, K. J. (1957). *Science*, **125**, 113.
(18) Eisenberg, F., Isselbacher, K. J. and Kalckar, H. M. (1957). *Science*, **125**, 116.
(19) Sidbury, J. B. (1957). *J. Clin. Invest.* **36**, 929.
(20) Schwartz, V. and Golberg, L. (1955). *Biochim. Biophys. Acta*, **18**, 310.
(21) Komrower, G. M. (1953). *Arch franç. Pédiat.* **10**, 2.
(22) Cusworth, D. C., Dent, C. E. and Flynn, F. V. (1955). *Arch. Dis. Child.* **30**, 150.
(23) Holzel, A. and Komrower, G. M. (1955). *Arch. Dis. Child.* **30**, 155.
(24) Holzel, A., Komrower, G. M. and Schwartz, V. (1957). In *Modern Problems in Paediatrics*, **3**, 359. S. Karger, Basel/New York.
(25) Enklewitz, M. and Lasker, M. (1933). *Amer. J. Med. Sci.* **186**, 539.
(26) Enklewitz, M. and Lasker, M. (1935). *J. Biol. Chem.* **110**, 443.
(27) Flynn, F. V. (1955). *Brit. Med. J.* **1**, 391.
(28) Touster, O., Hutcheson, R. M. and Rice, L. (1955). *J. Biol. Chem.* **215**, 677.
(29) Touster, O., Mayberry, R. H. and McCormick, D. B. (1957). *Biochim. Biophys. Acta*, **25**, 196.
(30) Lasker, M., Enklewitz, M. and Lasker, G. W. (1936). *Hum. Biol.* **8**, 243.
(31) Schlesinger, W. (1903). *Arch. exp. Path. Pharmak.* **50**, 273.
(32) Silver, S. and Reiner, M. (1934). *Arch. Int. Med.* **54**, 412.
(33) Deuel, H. J. (1936). *Physiol. Rev.* **16**, 173.
(34) Bachmann, G. and Haldi, J. (1937). *J. Nutrit.* **13**, 157.
(35) Rynbergen, H. J., Chambers, W. H. and Blatherwick, N. R. (1941). *J. Nutrit.* **21**, 553.
(36) Edhem, G., Erden, F. and Steinitz, K. (1938). *Acta med. scand.* **97**, 455.
(37) Sachs, B., Sternfield, L. and Kraus, G. (1942). *Amer. J. Dis. Child.* **63**, 252.
(38) Lasker, M. (1941). *Hum. Biol.* **13**, 51.
(39) Govaerts, P. (1952). *Brit. Med. J.* **2**, 175.
(40) Lambert, P. P. (1954). In *CIBA Foundation Symposium on the Kidney*, ed. Lewis, A. A. G. and Wolstenholme, G. E. W. Churchill Ltd, London.

(41) Reubi, F. C. (1954). *Ibid.*

(42) Shannon, J. A. (1939). *Physiol. Rev.* **19**, 63.

(43) Hjarne, U. (1927). *Acta med. scand.* **67**, 422.

(44) Bowcock, H. M. (1929). *Ann. Int. Med.* **2**, 923.

(45) Houston, J. C. (1951). *Ann. Eugen., Lond.* **15**, 293.

(46) Dent, C. E. (1952). *J. Bone Jt. Surg.* **34**B, 266.

(47) Hockwald, R. S., Arnold, J., Clayman, C. B. and Alving, A. S. (1952). *J. Amer. Med. Ass.* **149**, 1568.

(48) Dern, R. J., Beutler, E. and Alving, A. S. (1955). *J. Lab. Clin. Med.* **45**, 30.

(49) Szeinberg, A., Sheba, C., Hirshom, N. & Bodonyi, E. (1957). *Blood*, **12**, 603.

(50) Beutler, E., Dern, R. J., Flanagan, C. L. and Alving, A. S. (1955). *J. Lab. Clin. Med.* **45**, 286.

(51) Flanagan, C. L., Beutler, E., Dern, R. J., and Alving, A. S. (1955). *J. Lab. Clin. Med.* **46**, 814.

(52) Beutler, E., Robson, M. J. and Buttenwieser, E. (1957). *J. Lab. Clin. Med.* **49**. 84.

(53) Rall, T. W. and Lehninger, A. L. (1952). *J. Biol. Chem.* **194**, 119.

(54) Beutler, E., Robson, M. and Buttenwieser, E. (1957). *J. Clin. Invest.* **36**, 617.

(55) Carson, P., Flanagan, C. L., Ickes, C. E. and Alving, A. S. (1956). *Science*, **124**, 484.

(56) Dern, R. J., Beutler, E. and Alving, A. S. (1954). *J. Lab. Clin. Med.* **44**, 171.

(57) Beutler, E., Dern, R. J. and Alving, A. S. (1954). *J. Lab. Clin. Med.* **44**, 439.

(58) Childs, B., Zinkham, W., Browne, E. A., Kimbro, E. L. and Torbert, J. V. (1958). *Johns Hopk. Hosp. Bull.* **102**, 21.

CHAPTER 6

THE HUMAN HAEMOGLOBINS

In 1949 Pauling and his colleagues [1] made the important discovery that the formation of an abnormal haemoglobin represented the biochemical basis of the condition known as sickle-cell anaemia. This finding opened up a whole new field of investigation in human biochemical genetics, and it has been intensively developed during the past few years. As a result a series of different genetically determined types of haemoglobin are now known and the study of their modes of formation and their structures has become of considerable importance in relation to the general problem of the part played by genes in protein synthesis, and of the biological significance of individual variations in protein structure in human populations.

The sickle-cell phenomenon

The red blood cells of certain individuals possess the peculiar property of undergoing a reversible alteration in shape in response to changes in the partial pressure of oxygen. When the oxygen tension is lowered these cells change from their normal biconcave form to elongated filamentous and sickle-shaped forms. The peculiar 'sickled' shape that these cells assumed was first noted by Herrick in 1910 [2].

Most individuals whose erythrocytes can be induced to sickle appear to be perfectly healthy and to suffer no ill-effects. Occasionally, however, the phenomenon is associated with a fairly severe form of haemolytic anaemia which is often fatal in childhood or adolescence. The former class of people are said to have the sickle-cell trait, and the latter to suffer from sickle-cell anaemia. Provided the oxygen tension is reduced sufficiently all the erythrocytes in both classes of individual can be shown to sickle. However, a considerably greater reduction in the partial pressure of oxygen is required for a major fraction of the trait cells to sickle than for the 'anaemia' cells to do so [3].

The excessive haemolysis in sickle-cell anaemia has been shown to be due to an intracorpuscular rather than an extracorpuscular defect. Thus 'trait' cells survive like normal cells when transfused into the circulation of sickle-cell anaemic individuals. Sickle-cell anaemic cells, however, consistently show a markedly shortened life span [4,5].

The genetics of sickling

The sickle-cell trait is common among negro populations in Africa and the United States. In 1923 Taliaferro and Huck[6], from a study of a large Negro family containing many individuals with the sickle-cell trait, came to the conclusion that the condition was inherited as a simple Mendelian dominant character. At this time little distinction was made from the genetical point of view between the asymptomatic individuals with the 'trait' and those with frank haemolytic anaemia. Both were known to occur in the same families and it was assumed that the condition produced by the abnormal gene in heterozygotes was extremely variable and the two types of cases simply represented extremes of a continuous distribution. This view was widely accepted until in 1949 Neel[7], working in the United States, and Beet[8] in Africa, put forward the hypothesis that the sickle-cell trait and sickle-cell anaemia occurred respectively in individuals heterozygous and homozygous for the same abnormal gene. The 'trait' individuals carry the gene only in single dose, the 'anaemia' individuals have it in double dose. Neel[9] subsequently published detailed findings in a series of some seventy-five families, and for the most part these afforded strong evidence for the hypothesis, which is now generally accepted.

The hypothesis that the sickle-cell trait and sickle-cell anaemia are related as heterozygote and homozygote requires that both parents of patients with sickle-cell anaemia should show the sickle-cell trait. In Neel's original survey, one or both parents of sixty-one sibships in which sickle-cell disease was segregating were tested. In thirty-three instances both parents could be tested and in twenty-eight only one. All except one of these ninety-four parents was found to have the sickle-cell trait. This clearly provides strong support for the hypothesis and subsequently two larger series studied in Africa and involving more than 500 cases have given similar results[10,11]. The proportion of exceptions here, after allowing for illegitimacy, appears to have been about 2 per cent. These occasional exceptions seem to be a real phenomenon and require special explanation. Neel pointed out that they could be attributed either to incomplete manifestation of the sickle-cell gene such that occasionally individuals carrying it fail to show the sickling phenomenon; or to the occurrence of a mutation at some stage in gametogenesis in the 'normal' parent; or to the occurrence of a haemolytic anaemia with sickling in consequence of the interaction of the sickle-cell gene with some other abnormal gene not itself producing sickling in the heterozygote. It is now known that the last possibility does in fact occur and can be the cause of certain apparent exceptions to the general pattern of inheritance. Whether it can account for all the observed exceptions is, however, still uncertain.

Other requirements of the genetical hypothesis are that among the children of parents both of whom have the sickle-cell trait, on the average one-half should also show the trait, one-quarter have sickle-cell anaemia and one-quarter be normal; that about half the children

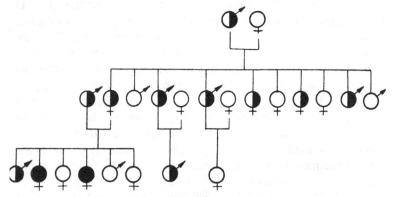

Fig. 39. Pedigree of sickle-cell disease. (After Neel.)

from matings between sickle-cell trait and normal individuals should show the trait; and that the offspring from the rare matings between sickle-cell anaemic individuals and normals should all have the sickle-cell trait. With few exceptions the distribution of the trait and anaemia in the seventy-five families studied by Neel fell into this pattern, and data collected since then has substantially confirmed this characteristic type of familial distribution (Fig. 39).

Sickle-cell haemoglobin

In 1949 Pauling, Itano, Singer and Wells[1] showed that the erythrocytes of patients with sickle-cell anaemia contained haemoglobin having a significantly different isoelectric point from the haemoglobin derived from normal individuals. The electrophoretic mobilities of the two haemoglobins were found to differ over quite a wide range of pH. For example, at pH 6·9 in phosphate buffer carbonmonoxyhaemoglobin from sickle-cell anaemic individuals migrated as a positive ion and the normal derivative as a negative ion (Fig. 40).

In individuals with the sickle-cell trait, a mixture of the two types of haemoglobin was found. Approximately 60 per cent of all the haemoglobin present was of the normal type and 40 per cent of all the haemoglobin present was of the abnormal type. Since all the erythrocytes in such individuals were known to sickle provided the oxygen tension was sufficiently low, it appeared likely that both types of haemoglobin were present in each cell.

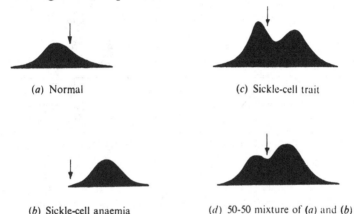

(a) Normal

(c) Sickle-cell trait

(b) Sickle-cell anaemia

(d) 50-50 mixture of (a) and (b)

Fig. 40. Electrophoretic patterns of carbonmonoxyhaemoglobins in phosphate buffer pH 6·9. (After Pauling et al.[1].)

Pauling and his colleagues pointed out that these findings could be readily interpreted in terms of the genetical hypothesis that sickle-cell anaemia and the sickle-cell trait occurred respectively in individuals homozygous and heterozygous for the sickle-cell gene. The normal allele of the gene could be regarded as controlling more or less directly some aspect of the synthesis of haemoglobin. The sickle-cell gene could lead to some peculiarity in this process, resulting in the formation of an abnormal type of haemoglobin molecule. In the heterozygote, both lines of synthesis proceed, the former being somewhat more efficient. In other words a direct relation between the genes present and the haemoglobins formed appeared to exist.

Perutz and Mitchison[12] shortly afterwards discovered a second important characteristic of this new and abnormal type of haemoglobin. They found that reduced sickle-cell haemoglobin was considerably less soluble than reduced normal haemoglobin (Fig. 41).

The oxyhaemoglobin derived from sickle-cell anaemic individuals, on the other hand, appeared to be equally soluble as that derived from normals. This immediately suggested a direct explanation of the phenomenon of sickling which occurs when erythrocytes containing the abnormal haemoglobin are exposed to an atmosphere of low

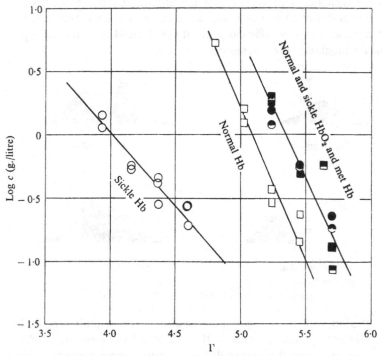

Fig. 41. Solubilities of normal and sickle haemoglobins plotted against ionic strength of phosphate buffer. (After Perutz and Mitchison (12).) ○, sickle haemoglobin (reduced); ●, sickle oxyhaemoglobin; ◓, sickle methaemoglobin; □, normal haemoglobin (reduced); ■, normal oxyhaemoglobin; ◪, normal methaemoglobin.

oxygen tension. The reduced haemoglobin might be expected to come out of free solution and the sickling to result from a consequent deformation of the red cell (13). Harris (14) showed that concentrated (15–25 g. per cent) sickle-cell haemoglobin solutions, free from any cell stroma, became increasingly viscous as the oxygen tension was decreased and eventually assumed a semi-solid gel-like state. Microscopically, spindle-shaped bodies 1–15μ in length could be observed, and these when examined under the polarising microscope were bi-refringent. They disappeared on reoxygenation of the solution and reformed again when the oxygen was removed. There were remarkable similarities in shape between these haemoglobin tactoids formed in stroma-free solutions of deoxygenated sickle-cell haemoglobin and intact sickled cells. Harris suggested that 'the sickled erythrocyte is in essence a haemoglobin tactoid thinly veiled and somewhat distorted by the cell membrane'. These observations have since been extended by Allison (15) and Harris and his colleagues (16) and it now seems clear that the phenomenon of erythrocyte sickling can be mainly attributed to the physical state of the haemoglobin in the erythrocytes and that the cell membrane and stroma play little if any direct part in the process.

In the homozygotes with sickle-cell anaemia the concentration of the abnormal haemoglobin in the red cells is sufficient to allow of an appreciable degree of sickling within the normal physiological range of oxygen tensions. Sickled cells are more fragile and more readily destroyed than normal cells, and this presumably accounts for the significantly shorter erythrocyte life span, and for the haemolytic process which is observed in sickle-cell anaemia. Furthermore the change in red cell morphology leads to an increased viscosity of the blood roughly proportional to the number of cells so altered (16). This probably on occasion results in an impeded blood flow in particular organs with resultant hypoxia and further sickling. A vicious circle may thus be set up which can lead to localised ischaemia, thrombosis, and infarction. This is probably the cause of the acute painful crises which often occur in sickle-cell anaemia.

In the heterozygotes with the sickle-cell trait the concentrations of the abnormal haemoglobin are too low to allow of sickling under ordinary physiological conditions, so that no ill-effects ensue. However, under special conditions such as those encountered in high-altitude flying, crises with complications such as splenic infarction may be precipitated.

Foetal haemoglobin in sickle-cell anaemia

The biochemical situation was shown to be rather more complex than had at first been envisaged, when, in 1951, Singer, Chernoff and Singer (17) found that in sickle-cell anaemia, but not in sickle-cell trait, there frequently occurred an appreciable amount of what appeared to be foetal haemoglobin.

Ever since the second half of the last century it has been known that the haemoglobin of the foetus is different from that of the adult. The most convenient method of differentiating between the two types of haemoglobin is based on the fact that foetal haemoglobin is much more resistant to alkali denaturation than is adult haemoglobin, and this fact is widely used in the quantitative estimation of foetal haemoglobin in mixtures. Foetal and adult haemoglobin also differ in other important respects. For example, they have a different ultra-violet spectral absorption, they are immunologically different, and there are quite marked differences in the aminoacid compositions, and in the nature of the N-terminal aminoacid residues. They also differ slightly in electrophoretic mobility, though a clear separation by electrophoresis is difficult to obtain unless rather special conditions are employed.

In the newborn some 60–80 per cent of the haemoglobin present is foetal in type. With the development of the infant the proportion of foetal haemoglobin gradually decreases so that by the end of the first year of life it has been practically completely replaced by adult haemoglobin. It is probable that the capacity to form foetal haemoglobin is not entirely lost in the adult, and its formation may go on at a very low level, so that traces (0–0·4 per cent) of it can occasionally be detected in the normal adult [18].

Singer and his colleagues [17], using the method of alkali denaturation, showed that in a series of typical cases of sickle-cell anaemia, irrespective of age, some 2–24 per cent of the haemoglobin present was foetal in type. In the sickle-cell trait, however, foetal haemoglobin was not present in appreciably increased amounts. Now although Pauling and his colleagues [1] had originally thought that all the haemoglobin present in sickle-cell anaemia was of the new abnormal type, this view had had to be modified as the material was extended. Wells and Itano [19] reported that in some cases of sickle-cell anaemia 5–20 per cent of a pigment behaving electrophoretically like normal haemoglobin was also present, and in other cases it seemed possible that small quantities of this material might have been obscured in the electrophoretic separation. It finally became clear that the alkali-resistant fraction found by Singer and his colleagues corresponded to the 'normal' component found by Wells and Itano. Thus at this point the position with respect to the different haemoglobins in sickle-cell anaemia, in the sickle-cell trait, and in normal individuals could be represented as shown in Table 21.

Table 21. *Distribution of normal, sickle-cell and foetal haemo-globin in sickle-cell anaemia and the sickle-cell trait*

	Haemoglobin		
	Normal adult	Sickle cell	Foetal
Sickle-cell anaemia	Absent	76–98 %	2–24 %
Sickle-cell trait	55–77 %	23–45 %	Absent
Normal	100 %	Absent	Absent

The finding of foetal haemoglobin in unusual amounts in sickle-cell anaemia, but not in the sickle-cell trait, led to the hypothesis that in the presence of factors suppressing normal adult haemoglobin synthesis, foetal haemoglobin synthesis tended to persist at an appreciable level. Such a concept is supported by the finding that increased foetal haemoglobin formation is not peculiar to sickle-cell anaemia but also occurs in certain other chronic anaemias the most notable of which is Cooley's anaemia or thalassaemia major where a substantial proportion of the haemoglobin formed may be foetal in type. This persistence of foetal haemoglobin synthesis can perhaps be thought of as some kind of non-specific compensatory mechanism. However, it should be noted that the amounts of foetal haemoglobin present in sickle-cell anaemia are rather variable from case to case, and Singer and his colleagues [17, 20] were unable to correlate the amounts present with either the clinical or haematological severity of the anaemia.

The proportion of abnormal haemoglobin in the sickle-cell heterozygotes

The proportion of sickle-cell to adult haemoglobin in different individuals with the sickle-cell trait is extremely variable. Values ranging from 22 per cent to 45 per cent for the sickle-cell haemoglobin component have been reported, and such variation is well outside the range attributable to experimental error. The distribution of the proportions of the two haemoglobins in different heterozygotes appears to be bimodal (Fig. 42). One mode is at about thirty-five per cent abnormal haemoglobin and the other at about forty-one per cent. It is possible as suggested by Itano [21] that the distribution may be actually trimodal with a third mode at about twenty-six per cent. abnormal haemoglobin.

Wells and Itano[19] showed that in a small series of heterozygotes repeated samples taken on different occasions from the same person had substantially the same proportions of the two haemoglobins. Furthermore, the proportions appeared to be independent of age or sex, the values found in husbands and wives were not significantly correlated, and there were no obvious differences in individuals coming from different parts of the United States. Thus the variation cannot readily be accounted for in terms of any gross environmental differences.

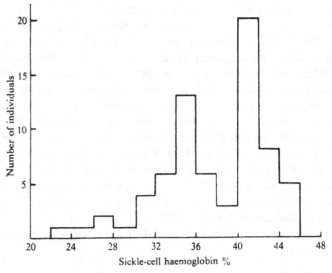

Fig. 42. Percentage of sickle-cell haemoglobin in different individuals with the sickle-cell trait. (After Neel *et al.*[22].)

It appears in fact that much of this variation is genetically determined. Neel, Wells and Itano[22] showed that with respect to the proportion of abnormal haemoglobin present in the heterozygous individuals, the variation between families was significantly greater than the variation within families. In other words, in some families the average percentage of the abnormal haemoglobin in the heterozygotes was significantly different from that in others. The exact interpretation of this is still uncertain. The possibility that there is more than one sickle-cell gene, each producing somewhat different amounts of the abnormal haemoglobin in the heterozygotes, could not readily be sustained on detailed examination of the pedigrees, because both low and high values could be found together in certain families in which one sickle-cell gene was segregating. Another possibility is that the situation may be produced by variations in the degree of activity of the normal allele of the sickle-cell gene, that is by the occurrence of a series of 'isoalleles' at this locus [21]. A third possibility is that the results could be produced by the occurrence in the populations studied of a common modifying gene or genes, which is capable in some way of influencing significantly the proportions of the two types of haemoglobins in the heterozygotes [22].

While the genetical basis of the common kind of variation in sickle-cell heterozygotes is obscure, a number of situations are known in which the presence of some other gene known in itself to influence haemoglobin formation specifically may produce profound modifications in the sickle-cell heterozygote. The first of such interactions to be recognised was the one with the gene causing the condition known as thalassaemia.

Thalassaemia sickle-cell disease

Thalassaemia major or Cooley's anaemia is a severe genetically determined microcytic hypochromic anaemia which is unresponsive to iron therapy and is frequently fatal at an early age. It has been found most commonly in populations living in countries in the northern Mediterranean area, or in people who originated there. It is now generally accepted that the affected patients are homozygous for a gene which in heterozygotes results in a very much milder type of abnormality [23]. The condition in the heterozygotes is called thalassaemia minor. Characteristically this is a mild or minimal microcytic anaemia occurring in the absence of iron deficiency and usually causing little or no clinical disturbance. However, the degree of haematological abnormality is extremely variable in these heterozygotes and this may occasionally give rise to difficulty in characterisation and classification, although using a battery of haematological criteria it is generally possible to arrive at an unequivocal conclusion in most instances.

The precise biochemical basis of thalassaemia is not understood. In the homozygotes a large amount of foetal haemoglobin is regularly found [17,24,25]. This may amount to 50 per cent or more of all the haemoglobin present. The remainder appears to behave as normal adult haemoglobin, and so far no abnormal type of haemoglobin has been identified. The situation is usually interpreted as due to some kind of defect in the normal synthesis of adult haemoglobin, resulting in a severe restriction in its rate of formation, and leading to a persistence of foetal haemoglobin synthesis at a very high level.

Table 22. *Percentage A_2 haemoglobin observed in sixty-five normal individuals and thirty-four individuals with the thalassaemia trait. (After Kunkel et al. 1957)*

Percentage A_2	Normal	Thalassaemia trait
1·6 –	4	—
2·0 –	13	2
2·4 –	28	—
2·8 –	19	—
3·2 –	1	1
3·6 –	—	1
4·0 –	—	4
4·4 –	—	6
4·8 –	—	4
5·2 –	—	5
5·6 –	—	5
6·0 –	—	3
> 6·4	—	3
Total	65	34
Mean percentage A_2	2·54	5·11
Standard deviation	0·35	1·35

In the heterozygote most of the haemoglobin present is of the normal adult type. There is, however, a certain difference from the situation encountered in normal individuals, which appears to be significant and characteristic of the condition. Kunkel and Wallenius[26] have shown, using a method of zone electrophoresis in a supporting medium of starch, that normal individuals regularly show a small fraction of haemoglobin which at pH 8·6 migrates towards the anode very much more slowly than the main fraction of normal adult haemoglobin. This slow-moving component (now referred to as haemoglobin A_2) usually amounts to about 2½ per cent of all the haemoglobin present. In thalassaemia minor this fraction is significantly increased (Table 22) and on the average about twice as much is found as in normals[27]. Besides this, small amounts of foetal haemoglobin may occur in thalassaemia minor. It is rather variable and rarely amounts to more than 5 per cent of all the haemoglobin present.

Silvestroni and Bianco [28] were the first to draw attention to a curious form of anaemia which combined features both of thalassaemia and of sickling. Numerous examples of this condition have since been recognised and the abnormality is now called thalassaemia sickle-cell disease. Clinically the condition closely resembles sickle-cell anaemia, but tends on the average to be somewhat less severe. Haematologically there is a microcytic hypochromic anaemia and the red cells show the sickling phenomenon. It is thought that the

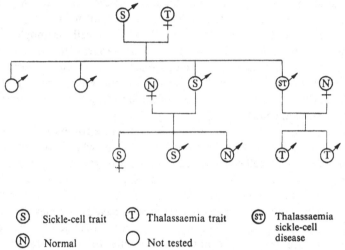

Fig. 43. Pedigree showing the segregation of thalassaemia minor and the sickle-cell trait in a family, and the occurrence of thalassaemia sickle-cell disease. (After Powell *et al.*)

condition arises because the patients are heterozygous both for the gene causing thalassaemia minor and also for the gene causing sickling. This hypothesis is supported by the fact that where the parents of such patients have been examined it has generally been found that one possessed the sickle-cell trait and the other had thalassaemia minor. More critical evidence that the affected individual is indeed a double heterozygote for the abnormal genes present in the parents was first obtained in a family reported by Powell, Rodante and Neel [29] (Fig. 43). The severely anaemic patient sickled and so could be presumed to carry the sickle-cell gene. His offspring by a normal both had thalassaemia minor, showing that in fact he must have carried the gene for this as well.

In thalassaemia sickle-cell disease it is usually found that some

60–80 per cent of the haemoglobin present is of the sickle-cell type and most of the remainder is normal adult haemoglobin. Small and variable amounts of foetal haemoglobin may also be found. Since this picture is believed to be due to the simultaneous presence of a single dose of the gene causing thalassaemia minor and a single dose of the gene responsible for the formation of sickle-cell haemoglobin, the findings are of considerable theoretical significance. In the sickle-cell trait only some 20–40 per cent of sickle-cell haemoglobin is found, so that it appears that the effect of the thalassaemia gene in this combination is to restrict the synthesis of normal haemoglobin to a relatively much greater extent than sickle-cell haemoglobin. Indeed, reports have been made of what appear to have been instances of thalassaemia sickle-cell disease in which no normal adult haemoglobin could be detected at all. Phenotypically the haemoglobin pattern was indistinguishable from that encountered in sickle-cell anaemia.

The situation is, however, probably even more complex. Zuezler, Neel and Robinson[30] refer to two families in which both thalassaemia and sickle-cell genes appeared to be segregating, and in which there occurred essentially asymptomatic individuals whose red cells sickled and also showed the characteristic features of thalassaemia minor. Three of the persons who appeared to have both genes showed only 36 per cent, 28 per cent and 22 per cent of sickle-cell haemoglobin respectively. These authors also refer to other families in which the findings were atypical in various ways. They go on to point out that the term 'thalassaemia minor' at present scarcely enjoys the specificity that may be attached to the sickle-cell trait or other conditions where a qualitatively distinct biochemical situation has been identified. 'Thalassaemia minor' may in fact include several genetically distinct entities each of which may interact differently with the sickle-cell gene. It is becoming clear that two urgent problems in this field are the detailed analysis of this possible genetical heterogeneity in thalassaemia, and the development of some specific biochemical test for this condition or group of conditions.

Haemoglobin C

Soon after the discovery of sickle-cell haemoglobin the study of certain families in which apparent exceptions to the general pattern of inheritance of the sickle-cell trait and sickle-cell anaemia occurred led to the identification of two further types of abnormal haemo-globin. These are now called haemoglobins C and D.

Haemoglobin C was discovered by Itano and Neel[31] when they examined electrophoretically, haemoglobin preparations obtained from members of two such atypical families (Fig. 44). In these families there occurred one or more children with a haematological picture of sickle-cell anaemia, but the disease was rather less severe than that usually encountered, and the situation was peculiar in that the erythrocytes of only one parent in each case could be induced to sickle. The other parent was apparently normal. When the haemo-globins from the exceptional parents who failed to show the sickling phenomenon was examined electrophoretically it was found that in each case two components were present. One of these corresponded to normal adult haemoglobin and the other represented an entirely new type of haemoglobin which migrated as a positive ion at pH 6·5 at a speed even faster than sickle-cell haemoglobin. The children with the anaemia were also shown to have this new haemoglobin, but here it occurred in combination with sickle-cell haemoglobin. This condi-tion is now called haemoglobin C sickle-cell disease, and represents a new and distinct haematological syndrome. It is in general less severe than classical sickle-cell anaemia, but haemolytic crises do occur, and they may be particularly marked in pregnancy. The individuals with a mixture of normal haemoglobin and haemoglobin C are said to have the haemoglobin C trait. This is asymptomatic.

From the manner in which the new haemoglobin was distributed in these families, it could be inferred that it was genetically deter-mined in much the same way as sickle-cell haemoglobin. That is to say, a single abnormal gene is necessary for its formation, and indivi-duals heterozygous for this gene and its normal allele form both haemoglobin C and normal haemoglobin. The patients with the anaemia in these families could be regarded as having received this new gene from one of their parents, and the sickle-cell gene from the other. In effect they were double heterozygotes and the presence of the two different abnormal genes resulted in the simultaneous formation of the two distinct abnormal haemoglobins. This inter-pretation has since been confirmed with the investigation of further families of this type. The homozygous state with respect to the haemoglobin C gene was not encountered in the original studies, but its existence was predicted and it was subsequently demonstrated[32, 33].

148 THE HUMAN HAEMOGLOBINS

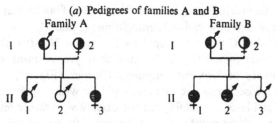

(a) Pedigrees of families A and B

			Haemoglobin components		
Family	Age	Sickling test	Pattern (see Fig. 44b)	Normal	Sickle	New component
AI 1	29	−	d	64·7	·	35·3
2	28	+	c	66·5	33·5	·
AII 1	6	−	d	66·4	·	33·6
2	4	−	a	100·0	·	·
3	3	+	f	13·0	39·0	48·0
BI 1	33	−	d	69·8	·	30·2
2	31	+	c	68·9	31·1	·
BII 1	12	+	e	·	47·0	53·0
2	10	+	e	·	50·0	50·0
3	8	−	a	100·0	·	·

Fig. 44. (a) Families described by Itano and Neel (1950) showing the occurrence of a new haemoglobin variant now known as haemoglobin C. ◑, sickle-cell trait; ◕, haemoglobin C trait; ◕, haemoglobin C sickle-cell disease; ○, normal. (N.B. the 'normal' haemoglobin component in A, II 3 is probably foetal.)

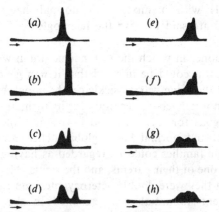

(b) Electrophoretic diagrams of carbonmonoxyhaemoglobins (in cacodylate buffer pH 6·5) from individuals in these families compared to the diagrams obtained from individuals known to be haematologically normal or to have sickle-cell anaemia or sickle-cell trait: (a) normal; (b) sickle-cell anaemia; (c) sickle-cell trait; (d) family A, I 1 and II 1: family B, I 1; (e) family B, II 1 and II 2; (f) family A, II 3; (g) mixture of (b) and (d); (h) mixture of (a) and (e).

It results in a mild anaemia, and as expected all or nearly all the haemoglobin present is haemoglobin C.

In neither haemoglobin C sickle-cell disease or homozygous haemoglobin C disease has any normal adult haemoglobin been identified. Variable though usually small amounts of foetal haemoglobin may be present. Individuals heterozygous for haemoglobin C and its normal allele tend to have some 25–40 per cent of haemoglobin C, the remainder being normal adult haemoglobin. In this respect they resemble sickle-cell heterozygotes where the proportion of abnormal to normal haemoglobin is very similar. In the double heterozygote (haemoglobin C sickle-cell disease) haemoglobin C and haemoglobin S occur in roughly equal amounts.

Reduced haemoglobin C does not exhibit the extremely low solubility characteristic of reduced sickle-cell haemoglobin. This explains why it does not cause sickling and presumably why the clinical consequences of the homozygous condition are so much less severe.

Haemoglobin D

Itano [34] in the study of another anomalous family of which two children appeared to have sickle-cell anaemia, but one parent failed to show the sickle-cell trait, was able to uncover a further type of gene-controlled haemoglobin. He found that electrophoretically the haemoglobin present in the anaemic children corresponded closely to that found in sickle-cell anaemia. In the mother and two sibs, none of whom showed the sickle-cell trait, there were nevertheless two electrophoretically distinct haemoglobin components. Respectively 42 per cent, 35 per cent and 49 per cent of their haemoglobins were found to migrate with the same mobility as sickle-cell haemoglobin, and the rest behaved as normal adult haemoglobin. Thus electrophoretically they could be thought to be sickle-cell heterozygotes, even though they failed to show the sickling phenomenon. The explanation of this anomaly emerged as a result of solubility studies. It was shown that the abnormal haemoglobin present in the electrophoretic mobility as sickle-cell haemoglobin could be clearly distinguished from it by the fact that its solubility in the reduced state was considerably greater than the solubility of reduced sickle-cell haemoglobin. Its solubility actually approximated to that of normal adult haemoglobin. It represented in fact a new molecular species of haemoglobin, and it seemed reasonable to infer from its distribution in the family that it was, like sickle-cell haemoglobin and haemoglobin C, determined by a single abnormal gene. The two anaemic individuals were presumably heterozygous both for this gene and for the sickle-cell gene. Although their haemoglobin behaved electrophoretically as a single component, it was possible to show by solubility studies that it represented a mixture of sickle-cell haemoglobin and the new haemoglobin variant, now known as haemoglobin D.

The investigations emphasise the important point that electrophoresis *per se* is likely to be insufficient to identify and characterise all the haemoglobin variants. Proteins of different structures may well show identical behaviour in electrophoresis.

Other haemoglobin variants

The earlier investigations of the abnormal haemoglobins were carried out by the moving boundary method in the classical Tiselius apparatus. This technique, while still probably essential for precise electrophoretic characterisation, is rather laborious and unsuited to large-scale family and population studies. The recognition that equivalent separations could be obtained by the very simple technique of paper electrophoresis gave a great impetus to the search for unusual haemoglobin variants. During the last few years this technique has been extensively used both in surveys of populations where for one reason or another abnormal haemoglobins were expected to be found, and in the investigations of atypical anaemias in which the occurrence of an unusual haemoglobin might be plausibly expected. As a result a whole series of new haemoglobin types has been recognised and there is no reason to believe that the rate of their discovery is slowing down (for recent review see Itano[35]).

The identification of many new forms of human haemoglobin immediately raised many knotty problems in nomenclature. Currently the recommendations of a group of workers in the field convened by the U.S. National Institutes of Health in 1953[36] to consider this question are generally adhered to. Normal adult haemoglobin is called haemoglobin A, and foetal haemoglobin is called haemoglobin F. In general the newly discovered haemoglobins, which so far appear to be variants of adult haemoglobin, are called by the other letters of the alphabet in order of their discovery. Exceptions are, however, made in cases where the newly discovered haemoglobin is associated with some well-recognised clinical condition. Thus sickle-cell haemoglobin, the first of the electrophoretically distinct haemoglobins to be discovered, is called haemoglobin S and not haemoglobin B. The letter B is omitted from the alphabetic series to avoid further confusion. So far, apart from S, C and D which have already been mentioned, haemoglobins designated as E, G, H, I, J, K and L have been reported as a result of electrophoretic studies. Besides these mention must also be made of an abnormal form of haemoglobin reported by Hörlein and Weber in 1948[37], in cases of a rather unusual type of methaemoglobinaemia. It was characterised by a peculiar form of absorption spectrum. It has been suggested that it should be called haemoglobin M (see p. 250).

Complications in the terminology are introduced by the probability that the haemoglobin occurring in normal subjects is heterogeneous. It has already been mentioned that Kunkel and Wallenius[26] separated it electrophoretically into a main component amounting to about 97·5 per cent of the total, and a small fraction of about 2·5 per cent, migrating much more slowly at pH 8·6. It has been suggested that these be referred to as haemoglobins A_1 and A_2 respectively. Normal adult haemoglobin may be even more heterogeneous than is implied by this, and evidence for other fractions has been obtained by several techniques; their exact significance is, however, uncertain. For example a further fraction referred to as A_3 moving somewhat more rapidly towards the anode at pH 8·6 may often be separated out of the main component of adult haemoglobin. It appears to account for some 4–12 per cent of the total haemoglobin, but unlike the A_2 fraction increases in amount in old samples[38]. It is probably derived in some way from the main A_1 component, but since it has been observed in freshly drawn samples the conversion may take place *in vivo* as well as *in vitro*.

The properties of the different haemoglobins

Absolute mobilities of individual haemoglobins in electrophoresis are difficult to determine. However, for most practical purposes the electrophoretic differences between the different haemoglobins can be expressed in terms of relative mobilities. Characterisation is usually made by electrophoresing appropriate mixtures of the unknown component with various known haemoglobins. Itano, Bergren and Sturgeon[39] list the relative mobilities of the various haemoglobins which have been examined by moving boundary electrophoresis at both pH 8·6 and pH 6·5 as follows.

At pH 8·6 in barbital buffer all the haemoglobins carry negative charges and migrate at various speeds towards the anode. Haemoglobin H has the highest mobility and the others follow in this order:

$$H > I > J > A > F > G > S = D > E > C.$$

In cacodylate buffer at pH 6·5 haemoglobin H still carries a negative charge. The others have positive charges and migrate

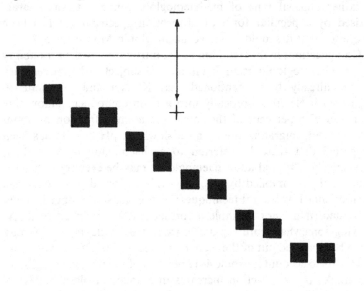

C E S D L G F A K J I H

Fig. 45. Diagrammatic representation of electrophoretic separation of different haemoglobins on filter paper at pH 8·6. (After Ager *et al.*[(40)].)

towards the cathode. Haemoglobin C has the highest mobility and the others follow in the order given:

$$C > S = D \geqq G > E > A > F > J > I.$$

Below pH 6·1 haemoglobin H also carries a positive charge and migrates towards the cathode.

The A_2 fraction of normal haemoglobin appears to have mobilities similar to haemoglobin E.

Very similar though not completely identical results have been obtained by studies using paper electrophoresis[(40)] (Fig. 45).

One point which emerges from these comparisons is that the relative mobilities of two haemoglobins towards the anode at alkaline pH is not necessarily indicative of their order of migration towards the cathode at acid pH. Characterisation relative to one another at more than one pH has become an essential part of the investigation of these substances.

Some of the haemoglobins have also been separated by elution from an ion-exchange resin, and the relative order of elution may be helpful in their characterisation. The relative order of elution of some of the haemoglobins [41] from the cation-exchange resin I.R.C. 50 has been found to be

$$H > F > I > J = A > E > S = D > C.$$

Certain of the new haemoglobins have only thus far been encountered in mixtures with normal haemoglobin and they have not been isolated in pure form. Apart from their electrophoretic and chromatographic behaviour little is known about the details of their other properties. However, it seems clear that none of them share the property so far peculiar to haemoglobin S of having an extremely low solubility in the reduced form. Consequently haemoglobin S is still specifically associated with the sickle-cell phenomenon. Similarly, although it is possible that variations in the rate of denaturation with alkali occur from one to another of these new haemoglobins, haemoglobin F is still peculiar in that its rate of alkali denaturation is extremely slow. The only other outstanding characteristic that has been reported among them is the apparently extreme instability of haemoglobin H. This is peculiar in being readily denatured under relatively mild conditions [42]. For example, practically complete denaturation occurs by a single freezing and thawing.

The structural peculiarity of the haemoglobin variants

Pauling and his colleagues [1] concluded from the behaviour of normal and sickle-cell haemoglobin in electrophoresis that the sickle-cell haemoglobin carried some two to four more net positive charges per molecule than normal haemoglobin over a pH range of about 1·5 pH units on either side of neutrality.

Dimethyl esters of the protoporphyrins were prepared from the haem of each of these haemoglobins and were found to be identical. It was therefore supposed that the difference must reside in the globins, and in fact Havinga and Itano [43] were able to demonstrate that the native globins prepared from normal and sickle-cell haemoglobins showed similar differences in electrophoretic mobility.

It soon became clear, however, that the marked differences in electrophoretic behaviour, and in the solubilities of the two haemoglobins, must depend on very small and subtle differences in molecular structure. X-ray diagrams obtained from crystals of sickle-cell and normal haemoglobin appeared to be identical in every detail[13]. Aminoacid analysis[44,45] failed to reveal any striking differences between the two proteins within the limits of error of the methods available, and similarly no consistent differences could be found when the N-terminal[46,47] or C-terminal residues[48], the primary amide groups[49] or the sulph-hydryl groups[50] were examined.

A specific chemical difference between the two proteins was eventually demonstrated by Ingram in 1956[51]. This was achieved be examining the peptides produced by hydrolysis of the proteins with trypsin. This enzyme attacks only those bonds which are derived from the carboxyl groups of lysine and arginine. There are nearly sixty of these in normal and sickle-cell haemoglobin, but since it is thought that each molecule is composed of two identical half molecules, the number of peptides obtained by the action of trypsin was expected to be about thirty, with an average chain length of ten aminoacids. The peptides were separated by a two-dimensional combination of paper electrophoresis and chromatography. About thirty peptides were obtained in each case as expected. The great majority of these appeared to behave identically in the two proteins. There was, however, one peptide spot in the sickle-cell haemoglobin digest which was not present in the normal haemoglobin digest, and similarly one peptide in the normal haemoglobin digest was not present in the sickle-cell haemoglobin digest. The anomalous peptide in the sickle-cell haemoglobin was somewhat more positively charged at pH 6·5 than the anomalous peptide in the normal haemoglobin. These results indicated that the difference between the two proteins probably lay in the aminoacid sequence in one small portion of the polypeptide chains.

Ingram[52] subsequently isolated the two anomalous peptides and determined their aminoacid sequences. The only difference between them was that the sequence in the sickle-cell peptide contained a valine residue in a situation which was occupied in the normal adult haemoglobin peptide by a glutamic acid residue. The other eight aminoacid residues in the two peptide sequences were identical in nature and in position. Furthermore aminoacid analysis of all the other peptides obtained by tryptic digestion indicated that these were probably all identical in the two molecules.

Haemoglobin has a molecular weight of about 67,000 and it is evidently composed of two identical half molecules each containing nearly three hundred aminoacid residues. Ingram concluded that the difference between normal adult haemoglobin and sickle-cell haemoglobin is simply that just one of these aminoacid residues is substituted by another. Glutamic acid contains a carboxyl group not present in valine and this is sufficient to account for the difference in electrophoretic properties of the two molecules. Presumably it also accounts for the solubility differences but how this occurs is not yet understood. It is remarkable that such a subtle difference in molecular structure should have such profound pathological consequences.

Haemoglobin A	—his—val—leu—leu—thr—pro—glu—glu—lys—
Haemoglobin S	—his—val—leu—leu—thr—pro—val—glu—lys—
Haemoglobin C	—his—val—leu—leu—thr—pro—lys—glu—lys—

Key: his = histidyl—   val = valyl—
     leu = leucyl—   thr = threonyl—
     pro = prolyl—   glu = glutamyl—
     lys = lysyl—

Fig. 46. Aminoacid sequences in anomalous peptides from haemoglobin S and C compared with the equivalent peptide in haemoglobin A. (After Hunt and Ingram.)

Hunt and Ingram [53] have now applied the same kind of analytical technique to haemoglobin C. Here they find that exactly the same aminoacid site in the molecule is involved. The glutamic acid residue in normal haemoglobin which is replaced by valine in sickle-cell haemoglobin is in haemoglobin C replaced by lysine. The relevant peptide sequence in the three molecules is shown in Fig. 46.

So far no similar analysis of the other haemoglobin variants has been reported. They will be awaited with great interest (see pp. 289 *et seq.*).

Genetics of the new haemoglobins

Apart from haemoglobin S and C, the genetical investigations on most of the other new haemoglobin variants has been limited to the detailed study of only a relatively small number of families. It appears probable, however, that with the exception of haemoglobin H, the other new haemoglobins that have been discovered can each be regarded as being determined by a single abnormal gene. In general, heterozygotes with the normal allele form a mixture of haemoglobin A and the particular abnormal haemoglobin. Such individuals are said to have the trait for the new haemoglobin and in all cases so far studied this appears to be asymptomatic. Homozygotes for each of these presumed genes have not yet been encountered in a number of cases. Where they have, it seems that all or nearly all of the haemoglobin present is of the appropriate type. Normal adult haemoglobin is absent, but small amounts of foetal haemoglobin may occur. Usually the homozygote suffers from some degree of anaemia associated with a more or less characteristic haematological picture.

With the rapid extension of the series of different genetically determined haemoglobins, it is apparent that the number of possible combinations of these genes which may occur in the same individual is becoming rather large. To these possibilities must also be added the combinations resulting from the simultaneous presence of one or other of these genes with the gene or genes responsible for the defect in haemoglobin synthesis occurring in thalassaemia. Many of these combinations may be expected to result in anaemia with more or less typical features. Thus the possibility is opened up of being able to characterise a whole series of previously ill-defined haematological conditions in terms of the character of the haemoglobin formed by the affected individual, and more specifically in terms of his genetical constitution. Some of the haemoglobin combinations that have been observed so far are listed in Table 23.

The genetics of haemoglobin H formation is rather obscure. It seems, however, to constitute an exception to the general pattern of inheritance encountered in the case of the other abnormal haemoglobins. Haemoglobin H was first described by Rigas, Koler and Osgood [42] in three sibs suffering from a thalassaemia-like anaemia. About 30–40 per cent of the haemoglobin present was of the abnormal type. The rest, apart from a small amount of foetal haemoglobin (2–4 per cent), appeared to be normal adult haemoglobin. Neither parent showed any haemoglobin H and in other respects their haematological pictures were unremarkable. A child of one of the affected patients had a blood picture consistent with thalassaemia minor, but showed no abnormality in haemoglobin composition. The same general kind of situation has also been encountered in other families where haemoglobin H has been demonstrated [43]. That is to say, it occurs only in association with a thalassaemia-like anaemia, neither parent of the affected patient may have the abnormal haemoglobin, but one or other parent and various other relatives may have what appears to be thalassaemia minor. It is evident that haemoglobin H is genetically determined and that its formation is in some way bound up with the segregation of a condition closely resembling, and perhaps identical with, thalassaemia minor. Possibly the individual must be heterozygous for thalassaemia minor, before the genetical factors determining haemoglobin H can find expression (54).

Table 23. *Examples of known haemoglobin combinations (note—In these examples the haemoglobin given in parentheses is not always found)*

A	Normal adult
A+F	Infants
A+F	Thalassaemia
S+F	Sickle-cell anaemia
A+S	Sickle-cell trait
A+S+F	Sickle-cell/thalassaemia
C (+F)	Hb-C disease
A+C	Hb-C trait
A+C+F	Hb-C/thalassaemia
S+C (+F)	Sickle-cell/Hb-C disease
D	Hb-D disease
A+D	Hb-D trait
S+D (+F)	Sickle-cell/Hb-D disease
E (+F)	Hb-E disease
A+E	Hb-E trait
E+F (+A?)	Hb-E/thalassaemia
G	Hb-G disease
A+G	Hb-G trait
A+I	Hb-I trait
A+H	Hb-H trait
A+J	Hb-J trait

The genetical relationships between the different genes determining haemoglobin formation

It is clear that a whole series of different abnormal genes exists in human populations which may in one way or another influence the character of haemoglobin synthesis. Any one individual may possess at least two of these genes, and the precise genetical structure of such compound heterozygotes is likely to be of considerable importance in understanding the exact role that these genes play in controlling haemoglobin formation, and the manner in which they interact one with another.

Two main types of situation can be envisaged. Any pair of these genes may be alleles, or they may occur at different chromosomal loci. If all the genes resulting in specific abnormalities in haemoglobin synthesis were alleles, that is to say alternative forms occurring at a single chromosomal locus, then any one person could possess only two such abnormal genes, one of which was derived from one of his parents, and one from the other parent. If the abnormal genes were each at different chromosomal loci, then many more possible

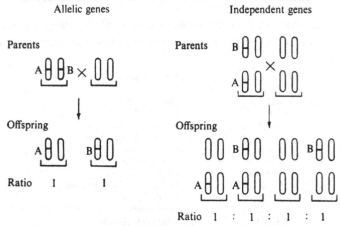

Fig. 47. Diagrammatic representation of the segregation of two mutant genes A and B according to whether they are allelic or at independent chromosomal loci.

combinations could exist, because any one individual could be heterozygous or homozygous for any number of them. In fact it seems possible that the true situation lies somewhere between these extremes. More than one different locus is probably involved, and at each locus there may occur several abnormal alleles. Formally such a situation would be essentially the same as that which controls the multiplicity of blood group antigens on the red cell surface.

In practice a decision about the different possibilities is likely to be arrived at mainly by the study of families in which more than one of these genes is segregating, and in which certain critical types of mating have taken place. One such informative type of mating is that between an individual heterozygous for two of these genes and a normal individual. The distinction between the hypothesis of allelism and of separate loci according to the progeny found from this type of mating is illustrated in Fig. 47. If the two abnormal genes are alleles, the children would be either heterozygous for one of them or heterozygous for the other. They would not be double heterozygotes or normals. Thus neither of the parental combinations should be found among the offspring. On the other hand, if the abnormal genes are at different loci, all the four types of possible combination can be expected among the offspring in approximately equal proportions. Because of the small size of human families it will in general be necessary to examine a number of such matings before one could expect to be certain of the answer.

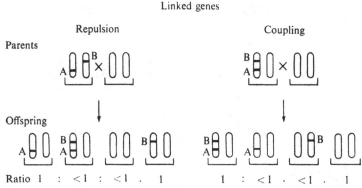

Fig. 48. Diagram showing the segregation of mutant genes A and B assuming that they occur at different loci on the same chromosome (that is, are linked).

The situation may be further complicated by the possibility that two or more of the different loci involved may be linked, that is to say occur on the same chromosome. An individual doubly heterozygous for two such linked genes could either have them in the coupling phase, that is on the same member of the pair of homologous chromosomes, or in the repulsion phase, that is on different members of the pair of homologous chromosomes. In these circumstances, the outcome of particular matings between double heterozygotes and normals will depend on whether the abnormal genes are in coupling or repulsion, and also on how close is the linkage. Close linkage and repulsion, for example, tends to simulate multiple allelism (Fig. 48).

A number of families have now been observed which give some information concerning the probable genetical relationship between the genes determining haemoglobins S, C and G.

Ranney[55] found that in five children who were offspring of three matings between individuals with haemoglobin C sickle-cell disease and normals, all had either the haemoglobin C trait or the sickle-cell trait, and none were normal or had haemoglobin C sickle-cell disease. Smith and Conley[56] found the same in four children who were very probably the issue of this type of mating. Singer and his colleagues[57]

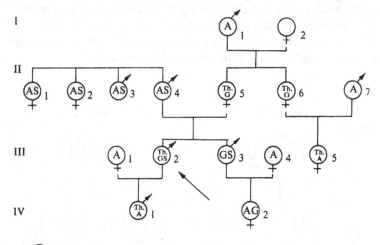

O Not tested

(A) Normal and only haemoglobin A detected

(Th./A) Thalassaemia trait and only haemoglobin A detected

(Th./G) Thalassaemia trait and only haemoglobin G detected

(Th./GS) Thalassaemia trait and only haemoglobins G and S detected

(AS) Sickle-cell trait, haemoglobins A and S detected

(AG) Haemoglobin G trait, haemoglobins A and G detected

Fig. 49. Occurrence of haemoglobins S and G, and also thalassaemia in the same family. (After Schwartz *et al.*)

found that among the offspring of a mating between a father with haemoglobin C sickle-cell disease and a mother with thalassaemia minor, two children had the sickle-cell trait, one had sickle-cell thalassaemia disease, and one had haemoglobin C thalassaemia disease. The absence of either parent combination in the children in these families suggests as far as it goes that the genes for haemoglobin S and for haemoglobin C are allelic.

One extremely interesting family has been described [58] in which the genes for haemoglobin S, haemoglobin G, and thalassaemia were evidently segregating. The pedigree is shown in Fig. 49. The propositus appeared to be heterozygous for each of these three genes. His child by a normal person had neither haemoglobin S nor haemoglobin G, so that the genes determining these haemoglobins are evidently not alleles. The propositus apparently received the gene for thalassaemia and also the gene for haemoglobin G from the same parent. Evidently then these two genes are not allelic.

Smith and Torbert [59] have described a family in which the sickle-cell gene and also a gene determining another haemoglobin variant which they refer to as Hopkins 2, were segregating. Hopkins 2 has a similar mobility to haemoglobin J but the identity of the two haemoglobins has not yet been established. One critical mating in this family between a mother with both haemoglobins S and Hopkins 2, and a normal father gave rise to a child who also had both haemoglobin S and Hopkins 2. Presumably then the genes determining these two haemoglobins are at different loci.

Thus at present the data suggests that at least two chromosomal loci are concerned in haemoglobin synthesis, and that the genes for haemoglobins S and C are alleles at one of these loci.

The incidence of the haemoglobin variants

One of the most striking things about the genes which determine the different types of haemoglobin is their remarkable variation in incidence from population to population. The sickle-cell gene, for example, is particularly common in central Africa and extremely rare, if indeed it occurs at all, in northern Europe. Even in central Africa, where probably some 15–20 per cent of all the people living in a zone south of the Sahara and north of the Zambesi show the sickle-cell trait, there are marked variations in frequency from tribe to tribe [60]. In some communities it may be as high as 45 per cent and in others lower than 2 per cent. A high incidence of the sickle-cell trait has also been observed in certain scattered populations in northern and central Greece [61,62], and also among occasional communities in southern India [63,64]. Elsewhere, with the exception of individuals or population groups whose ancestors are known to have originated from one of these main foci, the gene appears to be remarkably rare. Thus, in the U.S.A. it is found in about 9 per cent of the Negro populations but is virtually absent among the so-called white population.

Haemoglobin C is also common in Africa, but here the main focus appears to be in the Gold Coast. Populations in this area may show frequencies of the haemoglobin C trait of 5 to 20 per cent [65,66,67], the higher values occurring in the northern parts of this region. As one proceeds away from here the incidence rapidly falls off and it seems to be virtually absent in the Congo and in east Africa. The distribution therefore appears to be highly localised, and somewhat different from that of the sickle-cell trait. Indeed, one curious feature of the situation is that among these populations in west Africa where both the haemoglobin S and the haemoglobin C genes occur, there is a negative correlation between the two gene frequencies [68]. With the exception of groups who may reasonably be thought to have originated in this region, the haemoglobin C trait appears to be extremely infrequent or absent in other parts of the world.

The haemoglobin E gene on the other hand is particularly prevalent in south-east Asia, notably in Siam, Burma and Malaya, where frequencies of the haemoglobin E trait of more than 10 per cent have been observed in several different populations [69,70,71]. An appreciable incidence of haemoglobin E has also been noted in Indonesia and in certain communities in Ceylon. It does not, however, seem to occur in Africa or in Europe.

The haemoglobin D trait has been observed with a frequency of the order of one per cent among Sikhs and Punjabis in north-west India [72]. In most other populations which have been studied so far, however, it is apparently rare, though occasional examples of haemoglobin D have been seen in so-called 'Caucasians'.

While the data on the incidence of many of these haemoglobin variants is still far from complete, the following broad features of the pattern of their distribution can be regarded as established. Several of them occur with quite appreciable and sometimes rather high frequencies in some human populations and are extremely rare if not entirely absent in others. Although more than one such variant may exist in the same population, nevertheless the main focus, or foci, of concentration appears to be somewhat different for each gene. In general they have been found in populations living in, or whose ancestors came from, tropical or subtropical regions. In other areas they seem to be extremely uncommon if not non-existent.

A similar patchy pattern of distribution also occurs with respect to the gene which determines the thalassaemia type of red-cell defect. This has been mainly found in Mediterranean countries, though it is by no means peculiar to this area. Nevertheless, even in one region, foci occur where the gene frequency is particularly high. For example, the incidence of thalassaemia minor is especially marked in the Po valley, Sardinia and Sicily, and this contrasts with the much lower frequencies in the rest of Italy (23).

Now the peculiar pattern of distribution of these genes raises many rather difficult problems in the field of population genetics. The most obvious one is the following. Individuals who are homozygous for a gene such as the sickle-cell gene or the thalassaemia gene suffer from a severe disease which is often fatal in childhood or adolescence. They therefore contribute on the average much less to the next generation than do other individuals. At each successive generation there must be a steady loss of the gene from the population from this cause. One may well ask how under the circumstances the gene should have become so common in certain areas, that some 10–40 per cent of the population may carry it. Clearly for a gene to have attained such high frequencies in any particular population, there must exist, or have existed in the past, some process tending to counteract the heavy pressure of natural selection against it. Furthermore, since the incidence of the gene varies greatly from population to population, one must also assume that this mechanism counteracting the selective pressure against the affected homozygotes must vary greatly in intensity from one place to another.

Mutation and balanced polymorphism

Two kinds of explanation can be advanced to explain this sort of phenomenon. The first would attribute the situation to unusually high rates of mutation. If fresh mutations of the normal gene to its abnormal allele occurred at a sufficiently high rate, this might be sufficient to offset the loss of the abnormal alleles in each generation due to the relatively early death and consequent relative infertility of the affected homozygotes. On this basis it would be necessary to postulate that the mutation rate varied widely from population to population, and was presumably in some way a function of the local environment.

The second kind of explanation invokes the concept of 'balanced polymorphism'. This demands that the heterozygotes, that is individuals who carry the abnormal gene in single dose, should have a higher effective fertility than the normal homozygotes. Such a situation might arise either because on the average relatively more heterozygotes survive to adult life and become parents than do normal homozygotes, or because matings involving heterozygotes are more fertile than matings involving only normal homozygotes. Under these circumstances the loss of genes due to infertility of the abnormal homozygotes could be balanced by the net gain of the abnormal genes in each generation due to the relatively increased effective fertility of the heterozygotes. Here it would be necessary to suppose that the selective advantage of the heterozygote would vary in degree in different places and presumably would not be present at all in areas where the gene was excessively rare.

These possibilities have been explored in greatest detail in the case of the sickle-cell gene, because here the problem is seen at its most extreme. The abnormal homozygote is probably more severely affected from the point of view of its biological fitness than in any other type of haemoglobinopathy, with the possible exception of thalassaemia, and the gene frequency reaches higher values in certain populations than are found for any of the others. It has therefore provided the most favourable situation for the investigation of this general problem.

Mutation

Theoretically the rate of mutation of the sickle-cell gene can be estimated from data concerning the incidence of the sickle-cell trait in a population, and the frequency with which it is found that only one parent of a patient with sickle-cell anaemia shows the sickle-cell trait, or neither parent of a sickle-cell individual shows the trait. In practice the problem is rather more difficult. The question of illegitimacy inevitably arises when unusual results are encountered in human genetics, and this makes it necessary in critical attempts to estimate mutation rates of the order of magnitude to be expected here, to restrict the argument to situations where the mother is the exceptional parent. That is to say situations where the mother of a child who appears to be homozygous for the sickle-cell gene does not herself give evidence of being heterozygous for it. Even then, there are a number of other possibilities which must be considered before the phenomenon can be reasonably attributed to mutation. One is the possibility that the exceptional mother may in fact carry the abnormal gene but for some reason fails to manifest the sickle-cell peculiarity. This might be due to the presence of a 'suppressor' or a 'modifying' gene. While it is clear that the failure of the sickle-cell gene to become manifest in an individual by the formation of haemo-globin S in appreciable amounts could only be a very unusual oc-currence, nevertheless experience in other branches of human genetics suggests that this kind of phenomenon might occur, and if so, though rare, could have a frequency of the same order of magnitude, or even greater, than the true mutation rate. Another possibility is that the exceptional mother may carry a gene for some other sort of haema-tological defect and that the apparently sickle-cell anaemic child is really not a homozygote but a double heterozygote having received this unusual gene from the mother and a sickle-cell gene from the father. Such possibilities can to some extent be excluded by studies on the relatives of the exceptional mother and by further detailed biochemical and haematological investigations of the mother and the child. It remains, however, rather difficult to be certain that any one individual case is in fact due to a mutation.

Nevertheless, as Vandepitte and his colleagues [10] have shown, it is possible by this kind of approach to arrive at an upper limit for the mutation rate of the gene in any particular population. This maximal estimate can then be compared with the mutation rate to be expected, if this were the main factor which determined the incidence of the gene in the population being investigated. These workers studied a population in the Belgian Congo where about 25 per cent of the population had the sickle-cell trait. They found that among 233 mothers of sickle-cell anaemic children, 231 showed the sickling phenomenon, and two failed to do so. The blood of the two exceptions revealed only normal haemoglobin by electrophoresis and there were no other detectable haematological abnormalities. This leads to an upper limit for the rate of mutation to the sickle-cell gene in this population of $1·7 \times 10^{-3}$ per gene per generation. This figure represents a value which, compared with estimates of mutation rates of other human genes, is very high. Nevertheless, it is still only about one-tenth of the rate which would be required to maintain the gene frequency in this population if one assumes that the heterozygotes are at no selective advantage. If, in fact, the loss of sickle-cell genes in this population due to early death of the sickle-cell homozygotes were entirely counterbalanced by mutation, then a mutation rate of about $1·6 \times 10^{-2}$ per gene per generation would have been required. This would have meant that Vandepitte and his colleagues should have observed about nineteen exceptional mothers in their series instead of only two. These results have been substantially confirmed by another independent survey (11) in this area where out of 247 mothers of sickle-cell anaemic children only three failed to show the sickle-cell trait. Thus it seems that the high incidence of the gene in these populations could hardly be explained solely in terms of mutation.

It must be emphasised that the estimate of the mutation rate ($1 \cdot 7 \times 10^{-8}$) obtained in this investigation represents only a possible upper limit. The real value may be very much less. Judging by the rarity of case reports of sickling in northern European populations, it seems that here the mutation rate is probably less than 1×10^{-5} per gene per generation. Presumably then one must accept the concept of very widely different mutation rates in different populations, or find some special explanation to account for the exceptional mothers.

Balanced polymorphism

Whether or not it turns out that the mutation rates in these African populations are greater than in the so-called 'Caucasians', it would appear from these results that we must look elsewhere for the main cause of the high population frequencies, and for the disparities between one population and another. In fact, it is now generally believed that the sickle-cell heterozygote may in certain environments be at a selective advantage compared with the normal homozygote, and that this has led to a situation of balanced polymorphism.

The general conditions under which balanced polymorphism may occur have already been discussed (see page 31). The heterozygote must be at some advantage in terms of biological fitness compared with either type of homozygote, and in fact the magnitude of this effect must be quite considerable if it is to explain the very high frequencies of the sickle-cell gene which occur in certain parts of Africa. Thus in some tribes the incidence of the sickle-cell trait is as high as 40 per cent. If the rather conservative assumption is made that the survival rate of the sickle-cell homozygote is on the average about one-quarter of that of other members of the population, then the heterozygotes must enjoy a selective advantage of about 25 per cent greater than that of the so-called 'normal' homozygotes, in order to maintain a balanced equilibrium (73).

In 1954 Allison [74], elaborating a suggestion put forward by earlier workers, advanced a general hypothesis to explain how such a situation might arise. He suggested that sickle-cell heterozygotes are less susceptible to malaria than are normal individuals. As a consequence, in areas where malaria is prevalent and death from malaria is an important cause of mortality in childhood, sickle-cell heterozygotes will have a greater chance of surviving to adult life than the normal homozygotes. They will, therefore, contribute more to the next generation and the relative gain in sickle-cell genes so produced would offset the loss of these genes from the greatly increased mortality of the sickle-cell homozygotes due to chronic anaemia. In areas where malaria does not occur, no such selective advantage of the heterozygotes would be present and the frequency of the gene would be determined essentially by its mutation rate, which is assumed to be rather low.

Allison presented three types of evidence in favour of this hypothesis. In the first place he claimed that among children living in highly malarious areas the frequency of parasitaemia was lower in those with the sickle-cell trait than in the non-sicklers, and in those sicklers with parasitaemia, the parasite densities were on the average less than in the non-sicklers. Secondly he found large differences between sicklers and non-sicklers with respect to their susceptibility to experimentally induced malaria. Fourteen out of fifteen subjects who did not have the sickle-cell trait developed clinical malaria after inoculation, whereas only two out of fifteen individuals with the trait developed malaria. Finally he argued that there was a general correlation between the geographical distributions of malaria and of the sickle-cell trait. High frequencies of the trait were mainly encountered in regions where malaria was hyperendemic.

Since the publication of Allison's results a number of other workers have carried out investigations along the same lines in a variety of different populations. Much of this work has been concerned with the comparison of malaria parasite rates and densities between sickle-cell trait individuals and non-sicklers. While some of the results confirm those of Allison, others fail to do so, or do so only in part, and the resulting picture has become rather confused. However, it seems probable that, at any rate in young children prior to the development of an active immunity against malaria, a real difference in degree of parasitaemia between sicklers and non-sicklers exists [75].

So far only one attempt to repeat Allison's remarkable demonstration of a difference in susceptibility to experimental malaria has been made. This was carried out by Beutler and his colleagues in the U.S.A. (76). Only very slight differences were encountered between the sicklers and the non-sicklers in this experiment, and the authors regard them as of doubtful significance. It is of interest that the subjects in this investigation were either non-immune or only slightly immune as far as malaria was concerned, whereas Allison's subjects were all highly immune.

Raper (77) has brought forward evidence of a rather different kind in support of the malaria hypothesis. It is of particular interest because it indicates more directly how differential mortality from malaria may occur. He classified all the patients admitted to a children's ward at Kampala, into those with the sickle-cell trait and those without it, and then compared the sickling rate in different diseases. His results are shown in Table 24. The outstanding finding is the absence of sicklers among patients with cerebral malaria. In uncomplicated malaria, on the other hand, the rate was not very different from that in other conditions. Raper points out that the Lambotte-Legranges had previously observed the same phenomenon, and they, also, had concluded that the sicklers were in some way less susceptible to cerebral malaria. Raper also noted a low rate of

Table 24. *Incidence of sickle-cell trait among* 818 *consecutive admissions to a children's ward at Kampala (thirty-one patients with sickle-cell anaemia admitted during this period are not included).* (*After Raper*, 1956)

Disease group	Total	Number with sickle-cell trait	Incidence of sickle-cell trait
Miscellaneous	186	25	0·13
Pneumonia	118	18	0·15
Upper respiratory infections	59	13	0·22
Diarrhoea and vomiting	106	25	0·24
Poliomyelitis	26	4	0·15
Tuberculosis	37	8	0·22
Meningitis (purulent)	26	5	0·19
Malnutrition	77	11	0·14
Hookworm anaemia	30	2	0·07
Typhoid fever	17	6	0·35
Malaria (a) uncomplicated	83	13	0·16
(b) Cerebral	47	—	0·00
(c) Blackwater fever	6	—	0·00
Total admissions	818	130	0·16

sickling in hookworm anaemia, but here the figures were rather small, and not statistically significant.

Neel[78] has emphasized that the demonstration of a differential susceptibility to a particular disease is not by itself sufficient to establish that this is the sole, or even the main, cause of a balanced polymorphism. It is also necessary to show that it leads directly to a difference in viability or effective fertility which is quantitatively of the right order of magnitude. In this particular case this would involve the direct demonstration that in the appropriate population a sufficient fraction of all deaths were due to malaria, and these occurred predominantly in non-sicklers. Various estimates have been made of the mortality rates from malaria[78,79] which would be necessary to produce this phenomenon in different populations. So far no quantitative demonstration of the effect has been made.

Although there is in Africa a general correlation between hyper-endemic malaria and the incidence of the sickle-cell trait, there are nevertheless even here one or two areas where the results are markedly discrepant[80], and outside Africa there are many regions which are, or until recent times were, highly malarious, and in which no appreciable sickling occurs. It must be remembered that a high malarial rate in any one place is only one of a number of ecological features and disease patterns which will characterise it, and they will in general be roughly correlated one with another. It remains possible, therefore, that other quite different factors may be of significance in this context.

Two kinds of explanation have been put forward to account for the assumed failure of the malarial parasite to flourish to the same extent in people whose red cells contain significant quantities of sickle-cell haemoglobin as in people without it. One of these suggests that sickle-cell haemoglobin may be less readily metabolised by the malaria parasite than is normal haemoglobin[75]. The other suggests that a premature destruction of the parasitised red cells occurs because of a reduced intracellular oxygen tension and the induction of sickling[81,82]. The matter is still unsettled. It is of interest that, as far as can be seen, the differential susceptibility mainly occurs with respect to *Plasmodium falciparum*, and it is less marked and may be non-existent with *Plasmodium malariae*.

While the evidence is still in many respects incomplete there seems little doubt that the main features of the sickle-cell distribution must ultimately be explained in terms of balanced polymorphism. If so, it means that a change in the environmental situation which would result in an alteration in the selective advantage enjoyed by the heterozygote will lead to a progressive change in the gene frequency in subsequent generations. This could occur following changes in public health which might, for example, involve the eradication of malaria in a particular area. It would also be expected to occur as a result of the transfer of a proportion of the population to a new environment. This presumably occurred on a large scale with the transportation of African Negroes to the U.S.A. some 300 years ago. It seems likely that the selective advantage in favour of the heterozygotes does not operate in the U.S.A., and the incidence of the gene among the American Negro population is presumably falling. The exact rate of change is difficult to evaluate because of the lack of any certain knowledge about the proportions of slaves transported from different areas in Africa, and the gene frequencies obtaining there at the relevant times. Furthermore, some intermarriage with individuals of non-African descent has certainly taken place. The present incidence of the sickle-cell trait among Negroes in the U.S.A. is about nine per cent. Allison[73] considered it probable that the average incidence of sickling in the areas from whence they originally came was at least 22 per cent, and that not more than one-third of the genes in the present Negro population have been introduced from outside. Thus a fall in frequency of the trait from about 15½ to 9 per cent may well have taken place in about twelve generations as a result of the loss of selective advantage of the heterozygotes.

Similar population movements of a less obvious character have no doubt occurred at various times in Africa itself and elsewhere. This, combined with the intermixing of populations, has presumably contributed in at least some degree to the distribution pattern of the gene as it is found today. Thus the present position will no doubt reflect anthropological inter-relations between populations as well as variations due to the differential selection of the heterozygotes in various areas. In practice it is rather difficult to evaluate the relative importance of these factors in any given situation in the absence of external evidence regarding population movements which may have taken place.

Other haemoglobinopathies

In principle the same kind of problems about the nature of the processes determining the gene distributions in different populations apply to all the other haemoglobin variants and also to conditions such as thalassaemia. In general the selective pressures against the abnormal homozygotes vary greatly from condition to condition. Haemoglobin C disease and haemoglobin E disease, for example, are significantly less lethal than haemoglobin S disease. Thalassaemia major, on the other hand, probably has at least as severe an effect on survival to adult life as does sickle-cell disease. These variations will influence the degree of selective advantage it is necessary to postulate for the heterozygote to maintain an equilibrium, or the level of the mutation rate necessary if this were the predominant factor.

Haldane in 1949 [83] made the suggestion that thalassaemia heterozygotes might be less susceptible to malaria and that this could have brought about a balanced polymorphism in some areas. Certainly, in Italy those areas where thalassaemia is particularly common have been, in the past, those areas where malaria was particularly prevalent. However, there is as yet no direct evidence to incriminate malaria in this connection. If indeed it turned out that both sickling and thalassaemia have been maintained at high frequencies in particular areas by differential susceptibility to malaria, then one would be faced by the problem as to why it was the thalassaemia gene in some areas and the sickle-cell gene in others which was particularly prevalent. Since most of the other abnormal haemoglobin genes turn up with appreciable frequencies mainly in tropical and subtropical areas, the idea of a heterozygous advantage due to a relative resistance to one or another type of tropical disease is an obvious one. Such possibilities remain to be investigated. At the same time a great deal more needs to be learnt about the mutation rates of these genes.

One final point should be mentioned. In most cases it is quite uncertain whether the particular frequency of a gene which is observed in a given population represents an equilibrium value, or whether the gene is increasing or decreasing in frequency at each generation. It is possible that in some cases the gene is spreading and in others the particular selective forces which once caused its prevalence are now no longer operating, and it is being steadily eliminated. The situation is further complicated in certain populations by the occurrence of more than one different gene leading to abnormal haemoglobin synthesis. Here one cannot be sure whether there is or has been some complex type of equilibrium or whether perhaps one of the variants is in the process of supplanting the other. These and many similar problems illustrate the obscurities in this field of population genetics. Many speculations are possible but it is rather difficult to produce convincing evidence in favour of one or another of the many alternative hypotheses.

REFERENCES

(1) Pauling, L., Itano, H. A., Singer, S. J. and Wells, I. C. (1949). *Science*, **110**, 543.
(2) Herrick, J. B. (1910). *Arch. Int. Med.* **6**, 517.
(3) Sherman, I. J. (1940). *Johns Hopk. Hosp. Bull.* **67**, 309.
(4) Singer, K., Robin, S., King, J. C. and Jefferson, R. N. (1948). *J. Lab. Clin. Med.* **33**, 975.
(5) Callender, S. T. E., Nickel, J. F., Moore, C. V. and Powell, E. O. (1949). *J. Lab. Clin. Med.* **34**, 90.
(6) Taliafero, W. H. and Huck, J. G. (1923). *Genetics*, **8**, 594.
(7) Neel, J. V. (1949). *Science*, **110**, 64.
(8) Beet, E. A. (1949). *Ann. Eugen., Lond.* **14**, 279.
(9) Neel, J. V. (1951). *Blood*, **6**, 389.
(10) Vandepitte, J. M., Zuelzer, W. W., Neel, J. V. and Colaert, J. (1955). *Blood*, **10**, 341.
(11) Lambotte-Legrand, J. and C. (1955). *Ann. Soc. belge Méd. trop.* **35**, 47.
(12) Perutz, M. F. and Mitchison, J. M. (1950). *Nature, Lond.* **166**, 677.
(13) Perutz, M. F., Liquori, A. M. and Eirich, F. (1951). *Nature, Lond.* **167**, 929.
(14) Harris, J. W. (1950). *Proc. Soc. Exp. Biol., N.Y.* **75**, 197.
(15) Allison, A. C. (1956). *Clin. Sci.* **15**, 497.
(16) Harris, J. W., Brewster, H. H., Ham, T. H. and Castle, W. B. (1956). *Arch. Int. Med.* **97**, 145.
(17) Singer, K., Chernoff, A. I. and Singer, L. (1951). *Blood*, **6**, 413, 429.
(18) Huisman, T. H. J., Jonxis, J. H. P. and Dozy, A. (1955). *Biochem. Biophys. Acta*, **18**, 576.
(19) Wells, I. C. and Itano, H. A. (1951). *J. Biol. Chem.* **188**, 65.
(20) Singer, K. and Chernoff, A. I. (1952). *Blood*, **7**, 47.
(21) Itano, H. A. (1953). *Amer. J. Hum. Gen.* **5**, 34.
(22) Neel, J. V., Wells, I. C. and Itano, H. A. (1951). *J. Clin. Invest.* **30**, 1120.
(23) Bianco, I., Montalenti, G., Silvestroni, E. and Siniscalco, M. (1952). *Ann. Eugen., Lond.* **16**, 299.

(24) Liquori, A. M. (1951). *Nature, Lond.* **167**, 950.
(25) Rich, A. (1952). *Proc. Nat. Acad. Sci., Wash.* **38**, 187.
(26) Kunkel, H. G. and Wallenius, G. (1955). *Science*, **122**, 288.
(27) Kunkel, H. G., Ceppellini, R., Muller-Eberhart, V. and Wolf, J. (1957). *J. Clin. Invest.* **36**, 1615.
(28) Silvestroni, E. and Bianco, I. (1946). *Haematologica*, **29**, 455.
(29) Powell, W. N., Rodante, J. G. and Neel, J. V. (1950). *Blood*, **5**, 887.
(30) Zuelzer, W. W., Neel, J. V. and Robinson, A. R. (1956). In *Progress in Haematology*. Grune and Stratton.
(31) Itano, H. A. and Neel, J. V. (1950). *Proc. Nat. Acad. Sci., Wash.* **36**, 613.
(32) Spaet, T. H., Alway, R. H. and Ward, G. (1953). *Paediatrics*, **12**, 483.
(33) Levin, W. C., Schneider, R. G., Cudd, J. A. and Johnson, J. E. (1953). *J. Lab. Clin. Med.* **42**, 918.
(34) Itano, H. A. (1951). *Proc. Nat. Acad. Sci., Wash.* **37**, 775.
(35) Itano, H. A. (1957). *Advances in Protein Chemistry*, **12**, 216. Academic Press, New York.
(36) *Blood* (1953), **8**, 386.
(37) Hörlein, H. and Weber, G. (1948). *Dtsch. med. Wschr.* **73**, 476.
(38) Kunkel, H. G. and Bearn, A. G. (1957). *Fed. Proc.* **16**, 760.
(39) Itano, H. A., Bergren, W. R. and Sturgeon, P. (1956). *Medicine*, **35**, 121.
(40) Ager, J. A. M., Lehmann, H., and Vandepitte, J. M. (1958). *Lancet*, **1**, 318.
(41) Huisman, T. H. J. and Prins, K. (1957). *Clin. Chim. Acta*, **2**, 307.
(42) Rigas, D. A., Koler, R. D. and Osgood, E. E. (1956). *J. Lab. Clin. Med.* **47**, 51.
(43) Havinga, E. and Itano, H. A. (1953). *Proc. Nat. Acad. Sci., Wash.* **39**, 65.
(44) Schroeder, W. A., Kay, L. M. and Wells, I. C. (1950). *J. Biol. Chem.* **187**, 221.
(45) Huisman, T. H. J., Jonxiz, J. H. P. and van der Schaaf, P. C. (1955). *Nature, Lond.* **175**, 902.
(46) Havinga, E. (1953). *Proc. Nat. Acad. Sci., Wash.* **39**, 59.
(47) Huisman, T. H. J. and Drinkwaard, J. (1955). *Biochim. Biophys. Acta*, **18**, 588.
(48) Huisman, T. H. J. and Dozy, A. (1956). *Biochim. Biophys. Acta*, **20**, 400.
(49) Dickman, S. R. and Moncrief, I. H. (1951). *Proc. Soc. Exp. Biol., N.Y.* **77**, 631.
(50) Hommes, F. A., Santema Drinkwaard, J. and Huisman, T. H. J. (1956). *Biochim. Biophys. Acta*, **20**, 564.
(51) Ingram, V. M. (1956). *Nature, Lond.* **178**, 792.
(52) Ingram, V. M. (1957). *Nature, Lond.* **180**, 326.
(53) Hunt, J. A. and Ingram, V. M. (1958). *Nature, Lond.* **181**, 1062.
(54) Motulsky, A. G. (1956). *Nature, Lond.* **178**, 1055.
(55) Ranney, H. (1954). *J. Clin. Invest.* **33**, 1634.
(56) Smith, E. and Conley, C. L. (1956). Cited in ref. 30.

(57) Singer, K., Josephson, A. M., Singer, L., Heller, P. and Zimmerman, H. J. (1957). *Blood*, **12**, 593.
(58) Schwartz, H. C., Spaet, T. H., Zuelzer, W. W., Neel, J. V., Robinson, A. R. and Kaufman, S. F. (1957). *Blood*, **12**, 238.
(59) Smith, E. W. and Torbert, J. V. (1958). *Johns Hopk. Hosp. Bull.* **102**, 38.
(60) Mourant, A. E. (1954). *The Distribution of Human Blood Groups*. Blackwell, Oxford.
(61) Choremis, C., Ikin, E. W., Lehmann, H., Mourant, A. E. and Zannos, L. (1953). *Lancet*, **2**, 909.
(62) Deliyannis, G. A. and Tavlarakis, N. (1955). *Brit. Med. J.* **2**, 299.
(63) Lehmann, H. and Cutbush, M. (1952). *Brit. Med. J.* **1**, 404.
(64) Shukla, R. W. and Solanki, B. R. (1958). *Lancet*, **1**, 297.
(65) Neel, J. V., Hiernaux, J., Linhard, J. Robinson, A., Zuelzer, W. W., and Livingstone, F. B. (1956). *Amer. J. Hum. Genet.* **8**, 138.
(66) Allison, A. C. (1956). *Ann. Eugen., Lond.* **21**, 67.
(67) Edington, G. M. and Lehmann, H. (1956). *Man*, **36**, 1.
(68) Allison, A. C. (1956). *Acta Genet.* **6**, 430.
(69) NaNakorn, S., Minnich, V. and Chernoff, A. (1954). *J. Lab. Clin. Med.* **44**, 903.
(70) Lehmann, H. and Singh, R. B. (1956). *Nature, Lond.* **178**, 695.
(71) Lehmann, H., Story, P. and Thein, H. (1956). *Brit. Med. J.* **1**, 544.
(72) Bird, G. W. G. and Lehmann, H. (1956). *Brit. Med. J.* **1**, 514.
(73) Allison, A. C. (1954). *Ann. Eugen., Lond.* **19**, 39.
(74) Allison, A. C. (1954). *Brit. Med. J.* **1**, 290.
(75) Allison, A. C. (1957). *Exp. Parasitol.* **6**, 418.
(76) Beutler, E., Dern, R. J. and Flanagan, C. L. (1955). *Brit. Med. J.* **1**, 1189.
(77) Raper, A. B. (1956). *Brit. Med. J.* **1**, 965.
(78) Neel, J. V. (1956). *Ann. Hum. Genet.* **21**, 1.
(79) Lehmann, H. and Raper, A. B. (1956). *Brit. Med. J.* **2**, 333.
(80) Neel, J. V. (1957). *New Engl. J. Med.* **256**, 161.
(81) Mackey, J. P. and Vivarelli, F. (1954). *Brit. Med. J.* **1**, 276.
(82) Miller, M. J., Neel, J. V. and Livingstone, F. B. (1956). *Trans. R. Soc. Trop. Med. Hyg.* **50**, 294.
(83) Haldane, J. B. S. (1949). *La Ricerca*. Scient. suppl., p. 3.

CHAPTER 7

THE BLOOD-GROUP SUBSTANCES

The ABO blood groups

The first human blood-group differences were discovered by Land-steiner at the beginning of the present century[1]. He found that when blood serum from one individual is mixed with red blood cells from other individuals, clear-cut and characteristic individual differences could be demonstrated. In some cases marked agglutination or clumping of the red cells was observed. In others the red cells were unaffected. On the basis of cross-agglutination tests of this sort it was soon found that one could differentiate sharply between four classes of people, according to whether they possessed on their red cells one, both, or neither of two antigenic substances. The antigenic substances are now called A and B and the appropriate antibodies anti-A and anti-B. The serum of an individual does not contain antibodies to the antigen present on his own red cells. With rare exceptions, however, it does contain anti-A or anti-B or both antibodies when the red cells do not carry the corresponding antigen. Thus the four classes of people may be specified as shown in Table 25. In the United Kingdom approximately 46·7 per cent of people are group O, 41·7 per cent group A, 8·6 per cent group B, and 3 per cent group AB. In general the relative frequencies of these four groups are found to differ from population to population.

Table 25. *The ABO blood groups*

Blood group	Antigens on red blood cells	Antibodies in blood serum
O	—	Anti-A and Anti-B
A	A	Anti-B
B	B	Anti-A
AB	A and B	—

Epstein and Ottenberg[2] were the first to suggest that these blood types were inherited and this was proved by Von Dungern and Hirszfeld in 1910[3]. Their hypothesis of the inheritance of these characters implied that the presence or absence of the antigens A and B were determined by two independent pairs of genes at different chromosomal loci. It was not until 1925 that the idea that only one locus was involved, and that the four blood groups were determined by three alternative or allelic genes, was put forward by Bernstein[4]. Bernstein's hypothesis has now been extensively substantiated. This was the first situation in human genetics where the occurrence of multiple allelism was convincingly demonstrated, and some of the arguments differentiating between the two hypotheses are of general interest.

Table 26. *Genotype and phenotype frequencies expected on the hypothesis that the ABO blood groups are determined by two gene pairs at different chromosomal loci.*

Phenotype	Genotype	Genotype frequency	Phenotype frequency
O	aabb	x^2y^2	x^2y^2
A	AAbb Aabb	$(1-x)^2y^2$ $2x(1-x)y^2$	$(1-x^2)y^2$
B	aaBB aaBb	$x^2(1-y)^2$ $2x^2y(1-y)$	$x^2(1-y^2)$
AB	AABB AaBB AABb AaBb	$(1-x)^2(1-y)^2$ $2x(1-x)(1-y)^2$ $(1-x)^2(1-y)2y$ $2x(1-x)2y(1-y)$	$(1-x^2)(1-y^2)$

The two-loci hypothesis postulated the existence of two gene pairs which can be written **A** and **a**, **B** and **b**. With respect to each pair three types of individual would be expected **AA**, **Aa** and **aa**, **BB**, **Bb** and **bb**. **A** was regarded as dominant to **a**, and **B** as dominant to **b**. That is to say, by using the two available antisera, anti-A and anti-B, capable of detecting the antigenic substances A and B respectively, all individuals carrying the **A** gene would be detected by the first antiserum and all carrying the **B** gene by the second. Where only the alternative genes **a** and **b** were present, as in the double homozygote **aabb**, neither antiserum would cause agglutination and so the individual would be classified as O. The four phenotypic classes observed in the general population would on this hypothesis correspond to the genotypes shown in Table 26. If the gene frequencies of **a** and **A** are respectively x and $(1-x)$, and if the gene frequencies of **b** and **B** are respectively y and $(1-y)$, then in homogeneous populations where there is more or less random mating, the four phenotypes should occur with the relative frequencies given in Table 26. From this it can be seen that the following relationship should hold:

(Frequency of O).(frequency of AB)=
(frequency of A).(frequency of B).

Bernstein pointed out that in fact this relationship failed to satisfy the frequencies of the four blood groups in quite a large number of the populations for which data were at that time available. He showed that a much more satisfactory fit with the observed frequent cies was given by the hypothesis that three allelic genes **A**, **B** and **O** at a single locus were the genetical determinants. If **A** and **B** were regarded as dominant to **O**, the four blood groups would on this hypothesis be made up of the genotypes shown in Table 27. If the gene frequencies of **A**, **B** and **O** were respectively p, q and r, where $(p+q+r) = 1$, then the relative frequencies of the four classes in a homogeneous random mating population would be as shown in Table 27. The three gene frequencies should be given by

$$r = \sqrt{(\text{frequency of O})},$$
$$q = 1 - \sqrt{(\text{frequency of O} + \text{frequency of A})},$$
$$p = 1 - \sqrt{(\text{frequency of O} + \text{frequency of B})}.$$

Table 27. *Genotype and phenotype frequencies expected if the ABO blood groups are determined by three allelic genes*

Phenotype	Genotype	Genotype frequency	Phenotype frequency
AB	**AB**	$2pq$	$2pq$
A	$\begin{cases} \textbf{AA} \\ \textbf{AO} \end{cases}$	$\left.\begin{array}{l} p^2 \\ 2pr \end{array}\right\}$	$p^2 + 2pr$
B	$\begin{cases} \textbf{BB} \\ \textbf{BO} \end{cases}$	$\left.\begin{array}{l} q^2 \\ 2qr \end{array}\right\}$	$q^2 + 2qr$
O	**OO**	r^2	r^2

If the hypothesis is correct, the values of p, q and r so obtained should satisfy the equation $p+q+r=1$. This indeed Bernstein showed to be the case, within the limits of sampling error (Table 28).

The familial distribution of the four blood groups must, of course, also be adequately accounted for in terms of the hypothesis. The critical families are those in which one parent is AB. Among the offspring of such parents no O children should be found, and among the offspring of O × AB parents no AB children should occur. Neither of these statements would be true if two loci were involved. Table 29 gives the relevant data from Wiener's [5] extensive review of the literature. Out of more than 3000 children only thirteen occur in the unexpected groups. This small proportion of discrepancies can be reasonably attributed to the combined effects of illegitimacy, technical errors in grouping, and, conceivably, mutation. According to the theory, an AB individual should produce equal numbers of

Table 28. *ABO blood-group frequencies and the estimated gene frequencies on Bernstein's hypothesis.* (*After Bernstein*, 1925)

Race	Number of people	Observed frequencies of groups				Theory of von Dungern and Hirszfeld		Theory of Bernstein. Estimated gene frequencies			
		O	A	B	AB	O × AB	A × B	p	q	r	$p+q+r$
English	500	0·464	0·434	0·072	0·031	0·0143	0·0312	0·268	0·052	0·681	1·001
French	500	0·432	0·426	0·112	0·030	0·0129	0·0477	0·262	0·074	0·657	0·993
Italians	500	0·472	0·380	0·110	0·038	0·0179	0·0418	0·237	0·077	0·687	1·001
Serbians	500	0·380	0·418	0·156	0·046	0·0175	0·0642	0·268	0·107	0·516	0·991
Greeks	500	0·382	0·416	0·162	0·040	0·0153	0·0674	0·262	0·107	0·618	0·987
Bulgarians	500	0·390	0·406	0·142	0·062	0·0241	0·0577	0·271	0·108	0·624	1·003
Arabs	500	0·432	0·324	0·190	0·050	0·0218	0·0616	0·209	0·129	0·660	0·998
Turks (Macedonia)	500	0·368	0·380	0·186	0·066	0·0243	0·0707	0·256	0·136	0·607	0·999
Russians	1000	0·407	0·312	0·218	0·063	0·0256	0·0680	0·210	0·152	0·638	1·000
Spanish Jews	500	0·388	0·330	0·232	0·050	0·0194	0·0766	0·213	0·153	0·623	0·989
Madagascans	400	0·458	0·262	0·237	0·045	0·0261	0·0621	0·168	0·154	0·675	0·997
Senegal Negroes	500	0·432	0·224	0·292	0·050	0·0216	0·0654	0·149	0·189	0·657	0·995
Annamese	500	0·420	0·244	0·284	0·072	0·0302	0·0636	0·161	0·198	0·648	1·008
Hindus	1000	0·313	0·190	0·412	0·085	0·0266	0·0783	0·149	0·291	0·560	1·000

A and B gametes. The table shows that this is the case, the deviation from equality being less than the standard error of sampling. Finally, in matings AB × AB, the sum of the homozygous offspring A and B should be equal, within the limits of sampling error, to the total heterozygotes AB. This result is also obtained.

Table 29. *Offspring of parents at least one of whom is blood group AB.* (*After Wiener*, 1943)

Parents	Children				Total
	O	A	B	AB	
O × AB	8	633	646	3	1290
A × AB	—	533	247	312	1092
B × AB	2	183	406	232	823
AB × AB	—	28	36	65	129

Total A gametes 1609; Total B gametes 1647. (In the children of the mating A × AB, the A children are derived from A gametes of the AB parent and the B and AB children from the B gametes and so on.)

Total homozygotes from AB × AB = 64. Total heterozygotes from AB × AB = 65.

A_1 and A_2

There are two fairly common subdivisions of blood group A. Von Dungern and Hirsfield[6] found that when anti-A serum from a group B blood was absorbed with certain group A red cells until it lost the capacity of agglutinating the absorbing red cells, the serum still agglutinated a high proportion of other group A and group AB bloods. The implication of this kind of experiment is that the A antigen is heterogeneous and consists of two; the distinct and separate A_1

and A_2. This is now generally accepted, though it has been suggested that the difference may be a quantitative rather than a qualitative one. At any rate it is possible, using the available antisera, to reclassify A individuals into the subgroups A_1 and A_2, and similarly AB individuals into A_1B and A_2B. There are two antibodies, α which reacts with both A_1 and A_2, and α_1 which is specific for A_1 and does not react with A_2. α_1 is found in sera of most group B individuals, and also in the sera of about 1–2 per cent of A_2 people and about 26 per cent of A_2B people.

The two subdivisions of A are inherited as discrete entities. Thus Wiener[5] found that in thirty-eight matings of $A_1B \times O$ parents there were fifty-five children of group A_1 and fifty-three of group B, while in sixteen matings of group $A_2B \times O$ parents there were thirty-seven A_2 children and twenty-seven of group B. Thomson, Freidenreich and Worsaae[7] suggested that Bernstein's original theory could be extended to account for subgroups of A by postulating four allelic genes A_1, A_2, B and O, and extensive family material has confirmed this hypothesis. Using the sera generally available, A_1 can be said to be dominant to A_2 and O, A_2 dominant to O, and B dominant to O. The combinations of the four alleles give rise to six phenotypes as shown in Table 30. Typical figures for the gene frequencies are those estimated by Ikin, Prior, Race and Taylor for southern England[8]. Here they were A_1 0·21, A_2 0·07, B 0·06 and O 0·66

Table 30. *Genotypes and phenotypes for the four alleles* A_1, A_2, B, *and* O

Genotype	Phenotype
A_1A_1 ⎫ A_1A_2 ⎬ A_1O ⎭	A_1
A_2A_2 ⎫ A_2O ⎬	A_2
BB ⎫ BO ⎬	B
A_1B	A_1B
A_2B	A_2B
OO	O

Secretors and non-secretors

Substances responsible for the specificities of the A and B blood groups are not peculiar to the red-cell surface. They may also be found in other tissues and can be identified in tissue extracts by the ability of such extracts to absorb specifically the corresponding antibody. Nearly all the tissues of the body (the main exception is the brain) have been shown to possess such specific activity.

In a similar manner the presence of such substances may also be identified in a wide variety of body fluids and secretions. These include saliva, tears, sweat, digestive juices, bile, milk, pleural, pericardial and peritoneal fluids and also amniotic fluid. Particularly rich sources are the fluids present in pseudomucinous ovarian cysts and meconium, the first stool of the new-born. However, not all people possess this capacity to secrete A and B group specific substances in this manner. Lehrs[9] and Putkonen[10] discovered that, while in most people of blood groups A, B, and AB, the appropriate specific substances could be readily demonstrated in the saliva, in other people of the same blood groups the saliva appeared to be completely deficient in these substances. The two classes of people became known as 'secretors' and 'non-secretors'. It was shown that the ability or inability to secrete the A or B group-specific substances in the saliva is a constant trait in any one individual, and that when the specific activity is absent from the saliva it is also absent from other body fluids or secretions. In European populations some 20–25 per cent of people fall into the non-secretor class.

The group-specific substances appear to occur naturally in two forms. One form is soluble only in organic solvents such as alcohol or chloroform. The other is soluble in water. The A and B material present in the red cells is in the alcohol-soluble form and it may also be found in this form in nearly all other tissues, irrespective of whether the person is a secretor or non-secretor. The water-soluble forms of A and B specific substances are found in the secretions, body fluids or tissue extracts from secretors.

Schiff and Sasaki[11] showed that the two classes, secretors and non-secretors, were genetically determined. The familial distributions of the characters could be readily explained on the hypothesis that the non-secretors were homozygous for a 'recessive' gene. Its dominant allele determined the character 'secretor'. The secretor-non-secretor dimorphism appears to be determined by genes completely independent from those determining the ABO blood-group characters, and evidently two different loci are involved. The presence or absence of either A or B group-specific substance in the saliva of an individual must therefore be regarded as being directly dependent on two sets of genes at different loci.

O and H

The original classification into the four blood groups A, B, AB and O, was based on the presence of the reactive antigen A or B on the red cells. Group O erythrocytes were identified as cells devoid of either of these two antigens. The question naturally arose as to whether group O represented simply an absence of A and B or whether there existed an O antigen for which as yet no specific antiserum had been discovered.

Schiff[12] first demonstrated that certain carefully selected and absorbed sera from normal cattle could cause selective agglutination of O red cells. Subsequently it was discovered that a high proportion of group O individuals also secreted a substance in the saliva which was able to neutralise the agglutinating action of the absorbed cattle sera on the O red cells. It was thought that such sera were true anti-O sera reacting with a group-specific substance O produced by Bernstein's O gene and secreted in the saliva of 'secretors' of group O. A number of sera with very similar properties were subsequently obtained from a series of very diverse and rather unexpected sources. These included sera from goats and chickens immunised with *Shigella shiga*, sera from rabbits immunised with O red cells and also with material isolated from pseudomucinous ovarian cyst fluids of group O individuals, sera from the eel *Anguilla anguilla*, and extracts prepared from the seeds of various plants[13]. Very occasionally human sera have been found with the same properties.

The exact nature of the specific character of these so-called 'anti-O' sera, however, remains obscure[13]. If they were specific for a substance O which was determined by Bernstein's O gene, a characteristic pattern of reaction would be expected. One would expect that homozygous O cells should be agglutinated, and so also would the cells of individuals heterozygous for the gene O. Thus among A individuals it should be possible to distinguish between heterozygotes of the genotype AO and homozygotes AA. Similarly it would be anticipated that BO individuals could be differentiated from BB ones. AB individuals, however, should not react nor should AB secretors have 'O' group-specific substance in their salivas. Extensive studies with various sera of this type have, however, failed to substantiate the characteristic pattern of reactions anticipated on this hypothesis. Apart from irregularities in the behaviour of A and B cells from known genotypes, saliva from secretors of A_1B genotype may contain not only A and B group-specific activity, but also the so-called 'O' group-specific activity. It has become clear, therefore, that many of the sera reacting preferentially with O cells cannot be detecting a product peculiar to Bernstein's O gene.

Morgan and Watkins[13] suggested that the substance with which the majority of these sera are reacting should be called H to indicate its heterogenetic origin. The amount of H present on red cells seems to be in some way a function of the other antigens present, and in general the agglutinability of red cells of different ABO blood groups with anti-H sera goes roughly in the order $O > A_2 > B > A_1$. Similarly varying amounts of H may be detected in the secretions of secretors of different ABO genotypes.

As will be seen, the chemical properties of H substance are very similar to those of the A and B substances and it would appear that they are intimately related in their modes of formation.

Lewis substance

In 1946 Mourant[14] found a new antibody in certain samples of human sera which agglutinated red cells of some 20 per cent of European adults. In very young infants, however, a very much higher proportion of individuals gave positive reactions[15] and it was soon found that the distribution of the substance giving this particular group-specific reaction, both on red cells and in the body secretions, had many unusual features. The substance which reacts with this particular antibody is now referred to as Lewis a (Le^a), and secretions or red cells giving the reaction are said to be $Le^a +$.

Although only about 20 per cent of European adults have red cells giving positive reactions for Le^a, the substance can be detected in the saliva of some 90 per cent of individuals from such populations[16,17]. Thus while all individuals having $Le^a +$ red cells secrete Le^a substance, a high proportion of individuals having $Le^a -$ red cells also secrete Le^a. In general, however, much higher concentrations of Le^a are found in the saliva when the red cells are $Le^a +$ than when they are not.

Another important feature of the distribution of Le^a concerns its relationship to the secretion and non-secretion of the A, B and H substances[18,19,20]. All adults who have $Le^a +$ red cells appear to be non-secretors of the ABH substances. The great majority of adults with $Le^a -$ red cells are secretors of ABH substances. Thus secretors of ABH do not have Le^a on their red cells. Most, but not all, of them, however, secrete Le^a substance in their saliva.

The Le^a substance as it occurs on the red-cell surface appears to be present in a very different form from the A and B antigens on the red cells. The A and B substances seem to be part of the structure of the red cell membrane. They persist throughout the life of the cells, not only under normal conditions but also after transfusion into the circulation of a recipient with a different set of red cell antigens. Furthermore, the A and B group-specific substances characteristic of the recipient do not appear on the transfused red cells. Le^a behaves rather differently from this. It has been shown that repeated washing of red cells which are Le^a+ leads to a diminution in their Le^a reactivity[19], and that the washings inhibit anti-Le^a serum[21]. Furthermore, it has been found that under appropriate conditions Le^a− cells appear to take up Le^a from serum with which they have been incubated, and Le^a+ cells may lose their reactivity on incubation with certain sera not containing the substance[22]. Similar transformation of the Lewis character of the red cells may also be obtained by appropriate transfusion experiments. It seems possible, therefore, that Le^a is primarily an antigen characteristic of secretions, and that the red cells simply take it up *in vivo* when the concentrations present in the circulating plasma are sufficient, and possibly other special conditions are fulfilled.

There seems little doubt that the occurrence of Le^a is genetically controlled. The exact mechanism of its inheritance is still not definitely settled. Originally it was thought, on the basis of the familial distribution of individuals with red cells showing an Le^a+ reaction, that such individuals were homozygous for a gene which as far as the appearance of the antigen on the red cells was concerned was effectively recessive. The discovery that a high proportion of young infants also gave positive red cell reactions led to the suggestion that in infancy expression of the character in heterozygotes was possible, but that later this potentiality was lost. Similarly the occurrence of Le^a in the secretions of adults whose red cells were Le^a− was thought to be due to a partial manifestation of the character in heterozygotes. However, not all the data can be satisfactorily explained in this way. For example, the relative proportions of the presumed heterozygotes to homozygotes do not fit the hypothesis very comfortably. Furthermore, the high correlation between non-secretors and the occurrence of Le^a+ red cells requires explanation. Classifying individuals as

$Le^a +$ or $Le^a -$ on the basis of their red cell reactions is, with a few exceptions, effectively the same as classifying them for the capacity to secrete or not secrete the ABH substances. Since non-secretor status has the familial distribution of a character determined by a recessive gene, either identity or at least some very intimate relationship between the genes for non-secretor and Le^a would have to be postulated on this hypothesis.

Table 31. *Occurrence of Le^a substance on red cells and in saliva, in individuals who are of different Lewis genotypes and who may be secretors or non-secretors of ABH substances. It is assumed that the Le^a gene determines the formation of Le^a substance. The Le^- gene is its allele and does not lead to Le^a substance formation. (After Cepellini, 1954)*

Lewis genotype	ABH secretor status	Le^a substance	
		on red cells	in saliva
$Le^a Le^a$	Secretor	−	+
	Non-secretor	+	+ +
$Le^a Le^-$	Secretor	−	+
	Non-secretor	+	+ +
$Le^- Le^-$	Secretor	−	−
	Non-secretor	−	−

An entirely different hypothesis has been proposed by Ceppellini [17]. He suggests that Le^a is formed when an individual is either homozygous or heterozygous for a gene present at a locus quite different from either the ABO locus or the secretor-non-secretor locus. The amount of Le^a formed, and whether or not it occurs on red cells, depends, he suggests, on the ABH secretor status of the individual. Thus individuals who are homozygous for the gene causing non-secretion of the ABH substances, will, if they carry the Le^a gene, form relatively larger amounts of Le^a in their secretions and body fluids and will also exhibit Le^a on their red cells (Table 31). Suppression of ABH synthesis leads, as it were, to an increased Le^a synthesis. Individuals who are ABH secretors, and who also carry the Le^a gene, form relatively smaller amounts of Le^a, and although this can be detected in the secretions it does not, except in young infants, become attached to the red cells. Formally the hypothesis can be regarded as postulating an interaction between the Le^a gene and the secretor-non-secretor genes. This hypothesis fits well with the concept that the presence of Le^a on red cells is largely a function of its concentration in the body fluids and secretions.

A further complication is provided by the curious distribution of another material called Lewis b (Le^b), an antiserum for which was first found by Andresen in 1948 [23]. This substance is not found on red cells which are Le^a+. It is, however, found in the majority of cases where the red cells are Le^a−. It does not occur in the saliva of individuals who are non-secretors and have Le^a+ red cells. It is, however, present in association with Le^a and ABH substances in the saliva of many secretors. Because of the limited supplies of suitable antisera this material has been studied less extensively than Le^a. While its formation is obviously tied up closely with the secretor-non-secretor status of the individual with respect to the ABH substances, and also with the formation of Le^a, its exact genetical basis remains obscure.

It seems probable from all this that at least three loci are commonly concerned in determining the group-specific character of the water soluble mucoid substances secreted in the saliva and other body fluids. These are the ABO locus, the secretor-non-secretor locus, and the Lewis locus. In the great majority of people one or another, or a combination of substances with specificities designated as A, B, H, Le^a and Le^b occur. There remains a small proportion of people (about 1–2 per cent) who do not appear to have any of these materials in their secretions. They would be classified as non-secretor ABH, Le (a−b−). It seems possible that in these individuals mucoids with as yet unidentified group specific character may be formed.

Modifying genes

Genes that can be detected only by their effects on the expression of other genes are sometimes referred to as 'modifying' genes. A study of such effects is likely to be of considerable importance in understanding the biochemical basis of gene action, and interpreting the variation of genetically controlled characters. The so-called secretor-non-secretor genes can be regarded as typical examples of such 'modifiers'. In individuals who are homozygous for the non-secretor allele the formation of A, B and H group-specific substances in the water soluble form is effectively suppressed. The formation of A, B or H antigens on the red cells is, however, not interfered with. Thus the 'non-secretor' gene in the homozygote modifies in a characteristic manner the mode of expression of the **ABO** genes.

A number of other modifying genes which influence the expression of the **ABO** genes appear to exist, though they seem to be rather rare in most populations (24). The effect of one of these genes was first observed in three individuals living in Bombay (25). Both the red cells and serum were peculiar. The red cells were not agglutinated by anti-A, anti-B or anti-H. The serum contained not only anti-A and anti-B, but also anti-H in quite high titres. The red cells were Le^a+ and Le^a was found in the saliva. There were, however, no A, B, or H substances detectable in the saliva. The genetical basis of this so-called 'Bombay' phenotype was uncovered when a family in

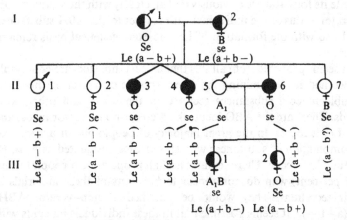

Fig. 50. Unusual segregation of ABO phenotypes in a family due to the occurrence of the 'suppressor' gene x. Individuals homozygous for x form no A, B or H substances, and have anti-A, anti-B, *and* anti-H antibodies in the plasma. (After Levine *et al.*) ◐, heterozygous for 'suppressor' gene (**Xx**); ●, homozygous for 'suppressor' gene (**xx**); Se, secretor of ABH substances; se, non-secretor of ABH substances.

which three individuals showing this phenotypic pattern were segregating, was studied in detail by Levine and his colleagues (26). The pedigree is shown in Fig. 50. II$_3$, II$_4$ and II$_6$ all exhibit the peculiar 'Bombay' phenotype. The critical point is that one of the children of II$_6$ has B on her red cells though this antigen is apparently not present in either parent, and the other child of II$_6$ secreted H substance in the saliva though both parents were apparently non-secretors. All the findings in this family can be explained on the hypothesis that II$_3$, II$_4$ and II$_6$ are homozygous for a rare gene x which suppresses the formation of B and H substances both in their alcohol-soluble form in the red cells, and in their water-soluble form in the secretions and body fluids. The fact that the parents of the anomalous individuals were first cousins strongly supports the concept that these individuals are homozygous for a rare recessive gene. The heterozygotes Xx, (I_1, I_2, III_1 and III_2) are evidently unaffected by the unusual gene. Because the appropriate critical matings have not yet been observed, it is not so far possible to say whether the formation of A substance would be suppressed in individuals homozygous for x.

Another rare modifying gene y has also been described. In homozygotes this inhibits the development of the A antigen on the red cells, and partially depresses its formation in the secretions [27]. The expressions of B and H are evidently not influenced by yy.

The isolation and properties of the group specific substances

The earliest attempts to isolate the specific blood-group substances used erythrocytes as starting material. Active material could be extracted with ethanol and other organic solvents. It appeared to be carbohydrate in nature but the yields were low and the native substances were never satisfactorily purified. The isolation of group specific substances from erythrocytes is particularly difficult because they appear to be bound in some way to the lipid and possibly the protein constituents of the red cell membrane, and it has not proved easy to separate in quantities sufficient for characterisation. As a result very little is known, even today, about the exact chemical nature of the group-specific materials on the red-cell surface.

The discovery of the water-soluble forms of these substances in tissue extracts and secretions opened the way to their isolation in reasonable quantities and in a comparatively homogeneous and pure state. Saliva and gastric juice were found to be the most potent sources of these materials from normal human subjects, and these particular secretions have been extensively exploited as starting materials by Kabat and his colleagues [28]. Morgan and Van Heyningen [29] discovered that pseudomucinous ovarian cysts were a particularly rich source of the group-specific substances. These pathological growths occur not infrequently. They may contain a few hundred ml. to several litres of fluid, and a single cyst may contain several grams of the group-specific substances. Animal sources have also been used as starting material. It has been possible, for example, to prepare from pig gastric mucin substances with serological specificities corresponding to human blood group A and H specificity.

The substances appear to be complex, high molecular weight mucopolysaccharides. Mild procedures must be used throughout their isolation because irreversible changes, often with an alteration in immunological properties, may be readily produced. The main problem is to devise satisfactory criteria for establishing the homogeneity and purity of the final product. Physical, chemical, and immunological methods have been variously used for this purpose. It is, however, often still difficult to assess how far minor variations in the products are due to some degree of degradation during preparation or to inhomogeneity, and how far they reflect real differences in the original native specific mucoids [30,31].

Table 32. *Typical analytical figures for preparations of human blood-group substances. (After Morgan, 1956)*

Substance	Nitrogen (%)	Acetyl (%)	Hexosamine* (%)	Reduction† (%)	Fucose (%)
A	5·7	9·0	37	56	18
H	5·3	8·6	31	54	13
Le*	5·0	9·9	32	57	12
B	5·7	7·0	20	50	18

* As glucosamine base.   † In terms of glucose equivalent.

Morgan and his colleagues [30–6] have now been able to obtain substantially homogeneous preparations of substances with group specific activity corresponding to A (from ovarian cysts of A_1 secretors), B (from ovarian cysts of B secretors), H (from ovarian cysts of O secretors), and Le^a (from ovarian cysts of non-secretors $Le^a +$). Despite the clear-cut differences in immunological specificity of these substances, their general properties and overall constitution and structure appear to be remarkably similar. They are all mucopolysaccharides (Table 32) made up of sugars, aminosugars and aminoacids. The molecular weights are of the order of 3×10^5 or larger. Two sugars and two aminosugars appear to be characteristic of these substances and are regularly present. They are D-galactose, L-fucose, D-glucosamine and D-galactosamine. At least eleven aminoacids occur. They include lysine, arginine, aspartic acid, glutamic acid, serine, threonine, glycine, alanine, valine, proline, leucine and or isoleucine. One curious feature is the relatively high proportion of threonine in the aminoacid complex.

No qualitative differences in composition have been detected between the substances with different serological specificities. There may, however, be some quantitative differences. For example, the ratio of glucosamine to galactosamine appears to vary somewhat from preparation to preparation. Thus for group A substance values for this ratio varying from 0·7 to 1·6 have been obtained, for Le^a and B substances the ratio is nearer to 3, and for H substances ratios from 2·7 to 12·7 have been found. In most specimens the glucosamine content is of the order of 16 to 20 per cent, and most of the variation in the ratios of the two aminosugars appears to arise from differing quantities of galactosamine present. These results were obtained on substances prepared from ovarian cysts. However, similar variations have been found in materials obtained from saliva. The aminosugars are thought to occur in the intact macromolecule as N-acetyl derivatives.

Studies of the degradation of these mucopolysaccharides under a variety of conditions [30], such as mild acid hydrolysis, mild alkali hydrolysis, oxidation with periodate and hypoiodous acids, and enzymic degradation, have all served to emphasise the basic similarities in the overall structures of the substances despite differences in serological specificity. They have also made it possible to build up at least a rough picture of the general structural arrangement of the macromolecule.

Mild acid hydrolysis, for example, results in the selective release of fucose and this reaches a maximum value equivalent to about 80 per cent of the total fucose originally present. This treatment also results in a progressive increase in cross reactivity with pneumococcus type XIV antibody, and does so independently of the character of the original blood-group activity. It has been suggested that this is due to the uncovering of N-acetyl hexosamine-galactose chains which make up major structures within the polysaccharide moieties of all the group-specific substances, and are similar in pattern to the N-acetyl-glucosamine-galactose structures of the pneumococcus type XIV specific polysaccharide [28,30].

Characteristically, the group-specific substances are readily degraded by extremely mild treatment with alkali. There seems to be no preferential liberation of any one structural unit, and the hydrolysis proceeds steadily and evidently in much the same manner throughout the disintegration of the substance. Studies of the products produced in the course of this hydrolysis suggest the disintegration of the macromolecules with mild alkali treatment can probably be attributed to the hydrolysis of glycoside linkages in alkali-labile, aminosugar-containing chains (37). Only a part of the N-acetyl hexosamine present seems to be concerned in this, and it seems probable that the hexosamines are linked in two different forms, one of which is alkali-labile, and the other relatively alkali-stable.

Oxidation of the reducing —CHO end groups has been achieved, using very mild conditions with hypoiodous acid. The analytical figures suggest that in each macromolecule of molecular weight of about 300,000 there are some fifty reducing carbohydrate end groups. The occurrence of such a high proportion of reducing end groups in this kind of large macromolecule is rather unusual, and Morgan suggests that it is probably due to the structural integration brought about by the aminoacid moiety of the molecule (30). After oxidation with hypoiodate, the A, B, and H substances retain their group specific serological activity, and so it appears that the reducing end groups are not essential for the immunological specificity.

Assembling all the evidence obtained from the degradation studies carried out under different conditions, Morgan has been able to put forward a hypothetical structure for the group substances which will account for many of the properties that they have in common (30). He suggests that the aminoacid and carbohydrate moieties of the molecule are closely integrated. The peptide chains are envisaged as being held together by carbohydrate chains which act as bridges, and at least two kinds of carbohydrate chain are postulated. An alkali-stable chain which contains galactose and N-acetylglucosamine units, and an alkali-labile N-acetyl hexosamine-rich chain. It is thought that the alkali-stable chains are probably responsible for the cross reacting pneumococcal type XIV activity which develops following treatment with weak acid. Possibly they are substituted in some of their free hydroxyl groups by L-fucose. The N-acetyl glucosamine and galactose units are probably joined here by the relatively alkali-stable 1·4 glycosidic linkages. In the alkali-labile chains the component aminosugars may be joined by 1·3 linkages.

Fig. 51 shows part of the hypothetical structure which is postulated. The peptides are indicated in the conventional manner, and the reducing or potentially reducing end groups of the carbohydrate chains by the sign →. The linkages readily hydrolysed by alkali are shown with a vertical dotted line. Hydrolysis of these alkali-labile bonds would lead to a break up of the macromolecule. A number of possible linkages are considered. For example, carbohydrate chain A is envisaged as being joined at its potentially reducing end to the

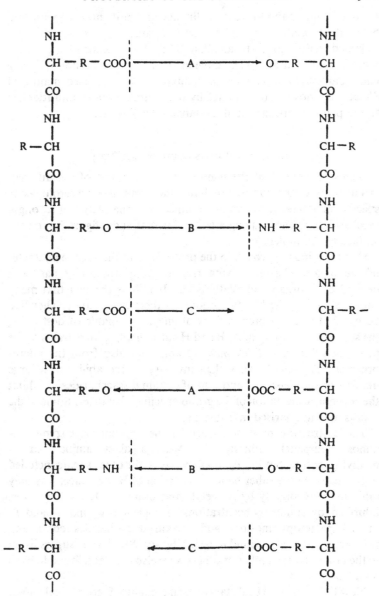

Fig. 51. A possible common macromolecular structure for the blood-group substances. (After Morgan [30].)

peptide chain by an O-glycosidic linkage and at its non-reducing end by an alkali-labile ester linkage. Carbohydrate chain B is considered as joined to the peptide by an alkali-labile N-glycosidic linkage at the reducing end and an alkali-stable ether linkage at the non-reducing end. Carbohydrate chain C is thought of as composed mainly of N-acetylaminosugar units joined by alkali-labile linkages and attached to the peptide through an alkali-labile ester linkage.

The chemical basis of group specificity

It seems probable that the main structural features of the different group specific mucoids are much the same, and that the serologically specific characteristics are determined by relatively short oligosaccharide sequences giving a particular spatial configuration on the surface of the molecule.

One ingenious approach to the problem as to the precise character of the oligosaccharides giving rise to group specificity has been devised by Morgan and Watkins[38]. It utilises the fact that many enzymes are inhibited by the product of their own activity. They had been able to obtain preparations of enzymes capable of destroying the serological activity of A, B and H substances, from extracts of the protozoan flagellate *Trichomonas foetus*, and also from the microorganism *Cl. welchii*. They then investigated the ability of a large number of simple sugars and also of certain disaccharides to inhibit the enzymic degradation of the group-specific substances. Some of the results are summarised in Table 33.

The destruction of A substance by the appropriate enzyme was almost completely inhibited by N-acetyl-galactosamine and its methyl glycoside, but hardly at all by any of the other sugars included in the test. On the other hand, destruction of B substance, was only inhibited very slightly by N-acetyl-galactosamine. It was, however, inhibited by similar concentrations of D-galactose, and α- and β-methyl galactopyranosides and certain disaccharides containing D-galactose were also found to be inhibitory. Besides the sugars listed in the table a large number of others were also tried and found to have no effect.

Now the A, B and H substances each contain L-fucose, D-galactose, N-acetyl-D-glucosamine, and N-acetyl-D-galactosamine, and one of these substances in each case inhibits the action of the corresponding enzyme. The implication is that when the serological specificity is

Table 33. *Percentage substrate remaining unchanged when the T. foetus enzyme acts on the A, B and H blood-group substances in the presence of different sugars. (After Watkins and Morgan, 1955)*

	Percentage unchanged substrate		
Sugar added	A substance	B substance	H substance
Control (no sugar added)	3	1	1
L-Fucose	3	1	50–100
D-Fucose	3	1	1
L-Galactose	—	1	3
D-Galactose	6	50–100	1
N-Acetyl D-glucosamine	1	1	1
N-Acetyl D-galactosamine	50–100	6	1
D-Glucosamine	3	1	1
D-Galactosamine	3	6	50–100
α-Methyl L-fucopyranoside	3	1	3
β-Methyl L-fucopyranoside	—	—	1
α-Methyl L-fucofuranoside	3	1	1
β-Methyl L-fucofuranoside	3	1	1
α-Methyl D-galactopyranoside	3	50–100	1
β-Methyl D-galactopyranoside	3	50–100	1
β-Methyl D-galactofuranoside	—	3	1
Lactose	—	50–100	1
Melibiose	—	50–100	1
Methyl-N-acetyl-galactosaminide	50–100	—	—

lost due to the enzymic action, the initial change in each case is the hydrolysis of a linkage involving the sugar which causes the inhibition. Thus it would follow that N-acetyl-D-galactosamine is a key unit in the oligosaccharide sequence responsible for A specificity, and that D-galactose, and L-fucose are involved in B and H specificity in an analogous way. In the cases of B and H substances direct evidence has been obtained that the main sugars liberated by the appropriate enzymes are galactose and fucose respectively. The inhibition by D-galactosamine of the enzyme decomposing H substance is, however, difficult to explain because this hexosamine is believed to be present in the N-acetylated form in the H specific mucoid, and yet N-acetyl galactosamine is without inhibitory effect.

Morgan and Watkins [39] have also been able to show that in the case of the haemagglutination reaction between O red cells and anti-H serum from the eel, a considerable degree of inhibition could be obtained with L-fucose but not with other simple sugars. This provides further evidence that L-fucose is the sugar most intimately concerned with H specificity. Analogous results have also been obtained by Kabat and his colleagues[40] studying the inhibition by various sugars of the precipitin reaction between the blood-group substances and their appropriate antibodies. Thus for the A-anti-A system appreciable inhibition with N-acetyl-galactosamine but not with other simple sugars could be obtained. Similarly for the B-anti-B system it was found that D-galactose was the only sugar of the four monosaccharides present in the blood-group substances which produces any inhibition.

Extension of these studies by using small oligosaccharides of known constitution, obtained either synthetically or from partial hydrolysates of the group-specific substances, may be expected to yield a great deal more information about the characteristic arrangements of sugars responsible for the group specificities. Thus Coté and Morgan[41] have isolated several disaccharides from a partial hydrolysate of A substance, and have shown that one of these, o-α-N-acetyl D-galactosaminoyl-(1 → 3)-galactose, is considerably more active than is N-acetyl-galactosamine in A-anti-A agglutination inhibition tests. It seems likely that this disaccharide represents a significant part of the oligosaccharide unit which is responsible for A specificity.

Another disaccharide isolated from A substance was o-β-D-galactopyranosyl (1 → 4) N-acetyl-D-glucosamine. This was found to be very active in inhibiting the marked reaction which develops between the group-specific substances after mild acid hydrolysis and the Type XIV pneumococcal antibody[42].

Le^a specificity has also been investigated by these methods[43]. An enzyme was obtained in an extract from *Trichomonas foetus* which inactivated Le^a substance, and it was found that this was inhibited with L-fucose. Thus in this respect Le^a activity appeared to resemble H activity. Since, however, the serological properties of the two substances were known to be quite distinct it seemed probable that other structural differences, such as the mode of linkage of the L-fucose or the nature of the sugars adjacent to it, must exist in the oligosaccharide sequences determining Le^a and H specificity. The matter was examined further by studying the inhibitory effects of a variety of oligosaccharides on the agglutination of Le^a (a +) red cells by human anti-Le^a serum. Some of the oligosaccharides used are illustrated in Fig. 52, and the main results obtained are indicated in Table 34. One compound, lacto-N-fucopentaose II showed considerable inhibitory activity, and a second compound, lacto-N-difuco-

Lacto-*N*-tetraose

    β-D-galactosyl-(1 → 3)-β-D-*N*-acetylglucosaminoyl-(1 → 3)-β-D-galactosyl-(1 → 4)-D-glucose

Lacto-*N*-fucopentaose 1

    β-D-galactosyl-(1 → 3)-β-D-*N*-acetylglucosaminoyl-(1 → 3)-β-D-galactosyl-(1 → 4)-D-glucose

       |

       | (1 → 2)

   α-L-fucosyl

Lacto-*N*-fucopentaose II

    β D-glactosyl-(1 → 3)-β-D-*N*-acetylglucosaminoyl-(1 → 3)·β-D-galactosyl-(1 → 4)-D-glucose

                   |

                   | (1 → 4)

               α-L-fucosyl

Lacto-*N*-difucohexaose

    β-D-galactosyl-(1 → 3)-β-D-*N*-acetylglucosaminoyl-(1 → 3)-β-D-galactosyl-(1 → 4)-D-glucose

       | |

       | (1 → 2) | (1 → 4)

   α-L-fucosyl   α-L-fucosyl

Fig. 52. Various oligosaccharides used in inhibition studies on the Le^a-anti-Le^a system. (After Watkins and Morgan.)

Table 34. *The amounts of Le^a substance and sugars giving inhibition with human anti-Le^a serum.* (*After Watkins and Morgan, 1957*)

Substance	Minimum amount of substance giving inhibition* (μg./0·1 ml.)
Human Le^a substance	0·04
L-Fucose	> 1000
D-Fucose	> 1000
α-Fucosyl-(1 → 2) fucose	> 1000
α-Fucosyl-(1 → 2)-galactose	> 1000
Fucosido-lactose	> 1000
Lacto-*N*-tetraose	> 1000
Lacto-difucotetraose	> 1000
Lacto-*N*-fucopentaose I	> 1000
Lacto-*N*-fucopentaose II	1
Lacto-*N*-fucopentait II	1
Lacto-*N*-difucohexaose	60

* One volume of inhibitor added to one volume of anti-Le^a serum.

hexaose, gave a significant but rather weaker effect. The others were inactive. A consideration of the differences in their structures suggests that the arrangement shown in Fig. 53 must be an important feature of the determinant grouping giving rise to Le^a activity.

In contrast to these findings it appears that neither lacto-*N*-fucopentaose II nor lacto-*N*-difucohexaose have any significant inhibitory action on the agglutination of O cells by eel anti-H serum (44). Thus although the determinant groupings in both H and Le^a probably include fucose the detailed organisation is likely to be quite different.

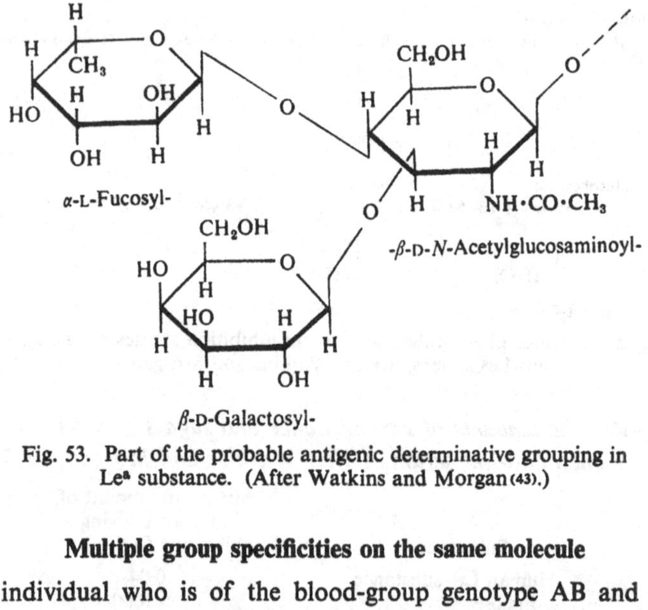

Fig. 53. Part of the probable antigenic determinative grouping in Le^a substance. (After Watkins and Morgan (43).)

Multiple group specificities on the same molecule

An individual who is of the blood-group genotype AB and is a secretor has secretions which show both A and B specific activity. The question arises whether these secretions contain mucopolysaccharide molecules each of which carry both the A and the B specific groupings, or whether they contain a mixture of macromolecules some of which have A and others of which have B specificity.

A and B substances once mixed cannot be separated by any of the conventional methods such as electrophoresis, ultracentrifugation, salting out, or alcohol fractionation. However, if a mixture of pure A and B substances, or a mixture of salivas from A secretors and B secretors is made up, it is possible to fractionate the two serological activities by precipitating one or the other group specific material with its appropriate anti-serum (45). Thus if anti-A is used, and the precipitate spun off, the B activity is found to remain in the supernatant, and the precipitate can be shown to contain only A reacting material. Similarly if B antiserum is used A remains in the super-natant and B appears in the precipitate. Now when secretions from individuals who are AB secretors are used in this test an entirely different result is obtained. When anti-A is the precipitating antibody virtually all the B activity is carried down in the precipitate with the A material, and the supernatant shows no B (Table 35). Similarly using anti-B serum, the A activity is found in the precipitate with the B activity, and the supernatant shows neither activity. The experi-ments indicate that in tissue fluids and secretions belonging to group AB secretors, a large proportion if not all the macromolecules showing blood-group specificity possess both A and B properties. In other words the heterozygote **AB** forms qualitatively different mucopolysaccharides from those found in individuals who are homozygous for either **A** or **B**.

Table 35. *Action of anti-A on an artificial mixture of A and B sub-stances, and on saliva from an AB secretor.* (*After Morgan and Watkins*, 1956)

		Precipitation with anti-A	
		Precipitate	Supernatant
A +	B	A	B
substance	substance		
	AB	AB	—
	saliva		

The same methods can be extended to investigate the situation when H activity is present in the secretions simultaneously with either A or B activity. So far the position has only been reported in A_2 secretors[46]. A_2 individuals are known to form relatively large amounts of H specific material. When saliva or ovarian cyst fluid from such individuals was treated with the appropriate anti-A sera, it was found that the precipitate contained both A and H activity. The supernatant, however, still showed some H activity although the A activity had been completely removed (Table 36). The result suggests that here at least two types of macromolecules are present, those with both A and H specificity, and those with only H specificity.

These findings are of some significance in relation to the general problem of the relation of H to A and B specificity. It has already been pointed out that there are good reasons for believing that H is not a specific product of the **O** gene. Morgan and Watkins[46] suggest that the present evidence indicates that H is a kind of basic substance on which the A and B genes somehow imprint their characteristic specificities. If this is so it would suggest that the genes A_1, A_2 and B act late in the synthesis of the group-specific substance and control the final stages only of the common precursor H substance into the strictly group-specific gene product. It is thought that the gene A_2 may be rather less effective than A_1 in bringing about the conversion of H to A. Consequently the substances formed in A_2 individuals may have more H character than those produced in A_1 individuals, and also a relatively higher proportion of H molecules may be left unchanged. When the genes A_1 and **B** act together one would expect a much more complete conversion of the precursor into a mucopolysaccharide possessing both A and B specificities, with relatively little remaining H properties. Both genes would presumably be influencing the same macromolecule, though possibly through the intermediary of individual specific enzymes.

Table 36. *Action of anti-A on an artificial mixture of A and H substances, and on saliva from an A_2 secretor. (After Watkins and Morgan, 1956)*

	Precipitation with anti-A	
	Precipitate	Supernatant
A + H substance substance	A	H
AH saliva	AH	H

Further support for this general concept has been provided by experiments in which A and B substances have been converted by enzyme action into materials devoid of their original specificity but now possessing H specific activity. In a very interesting experiment, for example, Watkins [47] has treated purified B substance with the B decomposing enzyme from *T. foetus*. This led to the appearance of H specificity and it was accompanied by the liberation mainly of galactose but also of smaller quantities of fucose and *N*-acetylhexosamine. The H active material so obtained was then treated with the H degrading enzyme. This led to the liberation mainly of fucose and small quantities of *N*-acetylhexosamine, and to the appearance of greatly enhanced serological reactivity with Type xiv pneumococcal antibody.

Preliminary experiments on salivas containing both A and Le[a] activities suggest that here also both types of serological property may be possessed by the same mucopolysaccharide molecule [31].

Concluding remarks

Although the A and B group characters were first recognised in red cells, it is now clear that substances with these and related group specificities are major constituents of all the normal mucilaginous secretions of the body. Quantitatively the amounts present in the secretions are very much greater than occur on the red cells. These mucopolysaccharides with group specificity are almost certainly essential for the normal working of the body, though it seems unlikely that the individualities in serological specificity that they exhibit result in any gross physiological differences between individuals of differing phenotypes. It is, however, possible that they may lead to rather subtle differences in functioning. There is, for example, a whole body of literature which suggests that individuals of different ABO and secretor genotypes may be more or less susceptible to certain disease processes such as gastric carcinoma and duodenal ulcer[48]. There is as yet no indication of how the rather minor structural differences between the various group-specific mucopolysaccharides could result in differences in susceptibility to such conditions.

The final structure of the specific mucopolysaccharides formed in the secretions and on the red cells in any given person is obviously dependent on a rather complex genetical situation. Alleles of at least three loci are probably involved. Thus the relative amounts of mucoids with A, B, H and Le^a specificities in any one individual will depend on his ABO genotype, his secretor status, and on whether or not he possessed the genetical factor determining Le^a. Besides these, other genes such as the modifying genes x and y may play a part, and whatever genetical factor is involved in Le^b formation must come into the picture. The problem of the precise manner in which these different genes influence the synthesis of the various mucopolysaccharides remains to be solved. At one time it was thought probable that the blood-group antigens could be regarded as direct and immediate products of genic activity. This seems less likely now. It appears more probable that various specific enzymes concerned in controlling the final stages of mucopolysaccharide synthesis may act as intermediaries between the genes and the group-specific substances.

REFERENCES

(1) Landsteiner, K. (1901). *Wien. klin. Wschr.* **14**, 132.
(2) Epstein, A. A. and Ottenberg, R. (1908). *Proc. N.Y. Path. Soc.* **8**, 117.
(3) Von Dungern, E. and Hirszfeld, L. (1910). *S. ImmunForsch.* **6**, 284.
(4) Bernstein, F. (1925). *Z. Indukt. Abstamm. u. VererbLehre*, **37**, 237.
(5) Wiener, A. S. (1943). *Blood Groups and Transfusion.* C. C. Thomas, Illinois.
(6) Von Dungern, E. and Hirszfeld, L. (1911). *Z. ImmunForsch.* **8**, 526.
(7) Thomsen, O., Friendenreich, V. and Worsaae, E. (1930). *Acta path. microbiol. scand.* **7**, 157.
(8) Ikin, E. W., Prior, A. M., Race, R. R. and Taylor, G. L. (1939). *Ann. Eugen., Lond.* **9**, 409.
(9) Lehrs, H. (1930). *Z. ImmunForsch.* **66**, 175.
(10) Putkonen, T. (1930). *Acta Soc. Med. 'Duodecim'*, A **14**, no. 2.
(11) Schiff, F. and Sasaki, H. (1932). *Klin. Wschr.* **34**, 1426.
(12) Schiff, F. (1927). *Klin. Wschr.* **6**, 303.
(13) Watkins, W. M. and Morgan, W. T. J. (1955). *Vox Sanguinis*, **5**, 1.
(14) Mourant, A. E. (1946). *Nature, Lond.* **158**, 237.
(15) Andresen, P. H. (1947). *Acta path. microbiol. scand.* **24**, 616.
(16) Grubb, R. (1951). *Acta path. microbiol. scand.* **28**, 61.
(17) Ceppellini, R. (1954). *V. Congr. Inter. de Trans. Sang.*
(18) Grubb, R. (1948). *Nature, Lond.* **162**, 933.
(19) Grubb, R. and Morgan, W. T. J. (1949). *Brit. J. Exp. Path.* **30**, 198.
(20) Race, R. R. and Sanger, R. (1950). *Blood Groups in Man.* Blackwell, Oxford.
(21) Brendemoen, O. J. (1949). *J. Lab. Clin. Med.* **34**, 538.
(22) Sneath, J. S. and Sneath, P. H. A. (1955). *Nature, Lond.* **176**, 172.
(23) Andresen, P. H. (1948). *Acta path. microbiol. scand.* **25**, 728.
(24) Editorial (1957). *Vox Sanguinis*, **2**, 2.
(25) Bhende, Y. M., Deshpande, C. K., Bhatia, H. M., Sanger, R., Race, R. R., Morgan, W. T. J. and Watkins, W. M. (1952). *Lancet*, **1**, 903.
(26) Levine, P., Robinson, E., Celano, M., Briggs, O. and Falkinburg, L. (1955). *Blood*, **10**, 1100.
(27) Weiner, W., Lewis, B., Moores, P., Sanger, R., Race, R. R. (1957). *Vox Sanguinis*, **2**, 25.
(28) Kabat, E. A. (1956). *Blood Group Substances.* Academic Press, New York.
(29) Morgan, W. T. J. and Van Heyningen, R. (1944). *Brit. J. Exp. Path.* **25**, 5.
(30) Morgan, W. T. J. (1956). In *Lectures on the Scientific Basis of Medicine.* 1954–5, **4**, 92.
(31) Morgan, W. T. J. (1958). In *Chemistry and Biology of Mucopolysaccharides*, ed. Wolstenholme, G. E. W. and O'Connor, M. Churchill, London.
(32) Morgan, W. T. J. and Wadell, M. B. R. (1945). *Brit. J. Exp. Path.* **26**, 387.

(33) Aminoff, D., Morgan, W. T. J. and Watkins, W. M. (1950). *Biochem. J.* **46**, 426.

(34) Annison, E. F. and Morgan, W. T. J. (1952). *Biochem. J.* **50**, 460.

(35) Annison, E. F. and Morgan, W. T. J. (1952). *Biochem. J.* **52**, 247.

(36) Gibbons, R. A., Morgan, W. T. J. and Gibbons, M. (1955). *Biochem. J.* **60**, 428.

(37) Knox, K. and Morgan, W. T. J. (1954). *Biochem. J.* **58**, v.

(38) Watkins, W. M. and Morgan, W. T. J. (1955). *Nature, Lond.* **175**, 676.

(39) Watkins, W. M. and Morgan, W. T. J. (1952). *Nature, Lond.* **169**, 825.

(40) Kabat, E. A. and Leskowitz, S. (1955). *J. Amer. Chem. Soc.* **77**, 5159.

(41) Coté, R. and Morgan, W. T. J. (1956). *Nature, Lond.* **178**, 1171.

(42) Watkins, W. M. and Morgan, W. T. J. (1956). *Nature, Lond.* **178**, 1289.

(43) Watkins, W. M. and Morgan, W. T. J. (1957). *Nature, Lond.* **180**, 1038.

(44) Kuhn, R. and Osman, H. G. (1956). *Z. Physiol. Chem.* **303**, 1.

(45) Morgan, W. T. J. and Watkins, W. M. (1956). *Nature, Lond.* **177**, 521.

(46) Watkins, W. M. and Morgan, W. T. J. (1956). *Acta Genet.* **6**, 521.

(47) Watkins, W. M. (1956). *Biochem. J.* **64**, 211.

(48) Roberts, J. A. F. (1957). *Brit. J. Prev. Soc. Med.* **11**, 107.

CHAPTER 8

THE PLASMA PROTEINS

The plasma proteins constitute an exceedingly complex mixture of many different protein species with diverse physiological functions. During the last two decades the application of developments in new methods of analysis of protein mixtures has served to emphasise this heterogeneity. These methods have also brought to light a number of inherited differences in the formation of certain of these proteins. Some of the variations thus revealed occur commonly in certain human populations, and allow normal individuals to be classified into more than one type, according to the particular properties of the specific proteins involved. This is the case, for example, with respect to the haptoglobin types discovered by Smithies, and the gamma globulin types discovered by Grubb and Laurell. Other variants occur more rarely, and have usually been discovered as a result of the detailed investigation of particular inherited pathological disorders. Here it is perhaps useful to differentiate between abnormalities in protein synthesis resulting in the complete or almost complete absence of one of the major fractions of the plasma proteins, such as albumin, γ-globulin or fibrinogen, and those abnormalities in which the synthesis is defective of a protein normally present in only very small amounts such as caeruloplasmin or anti-haemophilic globulin. In general while the former may be readily identified by standard procedures of protein fractionation such as electrophoresis, the latter usually require somewhat more specialised techniques for their characterisation. It is likely that so far only a small proportion of the variations occurring in those plasma proteins present in relatively small amounts have been uncovered, and one may anticipate rapid developments in this field as appropriate analytical techniques become available.

The haptoglobin types

Classical electrophoresis, either in free solution, or in a supporting medium such as filter paper, agar, or starch grains, results in a fractionation of human plasma proteins into six main groups;

Albumen, α_1, α_2, β- and γ-globulins, and fibrinogen. It is, however, known that this degree of resolution, though invaluable for many purposes, is nevertheless relatively coarse. Each of the main fractions with the possible exception of fibrinogen, is almost certainly hetero-geneous and represents a number of distinct protein species which happen to have similar mobilities in free solution at the particular pH at which the electrophoresis is carried out.

The development by Smithies[1] of a method of electrophoresis in a supporting medium of gelled starch has led to further resolution of certain of these fractions. The enhanced resolution is probably a consequence of the use of a supporting medium the pore size of which approaches the molecular dimensions of some of the proteins involved. Electrophoresis in starch gels appears, therefore, to com-bine resolution by 'true' free solution mobilities, with resolution according to molecular dimensions, at least over some of the ranges of molecular size present in the plasma proteins. Proteins of comparatively small size may be slowed relatively much less in the gels than proteins of larger size or greater dissymmetry, even though in free solution they may have the same mobilities. In consequence a more complex pattern of protein fractions is obtained and certain differences between individuals which are concealed in classical electrophoresis become apparent in this system.

Smithies found that when plasmas or sera from normal individuals were examined by this procedure, three distinct types of pattern might be recognised. They are illustrated in Fig. 54. The differences between these three types of pattern are due to the behaviour of a particular group of proteins which have been called haptoglobins, and the three types are now referred to as haptoglobin types 1.1, 2.1, and 2.2 (originally they were called I, IIA and IIB respectively)[2]. It should be noted that apart from these haptoglobins a number of other new protein fractions are revealed by this method of electro-phoresis. These include the 'pre-albumins', the 'post-albumins' and the 'fast' and 'slow' α_2 components. In general these other fractions occur more or less regularly in all sera and such variations as may exist are independent of the three types defined by the behaviour of the haptoglobins. Only a single haptoglobin component was observed in the type 1.1 sera and this migrated at about the same speed as the fast α_2 fraction under the experimental conditions adopted. In the types 2.1 and 2.2 sera, however, at least three haptoglobin com-ponents were seen in each case, using the ordinary methods of protein staining. They moved between the β fraction and the slow α_2 fraction and were originally referred to as $\alpha\beta$-components. However, in the 2.1 sera each of these three $\alpha\beta$ proteins had a mobility slightly greater than the corresponding ones observed in the 2.2 sera.

The particular fraction in classical electrophoresis to which these newly identified components belong has been determined by an elegant two-dimensional technique in which the serum proteins are first separated by conventional methods in filter paper, and are then resolved in the second dimension on a broad starch gel[3]. Using this

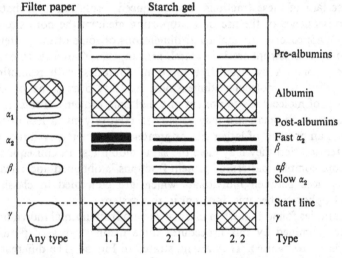

Fig. 54. Diagrams showing the three types of pattern obtained by electrophoresis of sera from different individuals in starch gel. (After Smithies.)

technique it was possible to show that the haptoglobins form part of the α_2 fraction of classical electrophoresis, and that this fraction also includes other distinct components, such as those referred to as fast α_2 and slow α_2 in the diagrams.

The haptoglobins are so called because they possess the distinctive property of forming stable complexes with haemoglobin. This is of considerable practical value in confirming the characterisation of the three types of individual because if some haemoglobin is added to the plasma prior to electrophoresis, the haptoglobin-haemoglobin complexes which are formed migrate in a characteristic manner which is different from that of the original haemoglobin-free material. Only a small amount of haemoglobin (100–150 mg. per cent) is required to saturate the binding capacity of the haptoglobins in normal serum and any excess haemoglobin migrates independently in the free state.

The resolution of the haptoglobin-haemoglobin complexes can be further enhanced by using certain special discontinuous buffer systems [4]. The pattern of the haemoglobin complexes can also be more readily distinguished if, instead of using a general protein-

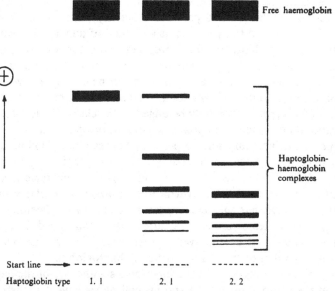

Fig. 55. Diagram showing the pattern of haptoglobin-haemoglobin complexes which may be obtained after electrophoresis in starch gel using a discontinuous buffer system (4) and visualising the complexes with a 'benzidine' reagent.

staining reagent to visualise the components, the haemoglobin complexed haptoglobins are specifically detected by a benzidine reagent. Combining the two methods one may obtain patterns illustrated in Fig. 55. Here the type 1.1 sera show a single fast-moving haptoglobin-haemoglobin complex, whereas the types 2.1 and 2.2 sera may each have six or more distinct haemoglobin-bound components. The fastest moving component in the type 2.1 sera appears to correspond in mobility to the single component found in the type 1.1 sera although quantitatively there is very much less of it present. The other haptoglobin-haemoglobin complexes in the 2.1 sera have each a distinctly different mobility from those found in the 2.2 sera.

The haptoglobin types are characteristic of the individual, and repeated examination of plasma samples from the same person invariably gives the same haptoglobin pattern. The types appear, therefore, to reflect real differences in the character of synthesis of this particular group of proteins.

Prior to the work of Smithies, Jayle and his colleagues in France [5] had already demonstrated that specific proteins binding haemoglobin exist in normal serum and had in fact coined the name haptoglobin to designate them. They showed that the haptoglobin-haemoglobin complexes exhibit marked peroxidase activity under certain conditions and had used this property as a method of quantitative estimation of haptoglobins. Furthermore, they had recognised that more than one form of haptoglobin might exist, and had been able to isolate the least common variety from the urine of a patient with the nephrotic syndrome. It was found to have a molecular weight of about 85,000, and it evidently belonged to the class of mucoproteins because it contained an appreciable amount of carbohydrate (about 17 per cent, including some 5 per cent hexosamine). This material has since been shown to correspond to the haptoglobin present in sera of Smithies type 1.1 [6]. The haptoglobins characteristic of Smithies types 2.1 and 2.2 evidently have larger molecular weights than this. Jayle has succeeded in isolating them from haemoglobin containing bulked serum as a mixture in their complexed form, and has estimated that on the average their molecular weights may be about twice that of the characteristic 1.1 haptoglobin.

The site of formation and the functional significance of the haptoglobins is still obscure. Jayle and his colleagues have demonstrated that the concentration of these proteins in serum is markedly increased in a variety of clinical disorders [5]. These include chronic and acute infections, rheumatoid arthritis, and malignant diseases. Their common feature is possibly the occurrence of some degree of tissue breakdown.

Laurell and Nyman [7] have studied their significance in relation to haemoglobinuria in a series of experiments involving the intravenous administration of haemoglobin solutions. It emerged that no free haemoglobin was present in plasma and no haemoglobinuria occurred until after the plasma haptoglobin binding capacity for haemoglobin was saturated. Furthermore, the haptoglobin-haemoglobin complexes, once formed, rapidly disappeared from the circulating plasma, and if sufficient free haemoglobin was infused the plasma could be completely depleted of haptoglobin within twenty-four hours. Provided the administration of haemoglobin had ceased, fresh haptoglobin began to reappear in the plasma during the next few days and soon reached its original concentration. Thus the haptoglobin concentration at any one time will to a large extent determine the apparent renal threshold for haemoglobin. Similar phenomena evidently occur during intravascular haemolysis [8].

Haptoglobins are only occasionally present in the plasma of the new-born. They gradually begin to appear during the first few weeks of life. Galatius-Jensen [9] has examined a series of young infants up to the age of six months, and has shown that by this time in only about 3 per cent of children could no serum haptoglobins be detected (Table 37).

Table 37. *Incidence of detectable haptoglobins in young infants (After Galatius-Jensen, 1957)*

Age	Number tested	Number with detectable haptoglobins	Proportion with detectable haptoglobins
At birth (cord blood)	34	4	0·12
1–2 months	71	34	0·48
2–4 months	147	128	0·87
4–6 months	104	101	0·97

An absence of serum haptoglobins may also sometimes be observed in adults. Very occasionally this can be attributed to the effects of intravascular haemolysis, with the consequent depletion of haptoglobins, in the manner described by Laurell and Nyman. In these instances the haptoglobins may be expected to reappear once the haemolytic process has ceased. This has in fact been observed in patients with pernicious anaemia. Here haptoglobins may be absent prior to treatment when an appreciable degree of haemolysis is going on. Once treatment has been started the haemolysis soon ceases and haptoglobins reappear in the circulating plasma. However, in a small proportion of adult Europeans (less than 1 per cent) no haptoglobins can be detected [9,10], although there is no indication of any haemolytic process going on and no haemoglobinuria. In certain African populations a much higher proportion of individuals may have no detectable haptoglobins [10]. The cause of this remains to be elucidated.

Family studies have shown quite conclusively that the three haptoglobin types defined by Smithies are inherited characteristics. Smithies and Ford Walker [11] put forward the hypothesis that they were determined by a pair of allelic genes Hp^1 and Hp^2, type 1.1

individuals being homozygous for the **Hp¹** gene, and type 2.2 individuals being homozygous for the **Hp²** gene, while type 2.1 individuals would represent the heterozygote **Hp¹Hp²**. On this hypothesis the expected results of different matings can be readily predicted and they are shown in Table 38. The hypothesis requires that no type

Table 38. (a) *Haptoglobin phenotypes and their corresponding genotypes.* (b) *Expected results of different matings.* (*After Smithies and Walker*, 1955)

(a)

Phenotype	1.1	2.1	2.2
Genotype	Hp¹/Hp¹	Hp²/Hp¹	Hp²/Hp²

(b)

	Children		
Parents	1.1	2.1	2.2
1.1 × 1.1	100 %	—	—
1.1 × 2.1	50 %	50 %	—
1.1 × 2.2	—	100 %	—
2.1 × 2.1	25 %	50 %	25 %
2.1 × 2.2	—	50 %	50 %
2.2 × 2.2	—	—	100 %

1.1 individuals should be derived from matings in which one or other parent is of type 2.2, and no type 2.2 individual should occur among the offspring of any individual of type 1.1. Extensive family studies carried out in several different laboratories have shown that these simple rules hold with only very few exceptions[9,12]. Also the numerical proportions of the three phenotypes among the offspring of different sorts of matings agree very closely with those theoretically expected (Table 39). Some of the occasional exceptions can be

Table 39. *Segregation of haptoglobin types in* 106 *families.*
(*After Galatius-Jensen*, 1957)

		Children haptoglobin type					
Parents		1.1		2.1		2.2	
Mating	No.	Obs.	Exp.	Obs.	Exp.	Obs.	Exp.
1.1 × 1.1	4	7	7.0	—	—	—	—
1.1 × 2.1	15	20	19·5	19	19·5	—	—
1.1 × 2.2	13	—	—	29	29·0	—	—
2.1 × 2.1	22	10	12·5	26	25·0	14	12·5
2.1 × 2.2	43	—	—	64	60·0	56	60·0
2.2 × 2.2	9	—	—	—	—	25	25·0
Totals	106	37	39·0	138	133·5	95	97·5

reasonably attributed to illegitimacy and in most cases it has been possible to confirm this by blood-group studies. There remain, however, certain rare exceptions where this does not seem to be the explanation. Thus in one large family(12) four 2.2 individuals were found among the offspring of two different matings in both of which the mother was of type 1.1. Here it seems possible that some rare modifying gene or unusual allele was segregating.

The hypothesis does not, however, provide any explanation for the occasional occurrence of a complete absence of serum haptoglobins in European populations and the rather high incidence of this phenomenon which has been observed in certain African populations. Such a deficiency of haptoglobins may be due to a failure in formation or to an excessive rate of destruction, and it is not unlikely that it can arise from several different causes. Several European families have been observed in which there was more than one apparently healthy individual in whom no serum haptoglobins could be detected, and this suggests that at least in some cases the phenomenon is genetically determined. If so it is probably caused by a 'suppressor' gene at some locus independent of that determining the three types of haptoglobin pattern.

Accepting the hypothesis of Ford Walker and Smithies that the allelic genes Hp^1 and Hp^2 determine the three haptoglobin phenotypes, it is possible to estimate the gene frequencies of the Hp^1 and Hp^2 genes in different populations. From this one can see how far the observed frequencies of the three phenotypes fit with expected

Table 40. *Incidence of haptoglobin phenotypes in different populations, and the expected incidence assuming a Hardy-Weinberg equilibrium. (Data of Harris, Robson and Siniscalco, 1958)*

Population		Total	Haptoglobin phenotypes			Estimated gene frequencies	
			1.1	2.1	2.2	Hp^1	Hp^2
England	Obs.	114	20	55	39	0·42	0·58
	Exp.	—	20·1	55·6	38·3	—	—
N. Italy (Berra)	Obs.	119	20	57	42	0·41	0·59
	Exp.	—	20·0	57·6	41·4	—	—
Naples	Obs.	93	10	44	39	0·34	0·66
	Exp.	—	10·8	41·7	40·5	—	—
Sardinia (Illorai)	Obs.	147	18	74	55	0·37	0·63
	Exp.	—	20·1	68·5	58·4	—	—
Sicily (Catania)	Obs.	107	16	53	38	0·40	0·60
	Exp.	—	17·1	51·4	38·5	—	—

frequencies in a Hardy-Weinberg equilibrium. The calculation is shown for several different populations in Table 40. The agreement between the observed and expected numbers is very good, and supports the hypothesis. The Hp^2 gene is commoner than the Hp^1 gene in all European populations which have been studied. However, it is probable that in Africa Hp^1 is much more frequent than Hp^2 [10,13].

If the hypothesis that a pair of allelic genes determine the three haptoglobin types is correct, then the situation illustrates two rather important points of some general interest. First of all it would mean that a single gene substitution can result in differences in synthesis of several distinct proteins, albeit with similar properties. Secondly, it would suggest that the heterozygote need not represent a mixture of the two groups of proteins found separately in the homozygotes, but may form a group of proteins qualitatively different from either. In both these respects the position differs strikingly from that encountered with the genes controlling the synthesis of the different types of haemoglobin.

β-Globulin types

Poulik and Smithies [3] have shown that the β-globulin fraction observed in conventional electrophoresis of human plasma may be separated into several distinct components by electrophoresis in starch gel. One of these components which they refer to as β-globulin C appears to be present in much greater quantities than the others in the great majority of people. However, in a survey of plasmas from Negro and Australian aboriginal subjects Smithies [14] found several individuals with a new β-component which he called β-globulin D. This occurred in about the same concentration as β-globulin C which was also present in these individuals. It moved somewhat more slowly than β-globulin C in the starch gel system. β-Globulin D was found in two out of the forty-nine American Negroes tested and five out of twenty-three Australian aboriginals. It was not observed in a large series of Canadians who were examined. On the other hand, in five out of 425 of the Canadian series another component referred to as β-globulin B was observed along with, and in about the same concentration as, β-globulin C [15]. β-Globulin B moved somewhat faster than β-globulin C.

The formation of β-globulins B, C and D appears to be genetically controlled and Smithies [15,16] has suggested that they may be determined by three allelic genes each of which is responsible for the formation of one of these three β-globulins. If this is so then the β-globulins C, D and B presumably represent alternative forms of the same protein species.

In a search for such β-globulin types in European and African subjects recently carried out in the author's own laboratory four unusual β-globulin patterns were encountered (17). In a series of 153 Africans from Gambia, four individuals were observed who had besides β-globulin C a slower-moving β-globulin component which in each case was present in about the same amounts as β-globulin C.

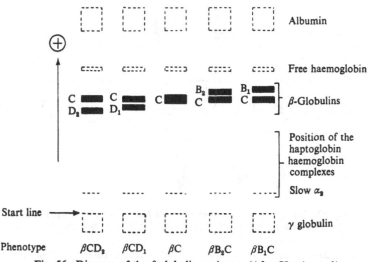

Fig. 56. Diagram of the β-globulin variants. (After Harris *et al.*)

In one of the individuals, however, the unusual β-globulin had a distinctly slower mobility than the unusual β-component in the other three. Since it is likely that one of these new globulin variants corresponded to the β-globulin D of Smithies they may be referred to for the present as β-globulin D_1 and D_2 respectively. The two new phenotypes in which they were observed may be referred to as β-CD_1, and β-CD_2 respectively (Fig. 56). In a series of 139 individuals from England no example of phenotypes β-CD_1 or β-CD_2 were observed. However, two individuals were encountered with an unusual β-component moving faster than β-globulin C. In both these cases the new component was present along with and in about equal amounts to β-globulin C. The mobility of the new fast-moving component was, however, different in the two individuals. Since one of them presumably corresponded to β-globulin B of Smithies, they can be referred to as β-globulins B_1 and B_2 and the corresponding phenotypes called β-B_1C and β-B_2C (Fig. 56).

It was possible to examine a number of the relatives of the individuals with phenotype β-B_1C and among them six further individuals were found with the same phenotype. The pedigree is shown in Fig. 57, and it seems reasonable to infer from it that the formation of β-globulin B_1 is genetically determined and that the individuals with the β-B_1C phenotype are heterozygous for the appropriate gene.

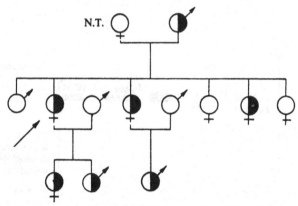

Fig. 57. Segregation of β-globulin B_1 in a family. (After Harris *et al.*)
β-Globulin phenotypes. O, βC; ◐, βB_1C; N.T. not tested.

It seems probable from all this that a whole series of genetically determined β-globulin variants can occur and the situation may well prove analogous to that found with respect to the genetically determined haemoglobin variants which have been so extensively studied in recent years.

The γ-globulin types

Grubb and Laurell[18,19] have demonstrated a curious inherited difference in the immunochemical character of the γ-globulin present in different people. To detect this difference they employ a rather complex serological system.

Certain sera obtained from patients with rheumatoid arthritis agglutinate Rh positive red cells which have been previously coated with 'incomplete' anti-Rh antibody. This agglutination was found to be inhibited by some normal sera but not by others. The inhibitor was shown to occur in the γ-globulin fraction and to be non-dialysable.

The presence or absence of this γ-globulin component which behaved as an inhibitor in the test system was found to be an inherited difference. The phenotype (designated Gm-) which did not have the inhibitor was shown to segregate in families in the manner of a Mendelian 'recessive' character (see page 18). This phenotype occurred with a frequency of about 40 per cent in a Swedish population, and with a frequency of only about 5 per cent in Esquimos.

Agammaglobulinaemia

It is believed that most antibodies circulating in the plasma are γ-globulins. It is not, however, known whether all γ-globulin molecules are capable of behaving as antibodies or whether they may possess other functions as well.

In 1952 Bruton [20] described a boy with a clinical history of severe and recurrent infections, an absence of circulating antibodies in the plasma, and an inability to produce antibodies in response to antigenic stimulation. Electrophoretic analysis of the plasma revealed a complete absence of γ-globulin. The other plasma proteins were present in normal amounts. The discovery that severe susceptibility to infection could be due to a fundamental inability to form antibodies, and that such a condition was readily demonstrable by the absence of γ-globulin in plasma-protein electrophoresis, led within a few years to the recognition of many other examples of this disorder and to an extensive investigation of the underlying disability.

It appears that two types of condition may occur with these characteristic features: a 'congenital' form which is usually recognised in early childhood and an 'adult' form which apparently develops later in life. The congenital form has frequently been observed in more than one member of the same family and is almost certainly genetically determined. Nearly all the cases described have been males. The adult form does not appear to be familial and is thought to be acquired in some way, though the environmental factors responsible for its causation are not known. Here both sexes appear to be equally affected.

In congenital agammaglobulinaemia the disease presents clinically as an extreme susceptibility to bacterial infection beginning usually during the second half of the first year of life, probably after the disappearance of passively transferred maternal γ-globulins. Repeated attacks of pneumoccal pneumonia, bacterial meningitis, bacterial infections of the middle ear, bacterial diseases of the paranasal sinuses and of the urinary and gastrointestinal tracts are common. The clear recognition of the characteristic features of this disease only in recent years is no doubt attributable largely to the development and extensive use of antibiotics, because few of these children would have survived the first year of life in the pre-antibiotic era.

Resistance to most virus infections is relatively much less impaired [21,22]. Diseases such as chickenpox, poliomyelitis, measles and influenza have not been found to occur excessively frequently nor have they been noticeably more severe. However, Bruton's original case did have mumps on three occasions, and Keidan and his colleagues [23] have described an infant girl with no circulating γ-globulin who died of generalised vaccinia following routine vaccination for smallpox. Usually, however, smallpox vaccination has been carried out successfully in these patients without complications.

In all cases of this condition the diagnosis is clearly established by electrophoresis of the plasma, either in free solution or in filter paper. Under these conditions virtually no γ-globulin is detected, but the other plasma proteins are present in essentially normal amounts.

Proof that the abnormality is one of defective synthesis rather than excessively rapid breakdown of γ-globulin has been provided by experiments in which γ-globulin was administered parentally to these patients and its rate of disappearance from the plasma observed [24]. Its half-life was either the same or even somewhat longer than that obtaining in normal subjects.

It is probable, however, that the failure in γ-globulin synthesis is usually not quite complete. Gitlin [25], using rabbit and horse antisera against γ-globulin in the extremely sensitive quantitative precipitin reaction, was able to show that very small quantities of γ-globulin were often present, though usually these could not be detected electrophoretically with any certainty. In general less than 25 mg. per cent was found in the congenital cases, and less than 100 mg. per cent in the adult 'acquired' form of the disease. There is usually about 1 g. per cent present in the normal subject.

Furthermore, Gitlin, Hitzig and Janeway [26], using a combined electrophoretic and immunochemical method of analysis, have been able to demonstrate the absence in agammaglobulinaemic plasma of at least two proteins other than γ-globulins, which occur in small amounts in normal plasma and migrate with the β-globulins. The functional significance of these two β-globulins is not known, but they have no apparent antigenic relation to γ-globulins. It may be that they are formed in the same site as γ-globulins, and that the underlying lesion in agammaglobulinaemia leads to a failure in their synthesis in the same way as it results in the failure of synthesis of the quantitatively much more important γ-globulins.

Extensive investigations of antibody formation have been carried out in these patients [22]. These have included a search for circulating antibodies to antigens known commonly to stimulate normal people, and also for the so-called 'natural antibodies' such as the iso-agglutinins to the blood-group substances. Attempts have also been made to induce antibody formation directly by injection of a wide variety of potent bacterial and virus antigens, and also to stimulate the formation of agglutinins to heterologous blood-group substances by the injection of 'mismatched' red cells.

It has been established quite clearly that in all cases there is a profound immunological handicap. In some instances this appears to be complete and the term 'immunological paralysis' has been suggested to cover the situation. In other cases some indication of a very low degree of antibody formation could be obtained and this has been called 'immunological paresis'. The response here, however, was certainly far less than that encountered normally. Of particular interest is the fact that although it has been repeatedly observed clinically that the major hazard in these patients is derived from bacterial infection and that most virus infections tend to be handled efficiently and with no more than normal risks, nevertheless very little, if any, antibody response could be elicited after injection of potent preparations of a number of different virus antigens such as those for poliomyelitis, influenza and mumps. In general little or no circulating antibodies could be produced in response to the very wide variety of antigenic stimuli applied.

Another facet of the immunological disturbance has been illustrated by the demonstration that skin from unrelated individuals has been transplanted on to subjects with agammaglobulinaemia and the grafts have taken successfully [27]. Such homotransplantation of skin between two different individuals does not normally succeed unless the subjects are identical twins. The rejection of homotransplants by the body is thought to depend on an immunity reaction against foreign antigens in the grafted tissues. Presumably this immunological response is not called forth in agammaglobulinaemia.

It is now generally believed that antibody formation mainly occurs in the lymph nodes, the bone marrow and the spleen, and that in these tissues the plasma cell represents the main cell-type where antibody formation and γ-globulin synthesis take place. Good [28] found that the lymph nodes in agammaglobulinaemia tend to be small, poorly developed, and have a relatively thin cortex with few germinal centres. They are deficient in plasma cells, though all the other cell types present in lymph nodes from normal subjects may be found. Similarly there is a marked deficiency of plasma cells in bone marrow from these patients. The difference in plasma-cell formation in agammaglobulinaemia as compared with the normal was shown up even more strikingly after antigenic stimulation. In normal children injections of appropriate antigens led to marked plasma-cytosis in the regional lymph nodes and in the bone marrow. In agamma-globulinaemia virtually no plasma-cell response was obtained at all. The absence of γ-globulin in the blood is presumably a reflection of this underlying defect in plasma-cell formation in the tissues.

Nearly all examples of agammaglobulinaemia in infancy or child-hood have occurred in boys. Not infrequently more than one child in the same sibship has been found to have the disease [21], and in some instances it has turned up in male cousins who were the off-spring of two apparently normal sisters [29]. Furthermore, there has sometimes been a history that maternal uncles or the male children of maternal aunts have died in infancy from severe infections, and they might reasonably be presumed to have suffered from the same disease. This familial distribution has led to the suggestion that the abnormality is determined by a rare, sex-linked gene whose effects are not manifest in the female heterozygotes. It is however, possible that more than one genetically distinct type of congenital agamma-globulinaemia may occur. For example, the female infant described by Keidan and his colleagues [23], was the offspring of two healthy parents who were first cousins. Here it seems likely that the defect was determined by a rare autosomal gene in double dose, and it is perhaps significant that the clinical features in this case were atypical.

So far there is no evidence that the adult form of agammaglobulin-aemia is genetically determined.

Analbuminaemia

Analbuminaemia is perhaps the most remarkable and unexpected variant in plasma protein synthesis to be discovered. Despite the virtually complete failure to form serum albumin, the clinical consequences are extremely mild.

The condition was first identified [30] in a 31-year-old female farm worker who suffered from slight oedema of the joints. She was able to work in the fields but complained of tiring sooner than her fellow workers of the same age. In the course of investigating her family it was discovered that her brother had precisely the same anomaly in protein synthesis, though he felt completely normal, was able to do heavy work on the land and had never suffered from oedema.

In both cases no serum albumin could be detected by conventional electrophoresis (Table 41). The α_1, α_2, β- and γ-globulins, however, were present at concentrations one and a half to two times those normally found. Fibrinogen was present in normal amounts. The total plasma protein concentration was about 5 g. per cent.

Table 41. *Concentrations of different serum protein fractions in two patients with analbuminaemia and their parents.* (*After Bennhold* et al. 1954)

		Serum proteins (gm. %)				
			Globulins			
	Albumin	α_1	α_2	β	γ	Total
Father	3·3	0·4	0·7	0·8	1·1	6·3
Mother	3·0	0·6	0·5	0·9	1·4	6·4
Son	—	0·5	1·1	1·5	1·9	5·0
Daughter	—	0·6	1·1	1·6	1·8	5·1

The question as to whether the low albumin concentration was due to an extensive rate of destruction or to a genuine failure in synthesis was settled by infusing albumin into the patient and following its rate of disappearance. In fact the rate of destruction of the infused albumin was considerably slower than in normal subjects.

It is probable that the defect in albumin synthesis is not quite complete. Using sensitive immunochemical techniques it was possible to detect albumin in concentrations of about 1·6 mg. per cent which represents 1/2200 of the normal concentration [31]. This probably explains why albumin infusions given therapeutically and designed to correct the plasma protein balance, failed to result in antibody formation and allergic reactions.

The only other findings of note were an increased blood sedimentation rate, and a marked hypotension of the order of 90/55 mm. Hg. This low blood pressure no doubt plays an important part in restricting the degree of disturbance in water balance which would be expected, and in minimising oedema. It is probable, however, that other factors also come into play and these remain to be analysed in detail.

Extensive investigation of the family of these two sibs failed to reveal any further examples of the disorder[31]. The parents were second cousins, and this strongly suggests that the defect is determined by a rare 'recessive' gene. So far no other families have been described in which this abnormality occurs, and in view of the widespread use of paper electrophoresis in clinical medicine and the very obvious character of the anomaly, it is clear that the abnormal gene responsible must be extremely rare.

Caeruloplasmin and Wilson's disease

In 1948 Holmberg and Laurell[32] isolated from serum a blue-coloured copper-containing protein which they called caeruloplasmin. Caeruloplasmin occurs in normal human plasma in concentrations of about 30 mg. per cent so that it constitutes roughly 0·5 per cent of the total plasma proteins. It has a molecular weight of about 151,000, and there are eight atoms of copper per molecule. Electrophoretically it migrates as an α_2 globulin. *In vitro*, it has been shown to exhibit oxidase activity towards a variety of substrates which include paraphenyline diamine and benzidine[33]. Its function *in vivo*, however, is not known, and considerable interest was therefore aroused when in 1952 Scheinberg and Gitlin[34] discovered that patients with Wilson's disease, or hepato-lenticular degeneration, have substantially lower concentrations of caeruloplasmin in their serum than do normal people.

Wilson's disease was first described in 1912[35]. It is a rare inherited disorder characterised by a progressive degeneration of the lenticular nucleus in the brain and by cirrhosis of the liver. The clinical manifestations usually develop during adolescence or early adult life, but there is considerable variation in the rate of progression of the disease and the relative preponderance of symptoms referable on the one hand to the nervous system and on the other hand to the liver. One curious and characteristic feature of the condition is the Kayser-Fleischer ring, a brown or greyish green zone of pigmentation developing at the limbus of the cornea.

An extensive family investigation by Bearn [36] leaves little doubt that the disease is determined by a rare 'recessive' gene for which the affected patients are homozygous. A remarkably high incidence of parental consanguinity (about 35 per cent) was observed. The segregation ratio in the sibships containing affected individuals agreed reasonably well with the theoretical expectations provided appropriate allowance was made for the variable age of onset of the clinical manifestations, and for the fact that the sibships were selected by known cases. Bearn found that in about 80 per cent of his cases signs or symptoms of the disease had developed by the age of thirty. So far there is no evidence that the heterozygotes are in any way peculiar, but they have not yet been investigated very intensively biochemically.

In Wilson's disease the amount of caeruloplasmin present in the plasma is on the average about 25 per cent of that normally found [34, 35]. This reduced concentration can be reasonably attributed to a diminished rate of synthesis rather than to an excessive rate of destruction, although so far it has not been possible to determine directly the half-life of caeruloplasmin in normal subjects. Scheinberg [38] has calculated on the basis of an observed half-life of caeruloplasmin in patients with Wilson's disease of about four days, that if the decreased serum caeruloplasmin were due to increased destruction it would be necessary to postulate a half-life of caeruloplasmin in the normal of well over 100 days. The magnitude of such a half-life is sufficiently greater than the reported half-life of other plasma proteins to make it intrinsically unlikely. Other evidence has been provided by studies following the administration of radioactive copper. In normal subjects the plasma radioactivity declines rapidly for the first few hours but then begins to rise, and even at twenty-four hours has still not reached a plateau. This secondary rise in normal people is due to incorporation of the radioactive copper in caeruloplasmin. This has been shown by immunochemical precipitation and by electrophoresis. Patients with Wilson's disease show a slower fall in plasma radioactivity but this decline continues and virtually no secondary rise is observed [39, 40].

There is probably considerable variation in the degree of failure in caeruloplasmin formation from case to case, judging from the concentrations which have been reported as occurring in the plasma in different patients (Table 42). In general the concentration of caeruloplasmin found does not appear to be correlated with either the age of the patient or the duration or severity of the clinical manifestations of the disease.

Table 42. *Distribution of serum caeruloplasmin concentrations in normal subjects and patients with Wilson's disease. Caeruloplasmin estimated immunochemically. (Combined data of Scheinberg and Gitlin* (34), 1952, *and Markowitz* et al.(37), 1955)

Caeruloplasmin mg. %	Normal	Wilson's disease
0 –	—	5
5 –	—	8
10 –	—	5
15 –	—	4
20 –	1	—
25 –	2	—
30 –	7	—
35 –	6	—
40 –	—	—
Total	16	22
Mean caeruloplasmin	33·0	9·4

The most specific method for detecting caeruloplasmin is probably immunochemical. It remains possible, however, that the 'caeruloplasmin' synthesised in Wilson's disease is in some way qualitatively different from that formed normally even though it may behave similarly immunologically.

Plasma caeruloplasmin deficiency is not the only aspect of copper metabolism which is disturbed in Wilson's disease. It has been repeatedly observed that the liver, brain and a number of other tissues of such patients when examined at post-mortem have been found to contain grossly abnormal amounts of copper (41,42,43). The increase is of the order of tenfold that found in control material.

The total copper in the plasma is significantly less than in normal subjects (43). However, if this is subdivided into the so-called 'direct reacting' copper, which represents copper circulating in loose combination with albumin, and the 'indirectly reacting' copper, which represents the copper present in caeruloplasmin, it emerges that while the caeruloplasmin fraction is greatly reduced, the loosely bound copper is considerably more than is found in normal individuals (Table 43). The copper in the cerebrospinal fluid is also increased and this is mainly of the 'direct reacting' type. An increased excretion of copper in the urine also occurs.

The overall picture then is of a generalised accumulation of copper throughout the body, associated with a specific defect in the formation of the copper containing plasma protein caeruloplasmin.

Table 43. *Mean plasma copper concentration in normal subjects and patients with Wilson's disease. (After Cartwright* et al. *1954)*

	Plasma copper (μg. %)	
	Normal	Wilson's disease
'Direct reacting' copper fraction	8	26
'Indirect reacting' copper fraction	108	24
Total copper	116	50

Careful measurement of the copper intake and output in these patients suggests that, in spite of the somewhat increased excretion of copper in the urine, they are in a state of positive copper balance (43). This seems to be due to an increased absorption from the gastrointestinal tract rather than to a decreased excretion of copper, for example, in the bile. Normally only a proportion of copper ingested is actually absorbed. It appears that in Wilson's disease this fraction is increased.

A group of findings referable to abnormalities in renal tubular function have also been demonstrated in Wilson's disease (44). These are less constantly present and rather variable in expression. They are thought to be secondary consequences of the disorder in copper metabolism. Generalised aminoaciduria associated with an increased excretion of aminoacid conjugates and perhaps peptides is common. The plasma aminoacid levels are not elevated and the aminoaciduria is evidently due to defective renal tubular reabsorption (45). Defective tubular reabsorption of glucose, uric acid, and phosphate have also been observed. The increased clearance of phosphate may result in reduced concentrations of plasma inorganic phosphate and this perhaps explains the occasional reports of the development of osteomalacia and spontaneous fractures in the disease. In general the renal damage appears to become progressively more marked as the patient grows older and the disease advances.

There is as yet no theory of the pathogenesis of Wilson's disease which adequately explains all the many diverse features of the condition. One attractive hypothesis, originally suggested by Scheinberg and Gitlin (34) and subsequently developed by Cartwright and his colleagues (43), suggests that the fundamental abnormality produced by the presence of the abnormal gene in double dose is a failure in caeruloplasmin synthesis. This is thought in some way to result in increased absorption of copper from the gastro-intestinal tract, and in consequence the loosely bound copper circulating in the plasma is increased, and copper is deposited in excessive quantities in the tissues. The deposition of copper in grossly abnormal amounts in the liver and brain can be thought to cause the characteristic degenerative processes that take place there and lead to the clinical symptomatology. Presumably the increased copper absorption goes on from birth, but the clinical manifestations only appear when the accumulation has been sufficient to cause severe structural damage. This evidently may take ten or twenty years. Deposition of copper in the kidney is presumed to lead to renal tubular dysfunction of a not very specific type, so that the reabsorption of a number of different metabolites such as aminoacids, glucose, phosphate and uric acid becomes impaired.

The main difficulty here, of course, is to explain why a defect in caeruloplasmin synthesis should give rise to an increased rate of copper absorption from the gut. No satisfactory reason for this has been provided, although it can perhaps be imagined that the increase in copper absorption represents part of an attempt to make more caeruloplasmin under unfavourable conditions. It is also possible that some precursor of caeruloplasmin may accumulate.

Quite a different concept of the disease has been presented by Uzman and his colleagues (46). They attribute the accumulation of copper in the tissues to the formation of certain tissue proteins with an unusually high affinity for copper. The low caeruloplasmin synthesis is regarded as a secondary effect due to the diversion of the available copper to the abnormal tissue proteins with an unusually high avidity for it. Incomplete tissue metabolism of these abnormal proteins is thought to lead to the formation of polypeptide residues also with a high affinity for copper. It is suggested that these chelated peptides are excreted in the urine and produce a concomitant aminoaciduria by competition for tubular reabsorption. Although these workers have brought forward some evidence suggesting the occurrence in Wilson's disease of an unusual protein fraction with a high affinity for copper in the liver, many of the other features of this hypothesis are somewhat speculative.

Blood coagulation and afibrinogenaemia

Fibrinogen normally occurs in plasma in amounts of 0·25–0·50 g. per cent. It is a long rod-like molecule approximately 700×40 Å with a molecular weight of about 330,000. When blood coagulates fibrinogen is converted to fibrin, which has a molecular weight of about 5,000,000, is insoluble, and forms the matrix of the clot. The process requires the presence of the enzyme thrombin. Evidently thrombin acts by splitting off from each fibrinogen molecule a negatively charged peptide of molecular weight 4000 to 8000. This leaves a less negatively charged molecule which is capable of rapid polymerisation through a series of intermediate forms to produce the large fibrin molecule.

The active enzyme thrombin is formed from its precursor prothrombin in plasma when coagulation is due to occur, as a result of a complex series of reactions involving a number of separate factors, each of which is necessary for the whole process to be carried through efficiently. These factors include such substances as antihaemophilic globulin, christmas factor, factor VII, factor V and several others (see page 224). They appear to be proteins present only in trace amounts in normal plasma, and unlike fibrinogen cannot be readily detected by conventional electrophoretic or other physico-chemical techniques. Their presence or absence in a given plasma must be inferred from the results of addition experiments in suitably designed *in vitro* clotting systems (for a full account see Biggs and Macfarlane [47]).

A whole series of genetically distinct disorders of coagulation have now been recognised, each of which can be apparently attributed to a specific deficiency of one or another of these various plasma proteins which are necessary for normal coagulation.

Among these disorders is the rare condition afibrinogenaemia which is characterised by the specific failure to synthesise fibrinogen. Clinically the haemorrhagic disorder here is similar to that encountered in the other hereditary diseases of blood coagulation. The outstanding feature is a marked tendency to bleed following small and apparently trivial injuries; death in early life due to severe haemorrhage is not uncommon. Characteristically no fibrinogen can be detected in the plasma and the defect is highly specific. All the other factors known to be necessary for normal coagulation are present, and the liver where fibrinogen is thought to be synthesised appears in other respects to be metabolically normal. That the defect is one of failure in synthesis has been shown by studies in the rate of disappearance of infused fibrinogen [48]. The rate of disappearance was substantially the same as that found in normal individuals. The half life is of the order of four to five days.

There is little doubt that the affected individuals are homozygous for a rare abnormal gene. This is indicated by the extremely high incidence of parental consanguinity. Out of twenty families reported in the literature and reviewed by Frick and McQuarrie, the parents were first cousins in five cases, and second cousins in two [49]. The condition is not infrequently encountered in more than one member of the same sibship. The segregation is sharp and the other relatives are clinically normal.

The question arises as to whether any deviation from normality can be recognised in the heterozygotes. In certain families, but not in all, both parents and some of the other relatives appear to have had fibrinogen concentrations rather lower than those usually encountered in the general population [49, 50]. The interpretation is difficult because the variation in the general population has not been clearly defined and because differences in the methods of estimation used may influence the values obtained [50]. Nevertheless, it seems probable that among the heterozygotes the synthesis of fibrinogen proceeds on the average at a slightly lower rate than occurs in random normal subjects. The distribution of plasma fibrinogen concentrations among heterozygotes, while largely overlapping the distribution in normals, may be expected to have a somewhat lower mean value. In practice only a proportion of such heterozygotes can be expected to be detected confidently, and the levels of fibrinogen even here will still be adequate for normal clotting to take place.

Haemophilia and Christmas disease

Until recently the term haemophilia was thought to denote a single disease entity, determined by a rare sex-linked 'recessive' gene. Characteristically there occurred a marked tendency to bleeding following apparently trivial injury. The whole blood coagulation time could be shown to be prolonged and there was a diminished consumption of prothrombin. Small amounts of normal plasma added *in vitro* restored the coagulation time to normal, and it was thought that the coagulation defect was due to an imperfect production of plasma thromboplastin as a result of a deficiency of some precursor substance, generally referred to as anti-haemophilic globulin. The abnormally slow formation of thromboplastin was believed to result in an inefficient conversion of prothrombin to thrombin and hence to a prolongation of the whole blood coagulation time. Other components known to be necessary for normal coagulation to take place such as prothrombin, fibrinogen, factor v and platelets could be shown to be normal, and circulating anticoagulants were not, in general, found to be present.

The familial distribution was typically that of a rare sex-linked recessive character (see page 27). In some 30 per cent of cases, haemophilia occurred in individuals from families where no previous history of the disease could be obtained and a large proportion of such sporadic cases could be plausibly attributed to mutation.

It is now known that at least two distinct sex-linked conditions are included in the cases which were classically referred to as haemophilia (51,52). It has therefore become necessary to define each disorder more precisely in terms of the underlying defect in blood coagulation. In both groups of cases excessive bleeding appears to be a consequence of the absence, or relative deficiency in the activity, of a specific factor normally present in plasma and necessary for efficient blood coagulation to take place. These factors are probably proteins, normally present in only trace amounts. In general normal plasma will correct the delayed coagulation of both types of disorder, and plasma from each of them will correct the coagulation of the defect in the other.

In the majority of cases which in the past have been designated as haemophilia, the deficient factor is a substance which retains the name antihaemophilic globulin. This disease is either still referred to simply as haemophilia, or as haemophilia A. In the other cases the material which is lacking is called Christmas factor or plasma thromboplastin component, and the disorder is referred to variously as Christmas disease, P.T.C. deficiency and haemophilia B. A number of other terms have also been suggested to designate the two conditions, but so far no final agreement on terminology has been reached. In England about 12 per cent of cases of 'classical haemophilia' which have been re-examined turn out to be examples of Christmas disease (53). It is probable, however, that in other European countries the proportion is significantly higher (53).

Although neither anti-haemophilic globulin or Christmas factor have been isolated, certain differences in their physical properties and behaviour in coagulation have been established. Some of these differences are summarised in Table 44.

Table 44. *Some properties of anti-haemophilic globulin and Christmas factor. (After Pitney and Dacie (54), 1955)*

Property	Anti-haemophilic globulin	Christmas factor
Stability on storage	Unstable	Stable
Adsorption to inorganic adsorbants	Not adsorbed	Adsorbed
Ammonium sulphate fractionation	Precipitated by 25 per cent amm. sulph.	Precipitated by 33–50 per cent amm. sulph.
Electrophoretic fractionation	In fibrinogen fraction	In β-fraction

In most cases it has been found that anti-haemophilic globulin deficiency and Christmas disease tend to run true to type in individual families. It seems reasonable, therefore, to conclude that two different mutant genes are responsible for these conditions. Both, however, appear to be sex-linked, and the question therefore arises whether they are alleles or whether two different loci on the X chromosome are involved. Brinkhous and Graham (55) have argued that, in view of the quite striking differences in properties between the two factors, we are probably dealing with two distinct protein species, and since antihaemophilic globulin occurs in normal amounts in Christmas disease, and Christmas factor in normal amounts in anti-haemophilic globulin deficiency, then it is probable that two quite distinct and independent loci are concerned. No doubt linkage studies with a common sex-linked marker, such as red-green colour-blindness, will eventually help to elucidate this question further.

The nature of the defect produced by the abnormal gene in these conditions is still uncertain. In both instances a gross deficiency in activity of the appropriate coagulation factor is observed. It appears more probable that this is due to a defect in the synthesis of the protein concerned rather than to the formation of some specific kind of inhibitor of its activity. However, it is possible that the peculiarity may represent not a complete failure in protein synthesis *per se*, but the formation of a protein similar to that normally present though differing from it slightly in its detailed structure and hence in its ability to perform the role of its normal counterpart in blood coagulation. Evidence that this may be the situation with respect to anti-haemophilic globulin deficiency in haemophilia has been provided by experiments in which, using an antiserum prepared against purified anti-haemophilic globulin, it was possible to detect significant amounts of a protein cross-reacting with this in haemophilic plasmas which lacked any anti-haemophilic globulin activity (56). It is a plausible hypothesis that a structural abnormality in the globulin might result in a change in its functional activity but not necessarily interfere with its reactivity with an antiserum prepared against its normal homologue.

It has long been recognised that in haemophilia there exists a very wide variation in the clinical severity of the disease from patient to patient, though in any one patient the degree of severity of the haemorrhagic tendency appears to stay more or less the same. At one extreme, repeated haemarthrosis with severe crippling and deep tissue haemorrhages following little or no provocation are common. At the other extreme, haemarthrosis and deep tissue haemorrhage may be very infrequent or absent, and excessive bleeding only occurs following definite injury (47). In clinically severe haemophilia, anti-haemophilic globulin activity appears to be either completely or almost completely absent from the plasma. In mild haemophilia, however, appreciable amounts of anti-haemophilic globulin may be demonstrable (53, 57). In general the mild forms of haemophilia tend to run true to type in individual families (58, 59) and this supports the suggestion first put forward by Haldane (60) that mild haemophilia is determined by a gene different from that determining the severer type. It seems probable that the genetical situation is even more complex and it has been suggested that a whole series of allelic genes may occur at this locus and result in different degrees of synthesis of anti-haemophilic globulin and consequently in different degrees of severity of the clinical condition (57, 59). It should be mentioned that variation in clinical severity has also been noted in Christmas disease, and this too may have a similar genetical basis.

A number of attempts using a variety of different methods have been made to find a test which would detect unequivocally among the female relatives of haemophilics those who are actually carrying the abnormal gene. Earlier claims to have achieved this have not been confirmed. Merskey and Macfarlane (61), for example, found that although occasional abnormal results were obtained in the group of 'known heterozygous' females, the majority fell within the range encountered among normal individuals. It seems possible that although on the average there may be a slight diminution in anti-haemophilic globulin formation in the heterozygotes, the distribution of concentrations overlaps the distribution occurring in normals very considerably, and the tests that have been used have little discriminative value.

Most of the heterozygotes tested appear to have been from families where the type of haemophilia segregating was of a severe or at least moderately severe type. In marked contrast to these findings are the results obtained by Graham and his colleagues (59) in the detailed investigation of a large family in which the type of haemophilia segregating in the males was extremely mild. Paradoxically, in this family a high proportion of the female heterozygotes tested had quite significantly low concentrations of antihaemophilic globulin in their plasma. On the average the concentration of anti-haemophilic globulin was found to be about 20 per cent of normal in the affected males, and about 50 per cent of normal in the heterozygous females. Using the same technique these workers failed to find any abnormality in a small series of heterozygous females from families in which severe haemophilia was segregating. It thus appeared that a gene responsible for mild haemophilia in the male produces a more profound effect in the female heterozygote than a gene responsible for the severe form of the disease.

So far, detailed studies of the female heterozygote in Christmas disease have not been published, but preliminary reports suggest that some deviation from the normal may occur (53).

Other coagulation defects

It has been recognised for many years that a number of inherited haemorrhagic disorders due apparently to some defect in the coagulation system occurred which could not be attributed to the effects of sex-linked genes. In the particular families in which they were found both females and males might be affected, and the familial distribution was not what would be expected assuming sex linkage.

Unusual variants have also been recognised as a result of peculiarities in the clotting tests which made it clear that they did not correspond to any of the previously identified types. In principle the argument involved in such investigations is the following one. When an individual is found to have a defect in blood coagulation, but the addition of his plasma or serum will correct the abnormality in coagulation in all other known types of clotting defect, and in turn the clotting defect in the patient is corrected by the addition of plasma or serum from each of the other types of recognised conditions, it is assumed that the patient's abnormality represents a new and previously undifferentiated clotting disorder. Furthermore, it is usually inferred that plasma from normal people contains a previously unrecognised factor necessary for blood coagulation to go on efficiently, and which is deficient in this new disease. This conclusion then leads to an attempt to define the role that the new factor plays in normal blood coagulation, to characterise its properties, and if possible to isolate it and study its chemistry.

A variety of new haemorrhagic disorders have now been discovered in this way. These include Owren's disease (parahaemophilia, factor v deficiency, Ac. globulin deficiency)[62], plasma thromboplastin antecedent deficiency[63], Hageman disease[64], factor VII (serum prothrombin conversion accelerator) deficiency[65], Stuart clotting disease[66], and a number of less clearly defined peculiarities. The role of the various factors in normal blood coagulation is still only incompletely understood[47], and only a little is known about their properties and chemical nature.

Most of the deficiencies of these various factors may evidently be genetically determined, and in some instances quite extensive family studies have been carried out. Where these have been combined with quantitative assays of the factor involved the results have been particularly rewarding. For example, the studies of the inheritance of factor v deficiency by Kingsley[67], and the analogous work on the Stuart factor deficiency by Graham and his colleagues[68], provide strong evidence for the view that in each case a single autosomal mutant gene is concerned. Individuals homozygous for the particular gene have a complete deficiency of the appropriate factor, while in heterozygotes a partial deficiency is produced (Fig. 58). In each of these cases the heterozygotes appear to have on the average about 50 per cent of the normal amounts of the factor, but they are extremely variable from one to another. Thus Kingsley observed values in these individuals as low as 24 per cent of the normal and as high as 68 per cent. While in most instances the heterozygotes appear to suffer from no ill-effects, the variation is such that the occasional heterozygotes may have sufficiently low a concentration of the factor present as to lead to overt haemorrhagic disturbances. In other heterozygotes the concentration of the factor may be so high as to fall within the limits of normal variability. Consequently not all the heterozygotes may be distinguishable unequivocably by the available methods.

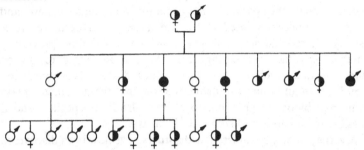

Fig. 58. Distribution of factor v activity in a family. (After Kingsley.) ○, normal factor v activity; ◑, partial factor v deficiency; ●, total factor v deficiency.

Serum cholinesterase variants

Attention was first directed to the occurrence of inherited differences in serum cholinesterase (pseudocholinesterase) formation, by the observation that certain individuals were unduly sensitive to suxamethonium, a muscle relaxant often used in anaesthesia. Many of these sensitive individuals have a low level of serum cholinesterase activity, and Lehmann and Ryan [69] found that a similar peculiarity not infrequently occurred among some of their immediate relatives who were otherwise healthy. Normally the effects of suxamethonium are limited because it is broken down by serum cholinesterase. These individuals with low serum cholinesterase activity evidently do not destroy it at the normal rate and are liable to develop a prolonged apnoea when it is administered in the usual doses.

Kalow and his colleagues [70,71,72] have examined the properties of the enzyme which is present in such suxamethonium-sensitive individuals, and have found that it differs markedly from that present in normal individuals in the degree to which its activity can be inhibited by the anti-cholinesterase substance dibucaine (percaine). Under standard conditions dibucaine produced about 79 per cent inhibition of the enzyme activity in normal subjects whereas in suxamethonium-sensitive individuals only about 16 per cent inhibition was obtained. They refer to the percentage inhibition with dibucaine as the dibucaine number (DN). They believe that the unusual DN in suxamethonium-sensitive individuals is part of an atypical pattern of substrate specificity and inhibition characteristics of the serum cholinesterase which is present, and suggest that this is due to the synthesis of an enzyme protein differing structurally in some way from that synthesised by most people. Thus the peculiarity which gives rise to suxamethonium sensitivity is attributed not to the formation of normal cholinesterase in smaller amounts than normal, but to the formation of a distinct enzyme protein with rather different catalytic properties from that of its normal counterpart.

Kalow and Staron[72] found that the distribution of dibucaine numbers in individuals in the general population was trimodal. Most individuals gave values clustering round a mode of about DN = 79. There was a second group (about 3 per cent of the population) clustering round a mode of about DN = 62, and also a third, rare, group with values of about DN = 16. People in this rare group probably occur with a frequency of the order of 1 in 1000 to 1 in 5000 of the population and it is to this group which individuals identified because of excessive sensitivity to suxamethonium belong. On the average the intermediate group gave somewhat lower values of total serum cholinesterase activity in the absence of inhibitor than did the main group, and the rare group showed still lower activity. However, it was not possible to discriminate sharply between the three groups on this basis alone because the distributions overlapped very considerably.

Family studies show that the three cholinesterase phenotypes defined by the dibucaine inhibition test are genetically determined. The simplest hypothesis is that there are two allelic genes. Individuals with DNs around 79 are homozygous for one of these, and those with DNs around 16 are homozygous for the other. The intermediate phenotype (DN around 62) would represent the heterozygotes. If this is so the gene frequency of the less common allele in the Canadian population studied by Kalow and Staron would be about 0·014. It is of interest that it can be calculated that if the two types of homozygote each form a structurally distinct enzyme protein with characteristic properties then the mean dibucaine number and the average total cholinesterase activity in the presumed heterozygotes correspond to what would be expected in a 50:50 mixture of the two enzyme proteins.

Most of the family data so far collected can be satisfactorily explained in this way (Fig. 59). However, at least one individual with

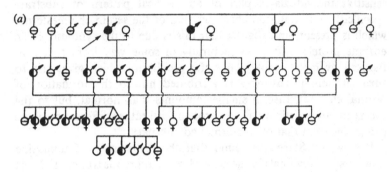

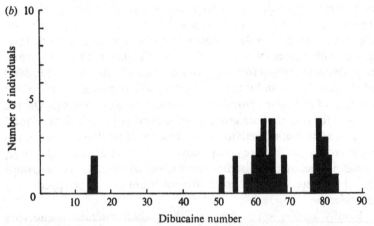

Fig. 59 (a) Segregation of usual, intermediate, and atypical serum cholinesterase dibucaine numbers in a family. (b) Distribution of the dibucaine numbers in the individuals in this family. (After Kalow and Staron[72].) ⊖, not tested; ◯, usual dibucaine number (71–85); ◑, intermediate dibucaine number (50–70); ●, atypical dibucaine number (10–20).

a very low DN (17·8) has been observed among the offspring of a mating where only the father was of the intermediate phenotype. This suggests that the situation can be more complex and that possibly more than two alleles occur.

REFERENCES

(1) Smithies, O. (1955). *Biochem. J.* **61**, 629.
(2) Smithies, O. and Walker, N. F. (1956). *Nature, Lond.* **178**, 694.
(3) Poulik, M. D. and Smithies, O. (1958). *Biochem. J.* **68**, 636.
(4) Poulik, M. D. (1957). *Nature, Lond.* **180**, 1477.
(5) Jayle, M. F. and Boussier, G. (1955). *Exp. Ann. Biochim. Med.* **17**, 157.
(6) Moretti, J., Boussier, G. and Jayle, M. F. (1957). *Bull. Soc. Chim. biol., Paris,* **39**, 593.
(7) Laurell, C. B. and Nyman, M. (1957). *Blood,* **12**, 493.
(8) Allison, A. C. and ap Rees, W. (1957). *Brit. Med. J.* **2**, 1137.
(9) Galatius-Jensen, F. (1957). *Acta Genet.* **7**, 549.
(10) Allison, A. C., Blumberg, B. S. and ap Rees, W. (1958). *Nature, Lond.* **181**, 824.
(11) Smithies, O. and Walker, N. F. (1955). *Nature, Lond.* **176**, 1265.
(12) Harris, H., Robson, E. B. and Siniscalco, M. (1958). *Nature, Lond.* **182**, 1324.
(13) Sutton, H. E., Neel, J. V., Binson, G. and Zuelzer, W. W. (1956). *Nature, Lond.* **178**, 1287.
(14) Smithies, O. (1957). *Nature, Lond.* **180**, 1482.
(15) Smithies, O. (1958). *Nature, Lond.* **181**, 1204.
(16) Horsfall, W. R. and Smithies, O. (1958). *Science,* **128**, 35.
(17) Harris, H., Robson, E. B. and Siniscalco, M. (1958). *Nature, Lond.* **182**, 452.
(18) Grubb, R. (1956). *Acta path. microbiol. scand.* **39**, 195.
(19) Grubb, R. and Laurell, A. B. (1956). *Acta path. microbiol. scand.* **39**, 390.
(20) Bruton, O. C. (1952). *Pediatrics,* **9**, 722.
(21) Janeway, C. A., Apt, L. and Gitlin, D. (1953). *Trans. Ass. Amer. Phycns,* **66**, 200.
(22) Good, R. A. and Varco, R. L. (1955). *Jnl-Lancet,* **75**, 245.
(23) Keidan, S. E., McCarthy, K. and Haworth, J. C. (1953). *Arch. Dis. Child.* **28**, 110.
(24) Gitlin, D. (1957). *Pediatrics,* **19**, 657.
(25) Gitlin, D. (1955). *Bull. N.Y. Acad. Med.* **31**, 359.
(26) Gitlin, D., Hitzig, W. H. and Janeway, C. A. (1956). *J. Clin. Invest.* **35**, 1199.
(27) Varco, R. L., MacLean, L. D., Aust, J. B. and Good, R. A. (1955). *Ann. Surg.* **142**, 334.
(28) Good, R. A. (1955). *J. Lab. Clin. Med.* **46**, 167.
(29) Porter, H. M. (1957). *Pediatrics,* **20**, 958.
(30) Bennhold, H., Peters, H. and Roth, E. (1954). *Verh. dtsch. Ges. inn. Med.* **60**, 630.
(31) Bennhold, H. (1956). *Verh. dtsch. Ges. inn. Med.* **62**, 658.
(32) Holmberg, C. G. and Laurell, C. B. (1948). *Acta chem. scand.* **2**, 550.
(33) Holmberg, C. G. and Laurell, C. B. (1951). *Scand. J. Clin. Lab. Invest.* **3**, 103.

(34) Scheinberg, I. H. and Gitlin, D. (1952). *Science*, **116**, 484.

(35) Wilson, S. A. K. (1912). *Brain*, **34**, 295.

(36) Bearn, A. G. (1953). *Amer. J. Med.* **15**, 442.

(37) Markowitz, H., Gubler, C. J., Mahoney, J. P., Cartwright, G. E. and Wintrobe, M. M. (1955). *J. Clin. Invest.* **34**, 1498.

(38) Scheinberg, I. H. Quoted in Bearn, A. G. (1957). *Amer. J. Med.* **22**, 747.

(39) Bush, J. A., Mahoney, J. P., Markowitz, H., Gubler, C. J., Cartwright, G. E. and Wintrobe, M. M. (1955). *J. Clin. Invest.* **34**, 1766.

(40) Bearn, A. G. and Kunkel, H. G. (1955). *J. Lab. Clin. Med.* **45**, 623.

(41) Glazebrook, A. J. (1945). *Edinb. Med. J.* **52**, 83.

(42) Cummings, J. N. (1948). *Brain*, **71**, 410.

(43) Cartwright, G. E., Hodges, R. E., Gubler, C. J., Mahoney, J. P., Daum, K., Wintrobe, M. M., Bean, W. B. (1954). *J. Clin. Invest.* **33**, 1487.

(44) Bearn, A. G., Yu, T. F. and Gutman, A. B. (1957). *J. Clin. Invest.* **36**, 1107.

(45) Stein, W. H., Bearn, A. G. and Moore, S. (1954). *J. Clin. Invest.* **33**, 410.

(46) Uzman, L. L., Iber, F. L., Chalmers, T. C. and Knowlton, M. (1956). *Amer. J. Med. Sci.* **231**, 511.

(47) Biggs, R. and Macfarlane, R. G. (1957). *Human Blood Coagulation and its Disorders*, 2nd ed. Blackwell, Oxford.

(48) Gitlin, D. and Borges, W. H. (1953). *Blood*, **8**, 679.

(49) Frick, P. G. and McQuarrie, I. (1954). *Pediatrics*, **13**, 44.

(50) Graham, J. B. (1956). *Amer. J. Hum. Gen.* **8**, 63.

(51) Biggs, R., Douglas, A. S., Macfarlane, R. G., Dacie, J. V., Pitney, W. R., Merskey, C. and O'Brien, J. R. (1952). *Brit. Med. J.* **2**, 1378.

(52) Aggeler, P. M., White, S. G., Glendenning, M. B., Page, E. W., Leake, T. B. and Bates, G. (1952). *Proc. Soc. Exp. Biol., N.Y.* **79**, 692.

(53) Biggs, R. and Macfarlane, R. G. (1958). *Brit. J. Haemat.* **4**, 1.

(54) Pitney, W. R. and Dacie, J. V. (1955). *Brit. Med. Bull.* **11**, 11.

(55) Graham, J. B. and Brinkhous, K. M. (1953). *Brit. Med. J.* **2**, 97.

(56) Shanberge, J. N. and Gore, I. (1957). *J. Lab. Clin. Med.* **50**, 954.

(57) Brinkhous, K. M., Langdell, R. D., Penick, G. D., Graham, J. B. and Wagner, R. H. (1954). *J. Amer. Med. Ass.* **154**, 481.

(58) Merskey, C. (1951). *Brit. Med. J.* **1**, 906.

(59) Graham, J. B., McLendon, W. W. and Brinkhous, K. M. (1953). *Amer. J. Med. Sci.* **225**, 46.

(60) Haldane, J. B. S. (1935). *J. Genet.* **31**, 317.

(61) Merskey, C. and Macfarlane, R. G. (1951). *Lancet*, **1**, 487.

(62) Owren, P. A. (1947). *Lancet*, **1**, 446.

(63) Rosenthal, R. L., Dreskin, O. H. and Rosenthal, N. (1953). *Proc. Soc. Exp. Biol., N.Y.* **82**, 171.

(64) Ratnoff, O. D. and Calopy, J. E. (1955). *J. Clin. Invest.* **34**, 602.

(65) Alexander, B., Goldstein, R., Landwehr, G. and Cook, C. D. (1951). *J. Clin. Invest.* **30**, 596.

(66) Hougie, C., Barrow, E. M. and Graham, J. B. (1957). *J. Clin. Invest.* **36**, 485.

(67) Kingsley, C. S. (1954). *Quart. J. Med.* N.S. **23**, 232.

(68) Graham, J. B., Barrow, E. M. and Hougie, C. (1957). *J. Clin. Invest.* **36**, 497.

(69) Lehmann, H. and Ryan, E. (1956). *Lancet,* **2**, 124.

(70) Kalow, W. and Genest, K. (1957). *Canad. J. Biochem. Physiol.* **35**, 339.

(71) Kalow, W. and Gunn, D. R. (1957). *J. Pharmacol.* **120**, 203.

(72) Kalow, W. and Staron, N. (1957). *Canad. J. Biochem. Physiol.* **35**, 1305.

CHAPTER 9

SOME MISCELLANEOUS INHERITED DISORDERS OF METABOLISM

The biosynthesis of haem and the porphyrias

The porphyrias are a group of metabolic abnormalities characterised by the excretion in abnormal quantities of substances which are either precursors or by-products in the biosynthetic pathways leading to the formation of haem. Haem is the prosthetic group of a number

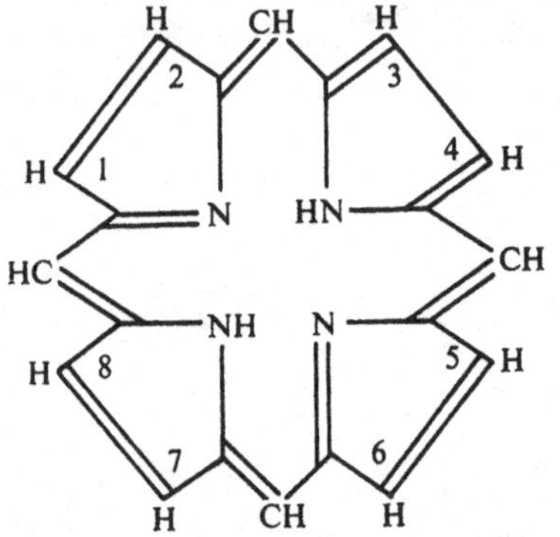

Substituents in the various positions of the porphyrin ring

Compound Position	1	2	3	4	5	6	7	8
Protoporphyrin IX	M	V	M	V	M	P	P	M
Coproporphyrin III	M	P	M	P	M	P	P	M
Uroporphyrin III	A	P	A	P	A	P	P	A
Coproporphyrin I	M	P	M	P	M	P	M	P
Uroporphyrin I	A	P	A	P	A	P	A	P

$M = —CH_3$; $V = —CH:CH_2$; $A = —CH_2COOH$; $P = —CH_2CH_2COOH$.

Fig. 60. Structures of various porphyrins.

of functionally important proteins which include haemoglobin, myoglobin, the cytochromes, and catalase. It seems to be the protein moiety of these substances which determines their characteristic functional properties. The haem is in nearly all cases the same, an iron complex of protoporphyrin. The particular isomer of protoporphyrin which forms the basis of haem is protoporphyrin IX. Its structure and also those of a number of other naturally occurring porphyrins are shown in Fig. 60.

During recent years considerable progress has been made in determining the biosynthetic pathways involved in the formation of haem [1] and the development of the subject has been very rapid. Two important landmarks were the discovery by Shemin and Rittenberg in 1945 [2] that the aminoacid glycine was specifically utilised in haem formation, and the isolation by Westall in 1952 [3] of porphobilinogen from the urine of a patient with acute porphyria. The structure of porphobilinogen was determined by Cookson and Rimington [4] and it was subsequently shown that this substance occupied a key position in the process of haem synthesis.

The sequence of events leading to the formation of porphobilinogen is believed to follow pathways indicated in Fig. 61 [1]. Glycine and an active form of succinate (possibly succinyl coenzyme A) appear to be the main precursors. δ-Aminolaevulic acid is an intermediate and the enzymic condensation of two molecules of this material gives rise to porphobilinogen.

Four molecules of porphobilinogen then go into the formation of haem. The precise sequence of reactions which takes place here is, however, not yet clearly elucidated. Rimington [1] has suggested the scheme shown in Fig. 62, where X denotes the intermediate and the number in front of it indicates the number of side chains with a carboxyl group that it possesses. Condensation of four molecules of porphobilinogen followed by stepwise decarboxylation and finally dehydrogenation and iron incorporation could lead to the formation of the haem. The X intermediates may be porphyrinogens, the reduced forms of the respective porphyrins. The porphyrins of the III isomeric series are thought to be derived from the intermediates in the manner indicated. It is thought that the pathway leading to the formation of the series I isomers may differ in that the free porphyrins themselves may lie on it. This is a very minor pathway in normal metabolism and cannot lead to haem formation.

Congenital porphyria

Congenital porphyria is a rare disorder characterised by severe photosensitivity beginning at or soon after birth and persisting throughout life. Exposure to sunlight results in erythema, bulla formation, and ulceration of the skin. Severe scarring and deformities may ensue.

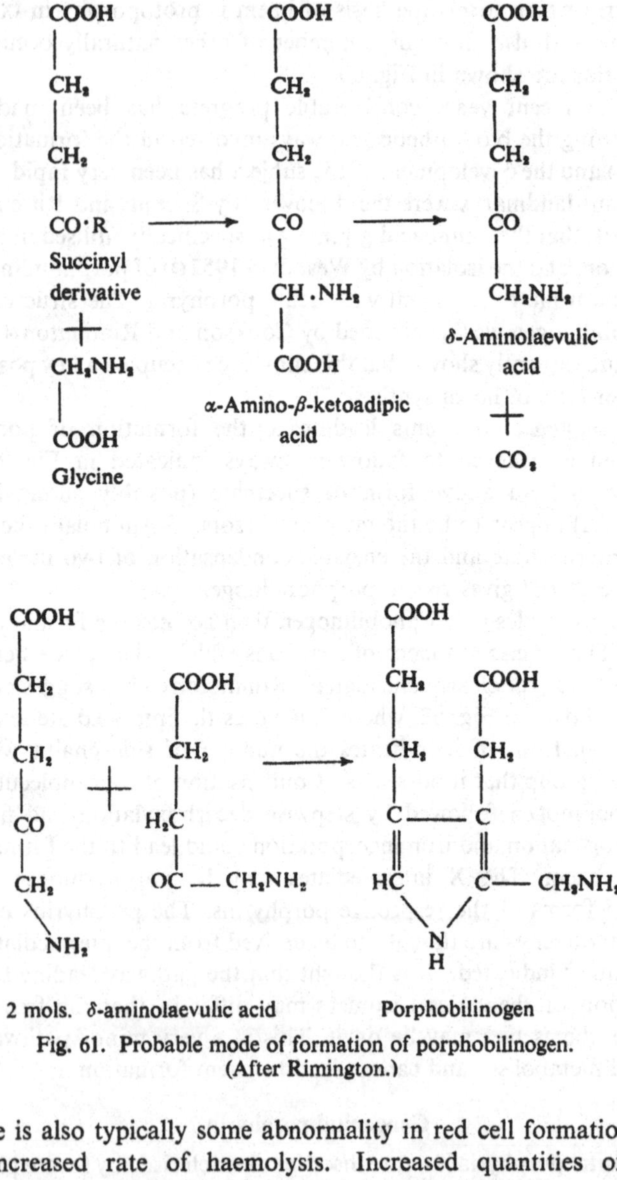

Fig. 61. Probable mode of formation of porphobilinogen.
(After Rimington.)

There is also typically some abnormality in red cell formation and an increased rate of haemolysis. Increased quantities of free porphyrins are formed, probably mainly in the bone marrow. These became distributed throughout the body and are particularly marked in the bones and teeth which are pigmented and show a characteristic red fluorescence in ultra-violet light. There is an increase in circulating porphyrins and a greatly elevated excretion of these substances in the urine. Typically the urine has a red colour due to the excessive amounts of porphyrins present.

The porphyrins formed in abnormal quantities in this disorder are predominantly, though possibly not exclusively, series I isomers. The urine contains uroporphyrin I (eight carboxyls) and coproporphyrin I (four carboxyls) in large amounts, and smaller quantities of other porphyrins with seven, six, and five carboxyl groups have also been detected (5, 6). There is, however, no abnormal excretion of porphobilinogen.

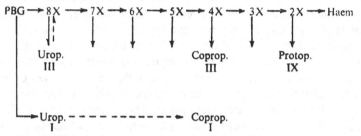

Fig. 62. Hypothetical scheme for the formation of haem from porphobilinogen (PBG). (After Rimington.)

Many of the features of congenital porphyria can be explained if it is assumed that there is some genetically determined abnormality in the enzymic conversion of porphobilinogen to types I and III porphyrins or porphyrinogens. Normally this process results in a great preponderance of type III isomers, and these are the precursors of haem. Type I isomers are usually only formed in very small amounts and seem to play no important part in normal metabolism. In congenital porphyria there seems to be a major defect in the balance of these two alternative pathways open to porphobilinogen, and considerably greater quantities than usual are deviated into the formation of type I porphyrins (6). These cannot be converted into haem or utilised in any other way. They accumulate in the body and are excreted in large amounts in the urine and the bile.

The photosensitive reactions are evidently caused by the presence of these porphyrins in the skin. The haemolytic tendency may be due to photosensitivity of red cells which contain abnormal amounts of porphyrin.

The excessive formation of porphyrins in this condition is believed
to occur mainly in the bone marrow. Schmid, Schwartz and Sundberg [7] examined marrow cells from such patients, using fluorescent
and absorption microscopy. They found that two distinct lines of red
cell precursors appeared to exist. In one line excessive quantities of
porphyrin were revealed in the normoblastic nucleus. In the other
line the normoblasts appeared to be quite normal. They thought that
the abnormal normoblasts formed excessive quantities of porphyrin
in their nuclei and that this might be released into the plasma during
red cell maturation. The apparent localisation of the metabolic error
to some but not other red cell precursors is a curious and somewhat
unexpected result. There is as yet no satisfactory explanation for it.

Another peculiar metabolic feature which has been observed in
congenital porphyria concerns the unusual pattern of stercobilin
formation. Stercobilin is the end-product of the breakdown of haem.
When ^{15}N-labelled glycine is fed to normal subjects and the ^{15}N
appearing in the excreted stercobilin is followed over a period of
time, a characteristic pattern of excretion of labelled stercobilin is
observed [8]. There are two main peaks. The major one occurs after
about 120 days and is attributable to the breakdown of haemoglobin
from erythrocytes after their normal life span. The other peak occurs
shortly after the administration of the labelled glycine. Its source is
not known with any certainty. but it may be derived from haem
synthesised in excess of globin and therefore not used in haemoglobin
formation. In one case of congenital porphyria investigated in this
way the pattern of appearance of ^{15}N-labelled stercobilin was found
to be quite different. The first peak was greatly exaggerated and the
second peak was relatively very much smaller than normal. Thus
a large part of the stercobilin must have been formed by some very
rapid process. The stercobilin was found to be the same as that
excreted normally and it could not have been derived from derivatives
of type I porphyrins. The precise explanation of this phenomenon is
at present quite obscure, and it is not at all clear how it is related to
the other pathological processes occurring in the disease.

The characteristic photosensitivity of congenital porphyria is
generally clinically manifest in the first few years of life. In the past
the disorder was confused with other forms of porphyria resulting in
photosensitivity developing later in life. These are now referred to
as porphyria cutanea tarda and evidently are metabolically and
genetically quite distinct. Congenital porphyria is probably much

less common than any of these other conditions. It occurs about equally frequently in the two sexes, and among the examples of the disorder recorded, an appreciable proportion have been familial. No systematic genetical studies have been carried out, but it is generally assumed that the disease is determined by a rare abnormal gene. The affected individuals are thought to be homozygous and as yet there is no indication of any metabolic abnormality occurring in the presumed heterozygotes. In a review of some thirty-four authentic reports of the condition, Schmid and his colleagues [7] found only one case in which parental consanguinity had been noted. This seems to be rather too low a proportion for such an extremely rare condition if the affected individuals are indeed homozygotes. Perhaps the possibility of parental consanguinity was not specifically inquired after in the majority of cases.

No example of both a parent and a child being affected has been recorded. In one instance an infant born of a mother with congenital porphyria was found to have unusual concentrations of porphyrins in the blood, urine, and meconium immediately after birth [9]. These disappeared within a few days and can probably be attributed to the transplacental passage of porphyrins from the mother to the foetus. The baby was subsequently quite normal.

Acute intermittent porphyria

The outstanding clinical features of acute intermittent porphyria are periodic attacks of peculiarly severe intestinal colic associated with neurological disorders which result in irregularly distributed though often widespread muscular paralyses, and mental disturbances. The attacks are often variable in character and either the abdominal or the neurological features of the condition may predominate. The attacks do not usually occur until adult life. There is no photo-sensitivity [10].

At post-mortem multiple patchy areas of demyelination have been observed, particularly in the peripheral motor nerves, but also to some extent in the central nervous system. It has been suggested that most of the clinical manifestations may be explicable in terms of widespread but rather irregular areas of acute nerve damage [11].

The characteristic biochemical finding in acute porphyria is the excretion in grossly abnormal amounts of porphobilinogen. An increased excretion of δ-aminolaevulic acid has also been observed and this is also probably typical of the disorder [12]. Most of the free porphyrins, however, which have at various times been reported in the urine of such patients were probably mainly formed secondarily from excreted porphobilinogen.

Porphobilinogen is generally not found in the urine of children before puberty even though they may subsequently go on to have attacks of acute porphyria with considerable porphobilinogen excretion [13]. In adults in remissions between attacks the porphobilinogen excretion usually persists though generally at a much reduced level. Adults may also be found who are excreting porphobilinogen but have not yet suffered an acute attack. They are presumably predisposed to do so and are said to have latent porphyria. They have usually been encountered among apparently healthy relatives of known cases [10]. On the other hand, in some instances it has apparently not been possible to detect increased porphobilinogen excretion in individuals known to have had typical acute attacks of the disease but who are at the time in a state of remission.

Porphobilinogen is regularly found in the liver of these patients at post-mortem [14]. Its concentration in the blood plasma is usually rather low, even when considerable amounts are being excreted in the urine. It is thought probable that most of the excess of porphobilinogen is formed in the liver, and that when the material is released into the circulation it is rapidly cleared by the kidneys [15]. There is little or no abnormal porphyrin formation in the tissues and this presumably explains the absence of photosensitivity.

The cause of this excessive accumulation of porphobilinogen is not known. There is no indication that there is any block in its subsequent conversion to haem and it seems more likely that it is being formed in excess of normal requirements for haem synthesis. This could be due to a defect in the further metabolism of δ-aminolaevulic acid along some other pathway, with its consequent accumulation and an increased formation of porphobilinogen, or alternatively there may be some abnormality of succinate glycine metabolism leading to an increased production of δ-aminolaevulic acid.

The cause of the neurological and other clinical manifestations of the disease is still quite obscure. Neither porphobilinogen or δ-aminolaevulic acid have any obvious pharmacological effects which might account for them [16, 17].

The acute attacks of the disease are often said to be precipitated or accentuated by the administration of barbiturate drugs. It is of interest, therefore, that some barbiturates have been shown to produce a form of porphyria when given experimentally to animals (18). The exact manner in which these drugs exert their effects, however, is not known.

Most of our knowledge of the genetics of acute porphyria is based on the extensive work of Waldenström in Sweden (10,13,19). He has studied over a long period a large number of families in which the abnormality was found to be segregating. The disease was frequently found in several generations of the same family, and was, in general, transmitted by an affected individual to a proportion of his or her offspring. There seems little doubt that the affected patients are heterozygous for a rare gene which in some way leads to an abnormality in δ-aminolaevulic acid and porphobilinogen metabolism. Such heterozygotes can in most cases be identified by the fact that in adult life they excrete porphobilinogen in greater or lesser amounts more or less continuously. Testing for porphobilinogen is, however, of little value in detecting such individuals in childhood, and may also fail to detect known heterozygotes in adult life. This accounts for occasional irregularities and 'skipping' of generations in the pedigrees.

The heterozygotes for this gene are predisposed to the development of acute attacks of the disease. The nature of the precipitating factor which induces these acute episodes is, however, not understood. Waldenström found the proportion of female to male cases to be about three to two in a series of more than 300 (10). This may indicate that females are somewhat more severely affected and are therefore more likely to be picked up. So far no report of an individual who might be regarded as homozygous for the abnormal gene has appeared.

Porphyria cutanea tarda

Probably several different metabolic disorders, not all of which are genetically determined, have been described under the name porphyria cutanea tarda (10). These conditions appear in general to exhibit clinical features resembling, in certain respects, those found both in congenital porphyria and also in acute intermittent porphyria. They seem, however, to be distinct both biochemically and genetically from either of these disorders.

In one group of cases an abnormal excretion of porphyrins both in the faeces and urine is associated with skin lesions developing in early adult life and attacks of abdominal colic. The skin lesions occur mainly on the exposed areas, and there may be obvious photo-sensitivity. Neurological disturbances are not common. When they do occur they tend to be milder than in acute porphyria. The clinical manifestations are variable and intermittent, and in the more acute phases there is often evidence of some degree of hepatic dysfunction.

Rimington and his colleagues [20,21] have drawn attention to a curious feature of this disorder, which they believe to be characteristic. During the phases of the disease when photosensitivity and abdominal colic occur, the urinary excretion of porphyrins is considerable. In clinical remission, however, the faecal porphyrins are greatly in-creased and the urinary porphyrins are reduced and are often within normal limits. In the urine it is mainly uroporphyrin and copro-porphyrin which are found in abnormal amounts, though a whole series of other porphyrins with seven, five, three and two carboxyl groups have also been detected in smaller quantities [6]. Porpho-bilinogen is generally absent, except possibly in the terminal stages of the disease. In the faeces it is mainly protoporphyrin and copro-porphyrin which are excreted in abnormal quantities. There is clearly a major disturbance in porphyrin metabolism which is quite unlike that found either in congenital or acute intermittent porphyria. Its nature, however, is quite obscure. It seems that the episodes of photosensitivity and other clinical manifestations are related to disturbances of liver function, which result in a failure to excrete the abnormal porphyrins being formed, into the faeces. They, therefore, accumulate, appear in the circulation, and are excreted in the urine.

The disorder is familial but probably a large proportion of affected individuals exhibit few obvious clinical signs or symptoms of the disease. The detection of predisposed individuals who are asympto-matic requires the analysis of faecal as well as of urinary porphyrins and this makes family studies somewhat inconvenient. However, in one large family investigated by Holti and his colleagues [22] (Fig. 63), nine individuals in several different generations were found to have an abnormal faecal porphyrin excretion. In all but the initial case, who was the most severely affected clinically, no abnormal urinary porphyrin excretion was detected.

What may be another form of porphyria, in which photosensitivity associated in various degrees with manifestations typical of acute intermittent porphyria, has been described in a large family occurring in South Africa [23]. This form of condition is said to be the com-monest type of porphyria encountered among Europeans in South

Africa (24). Its relation to other forms of porphyria is uncertain. The familial distribution suggests that the affected individuals are heterozygous for a rare abnormal gene.

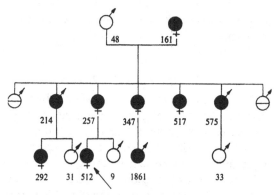

Fig. 63. Porphyria cutanea tarda. Faecal porphyrin excretion in part of a family described by Holti *et al.* Numbers=faecal porphyrins μg./g. dry weight. O, normal porphyrins; ●, raised faecal porphyrins; ⊖, not tested.

Hereditary coproporphyria

The excretion of large amounts of coproporphin III both in the faeces and urine, in the absence of any symptoms typical of other types of porphyria, probably represents another genetically distinct form of abnormal porphyrin metabolism. Berger and Goldberg (25) described a family in which a child aged ten was excreting very large quantities of coproporphyrin, and where both parents and also a paternal aunt excreted moderately increased but quite abnormal amounts of this substance (Table 45). The parents were first cousins. It seems likely that the parents and the affected aunt were heterozygous for a rare gene for which the child was homozygous.

Table 45. *Coproporphyrin excretion in family described by Berger and Goldberg*

	Urine coproporphyrin (μg./litre)	Faecal coproporphyrin (μg./g. dry wt.)
Upper limit of normal	100	15
Patient	5719	2082
Mother	500	525
Father	775	862

The child also suffered from rickets and from riboflavin deficiency. The associated finding of rickets was probably fortuitous, and in fact its improvement with appropriate therapy made no difference to the porphyrin excretion. It was thought possible, however, that the metabolic disorder was in some way connected with a predisposition to riboflavin deficiency.

Methaemoglobinaemia

Methaemoglobinaemia is a condition in which a substantial proportion of the circulating haemoglobin exists as methaemoglobin (Met Hb), that is pigment in which the haemoglobin iron is in the ferric state. Methaemoglobin is incapable of transporting oxygen.

It is thought that in the normal erythrocytes there is a steady formation of methaemoglobin going on. The cells, however, are capable of reducing it more or less as rapidly as it is formed. An equilibrium $Hb \rightleftharpoons Met\, Hb$ is set up, and in normal subjects this is well over to the left, so that less than half of one per cent of the pigment present in the erythrocytes is in the form of methaemoglobin. This intracellular reduction of methaemoglobin is believed to be coupled with glycolysis. In the glycolytic process coenzyme I (DPN) is reduced and is available for the reduction of methaemoglobin. Reduced coenzyme I, however, will only reduce methaemoglobin at a very limited rate and apparently in normal erythrocytes a flavoprotein which has been variously referred to as diaphorase I, coenzyme factor I, and methaemoglobin reductase acts as a hydrogen carrier between coenzyme I and methaemoglobin (Fig. 64)[26,27].

The occurrence of a substantial amount of methaemoglobin in the blood must be due to the formation of methaemoglobin at a rate exceeding the capacity of the reducing systems to remove it. This may arise in two ways. There may be a normal reducing system present but an excessively rapid rate of methaemoglobin formation. There may, on the other hand, be a normal rate of methaemoglobin formation but a defective reducing system. Both types of situation have been encountered in different forms of methaemoglobinaemia.

Methaemoglobinaemia .occasionally occurs as a result of the administration of certain drugs such as acetanilide, antipyrine, and phenacetin. It may also develop in infants as a result of the use of well water with a high nitrate content in the preparation of their food. In these instances the abnormality is due to an excessive rate of methaemoglobin formation, and it disappears within 24 to 72 hours after stopping the drug or changing the water supply.

There is, however, another group of methaemoglobinaemias which cannot be accounted for in this way. Here the abnormality is present at birth and persists unchanged, in the absence of specific treatment, throughout life. The quantity of methaemoglobin present in the blood

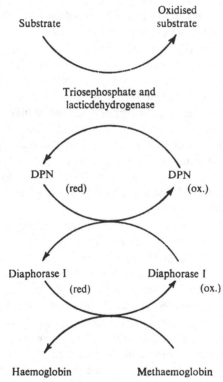

Fig. 64. Scheme for the reduction of methaemoglobin. (After Gibson.)

of such individuals usually amounts to several grams per cent, and may represent some 10–45 per cent of the total red cell pigment. There is usually a marked cyanosis, and there may be a compensatory polycaethaemia (28). In most cases the affected individuals seem to suffer no obvious physical disability and are able to lead quite normal lives. Sometimes, however, the abnormality has been found associated with severe mental defect (29, 30).

This condition of so-called 'congenital idiopathic' methaemoglobinaemia is not infrequently found in several members of the same family. It seems, however, that several biochemically and genetically distinct forms of the condition may occur, and not all of these have been clearly characterised.

In one group of cases studied by Gibson the enzymic situation in the red cell has been examined in some detail [27]. He found that where washed cells were suspended in saline containing glucose or lactate the rate of reduction of methaemoglobin was the same as in plain saline. In contrast to this, normal red cells showed a fourfold increase in the rate of methaemoglobin reduction when glucose or lactate was added. He further showed that this result was not due to the deficiency of enzymes normally concerned in glycolysis. In particular the triosephosphate and lactic dehydrogenases were present in normal amounts in the abnormal cells and similarly there were normal quantities of coenzyme I present. He concluded that the defect was probably due to a deficiency of diaphorase I activity, and indeed he was able to demonstrate a significant reduction of this activity in the abnormal cells. The defect, therefore, involved primarily the reducing system. The formation of methaemoglobin proceeded at a normal rate.

Another feature typical of many, though possibly not all, forms of methaemoglobinaemia was also demonstrated here. This concerns the character of the oxygen dissociation curve. Darling and Roughton [31] have shown that, in haemoglobin solutions containing methaemoglobin, there is a shift of the oxygen dissociation curve to the left, and it becomes less markedly inflected. In other words, the haemoglobin gives up less oxygen than is normal at a given oxygen tension. They interpreted this shift as being due to the presence in haemoglobin-methaemoglobin mixtures of molecules containing both ferrous and ferric iron in various atomic proportions. The same kind of shift in oxygen dissociation curve [29] has been found using blood from patients with methaemoglobinaemia. This phenomenon has a bearing on the mode of formation of the methaemoglobin, since it implies that the methaemoglobin is distributed widely throughout the corpuscles rather than segregated in certain ones. If there were two types of corpuscle in the circulation, one containing normal 'ferrous' haemoglobin and the other containing only methaemo-globin there would be no opportunity for the two pigments to inter-act, and so the oxygen dissociation curve would be normal in character.

A third feature of the condition is the therapeutic response to ascorbic acid and also to methylene blue. The effect of ascorbic acid is probably due to a direct reaction of the ascorbic acid with methaemoglobin (32). The response to methylene blue, which is more rapid and more complete, is thought to be due to a catalytic effect enabling methaemoglobin to be reduced by enzyme systems which are normally unable to bring this about. Gibson suggests that it opens up pathways involving coenzyme II (TPN) (27).

Most of the patients studied by Gibson were derived from a single family. Of nine brothers and sisters, five were affected. Neither parent had the condition nor was there any indication that it had turned up in any other relatives (33). The family came from a remote mountainous part of Ireland, and the antecedents of both parents had lived in the same village for generations so that they were likely to have been, in some degree, consanguineous. It was thought that the affected individuals might be homozygous for a rare recessive gene. A number of other examples of the condition occurring in only a single sibship in a given family have been described and these also, in spite of a paucity of reports of consanguinity, have usually been attributed to 'recessive' inheritance (28).

However, other workers have studied families in which the familial distribution of the disorder was clearly very different (34). Here it has been found in several generations, and an affected individual often transmitted the disorder to one or more of his children. Occasional 'skipping' of generations was also noted. It is extremely improbable that in these families the affected individuals are homozygotes. The pedigrees are more simply understood on the hypothesis that the affected people are heterozygous for a rare gene which, occasionally, fails to lead to a marked manifestation of the condition. In these families detailed enzyme studies have not been carried out, so that it remains possible that the condition here may be due to a different defect from that observed by Gibson. However, in other respects they had very similar features including a satisfactory response to ascorbic acid and methylene blue.

An entirely different kind of methaemoglobinaemia has been described by Hörlein and Weber (35). In this condition, 15–25 per cent of the pigment present in the red cells is in the form of methaemoglobin, but this methaemoglobin has a different absorption spectrum from normal methaemoglobin. By splitting the haem and globin components and recombining them with appropriate fractions from normal haemoglobin it was possible to show that the abnormality lay in the globin moiety of the molecule. The defect in the globin probably results in an excessive rate of methaemoglobin formation which the normal reducing systems cannot cope with. Administration of ascorbic acid or methylene blue failed to produce the striking therapeutic results achieved in the other forms of methaemoglobinaemia. A number of individuals in several different generations of the same family were affected in this way, and the peculiarity in globin synthesis can probably be attributed to the effect of a single gene, in much the same way as seems to be the case in other forms of abnormal haemoglobins. Further support for this interpretation has been obtained by Gerald and his colleagues (36) who have studied another family in which this same abnormality was segregating. They were able to separate the abnormal haemoglobin from normal adult haemoglobin electrophoretically, and they demonstrated that in the affected individuals both forms of haemoglobin were present. This abnormal haemoglobin is called haemoglobin M.

Congenital hyperbilirubinaemia

In 1952 Crigler and Najjar (37) described a new inherited syndrome characterised by very high concentrations of bilirubin in the blood plasma. They studied seven children who occurred in three different but interrelated sibships. The parents were in each case consanguineous and there seems little doubt that the affected children were homozygous for an extremely rare abnormal gene. Since then a further case has been observed in another sibship related to the original ones (38), and a further example of what appears to be the same disease has been found in a quite unrelated family (39).

In all these children marked jaundice appeared on the first or second day after birth and persisted throughout life. The concentrations of serum bilirubin were of the order of 15–40 mg. per hundred ml. and virtually all of this was of the indirect reacting or unconjugated type of pigment. There was no evidence of any excessive rate of red cell destruction.

All the interrelated patients studied by Crigler, Najjar and Childs, with two exceptions, developed spasticity and choreoathetosis after a few days or weeks of life and died within the first year. At postmortem marked staining of the damaged parts of the brain (kernicterus) was observed. The other two examples of the condition in this group appeared, however, to develop normally without any brain lesions. By the ages of six years and three years respectively (40), they seemed to be quite healthy, apart from the persistent jaundice. The isolated case showing similar hyperbilirubinaemia described by Rosenthal and his colleagues differed in that although neurological damage was present this did not develop until the child was three years old, although the jaundice had been present since birth.

Thus the clinical features of the condition may be remarkably variable. The early development of brain damage is analogous to that which may occur in haemolytic disease of the new-born due to antigenic incompatibility. It is presumably related to the lipophilic character of unconjugated bilirubin. The reason for the absence of neurological damage in two cases and its rather late development in another remains, however, quite obscure.

The formation of bilirubin from haemoglobin and its subsequent conversion in the liver to the water-soluble bilirubin glucuronide (conjugated bilirubin, direct reacting bilirubin) which is excreted in the bile, has been extensively studied in recent years (41). It appears that uridine diphosphate glucuronic acid acts as the glucuronyl donor, and that the enzyme glucuronyl transferase present in liver microsomes is necessary for the conversion of bilirubin to bilirubin glucuronide. This enzyme normally develops just at or shortly after birth.

Schmid and his colleagues (42) have found that the bile of these hyperbilirubinaemic children is colourless and contains only traces of conjugated bilirubin. Furthermore, the ability of these children to conjugate glucuronic acid with menthol, salicylic acid, and certain metabolites of hydrocortisone was markedly depressed. It seems probable, therefore, that the essential defect in hyperbilirubinaemia of this kind is a failure in the conjugation of bilirubin with glucuronic acid, possibly because of a deficiency of the enzyme glucuronyl transferase. It is likely that individuals who are heterozygous for the gene which in double dose results in the gross defect in conjugation may have a milder version of the same abnormality. Although they are not jaundiced, Childs (40) has found that the parents and some of the sibs of the affected patients may show some impairment in their ability to make glucuronic acid conjugates. This was much less in degree than that found in the affected homozygotes.

Acatalasaemia

An interesting condition which is evidently due to a genetically determined defect in catalase formation has been described by Takahara [43].
He studied nine patients in three different Japanese families. In each
family only a single sibship was involved and the parents were consanguineous. The defect was presumably inherited as an extremely
rare 'recessive' character.

The main clinical feature of these cases was the occurrence of
ulceration of the gums followed by varying degrees of oral gangrene
accompanied by the loss of the teeth. The biochemical abnormality
was first recognised when during the course of the surgical treatment
of one of the patients, hydrogen peroxide was applied to the operation wound. The blood oozing from the wound immediately turned
brownish black and there was no evolution of gas. Subsequently it
was shown that virtually no catalase activity could be detected in the
blood, and none was present in oral or nasal tissue removed by
biopsy. It was estimated that not more than 1 part in 1000 of the
catalase normally occurring could have been present in these patients.

Takahara suggested that the pathogenesis of the oral ulceration
and gangrene developed along the following lines. The gums are apt
to receive minor injuries during mastication. These afford suitable
sites for the proliferation of oral bacteria among which haemolytic
streptococci are commonly present and these are known to generate
hydrogen peroxide. In normal individuals the formation of hydrogen
peroxide at the site of these minor injuries is dealt with by the catalase
present, and little harm results. In individuals without catalase, however, it leads to further tissue damage, and also prevents adequate
local oxygenation by converting haemoglobin to methaemoglobin.
The bacteria tend to proliferate and this accentuates the sequence of
events, so that small ulcers gradually develop into larger lesions with
much necrosis but little inflammation.

Vitamin D resistant rickets

Classical rickets is nowadays a very rare disease, though fifty years
ago it was extremely common. This is largely due to the recognition
of the role of vitamin D in the prevention and cure of the disorder
and the consequent increase in the vitamin D content of diets given
to infants and young children. However, the eradication of classical

rickets has led to the recognition of a number of rather rare disorders of bone formation which resemble classical rickets very closely, but differ in that they fail to respond to doses of vitamin D normally effective in curing the disease. Such conditions have usually been referred to as vitamin D resistant rickets. In most cases it has been found that the bone lesions can be caused to heal, if vitamin D is administered to these patients in very large doses. The dose required is usually many thousand times greater than is normally necessary to cure classical rickets. It is frequently in fact very close to the dose which will produce vitamin D toxicity, so the assessment of the amounts required in any individual case to ensure healing but avoid toxic effects is often rather tricky.

There are a number of different kinds of resistant rickets and it has been possible to differentiate these from one another both on biochemical and genetical grounds[44,45], though a definitive classification still remains to be achieved.

The commonest type of condition which is encountered has been referred to by Dent as Type 1 resistant rickets[44]. It has a characteristic mode of progression. The infants appear normal at birth and grow and develop normally during the first year. After this, however, the child is noticed to be slow in attaining the usual milestones and unambiguous rachitic deformities become apparent. Some of the children do not come under medical observation until they are three or four years old, by which time the dwarfism, lateness in walking, abnormalities in gait, bow legs and so on have usually become very obvious. The X-rays show florid rickets.

Characteristically the plasma inorganic phosphate level is significantly lower than the normal. The plasma alkaline phosphatase is usually raised and the plasma calcium is within normal limits. There is no acidosis, no aminoaciduria, and no abnormality in the usual renal function tests; points which help to differentiate the condition from other forms of refractory rickets.

The general health of these patients is good and they survive to adult life. However, there is usually a considerable degree of deformity, and they have often been subjected to repeated osteotomies in order to correct this[46]. They are dwarfed, the limbs being very short in comparison to the trunk which is usually normal. In childhood aches and pains in the bones and a tendency to tire easily are common, but after growth has ceased these symptoms become less conspicuous and generally between the ages of twenty and forty the patients are quite fit except for any residual deformities. In later life pain and radiological signs of osteomalacia tend to appear and the patients may become quite crippled if not treated appropriately. The low plasma phosphate level persists throughout, though it may rise somewhat with consistent vitamin D therapy.

It has been suggested that the key biochemical abnormality in this condition is a specific defect in the renal tubular reabsorption of phosphate from the glomerular filtrate (44,47). Measurements of the maximal tubular capacity for phosphate reabsorption in these patients has shown that it is considerably reduced, averaging about half the normal values (48). Since under normal conditions the phosphate reabsorptive capacity is either saturated or near saturated, such a defect in reabsorption capacity would be expected to result in a significant reduction in plasma inorganic phosphate concentration. This in turn might influence the normal course of bone growth and development, and perhaps cause the rickets. The situation is, however, probably more complicated than this because Winters and his colleagues (48) have shown that certain relatives (usually females) of affected patients may exhibit a similar degree of reduced capacity of phosphate reabsorption with correspondingly low plasma inorganic phosphate levels, and yet have either no obvious bone disease at all or only minimal signs which can only be detected radiologically. It is possible that the deficient renal tubular reabsorption of phosphate may represent only one facet of a rather more complex disturbance of phosphate and calcium metabolism.

The disease is not infrequently found in several members of the same family, often in several different generations (45,46). Recently Winters and his colleagues (48) have reported the results of the investigation of a large group of related families in which many cases of resistant rickets occurred. They were able to carry out plasma phosphate determinations on some 166 individuals including twenty-five who had active rickets or residual deformities. They found that not only did the clinically obvious cases of resistant rickets show significantly low plasma inorganic phosphate levels, but so also did many of the apparently normal individuals. Individuals with hypophosphataemia were found in three different generations, and the characteristic appeared to be transmitted directly from parent to child. A peculiar feature of the familial distribution was that among the offspring of males with hypophosphataemia all the ten male children had normal plasma phosphate levels whereas all the eleven female children were

hypophosphataemic. Among the offspring of females with hypophosphataemia, eight out of fourteen males shared the same peculiarity,
and so did four out of thirteen females. They infer that in this family
the characteristic hypophosphataemia was determined by a rare sex-
linked gene. Both males and females carrying the gene showed hypc-
phosphataemia, but the occurrence of clinically obvious rickets
occurred much more commonly and was more severe among the
males than among the females. Estimates of tubular phosphate
reabsorption capacity in three clinically affected males and one female,
were not significantly different from those found in four hypophosphataemic females who had no bone deformities.

It remains to be seen whether other cases of resistant rickets are
also determined by a sex-linked gene. In most instances so far
studied the family histories are inconclusive. Whereas many examples
of a mother and son both having clinically obvious resistant rickets
have been reported, there appears to be as yet no unequivocal
example of a father and son being similarly affected. On the other
hand, preliminary studies of plasma phosphate levels among clinically
normal mothers of affected males suggest that while these may be on
the average somewhat lower than normal, the distinction between
hypophosphataemics and normals does not usually, in these families,
seem to be quite as clear cut as a peared to be the case in the data of
Winters and his colleagues.

If the sex-linked hypothesis is correct, one is faced with the problem
as to why some heterozygous females develop rickets as severely as
some males carrying the gene, and yet other heterozygous females
who apparently have as severe a defect in tubular phosphate reabsorption do not develop any bone lesions, or do so only minimally. However, similar difficulties arise with alternative genetical hypotheses,
such as that of an autosomal gene with incomplete manifestation, and
at the moment the sex-linkage hypothesis gives a better fit with the
available family data than does any other.

Hypophosphatasia

In 1948 Rathbun [49] drew attention to a severe osteodys rophic disorder which he called hypophosphatasia. It resembled in many
respects a severe form of rickets, but it was characterised by a marked
reduction in the level of serum alkaline phosphatase. Since then
many further examples of the same kind of bone disorder associated

with low serum alkaline phosphatase activity have been reported, and it has emerged that the syndrome is genetically determined. Despite the resemblance, in many respects, of the bone lesions to those found in rickets, the disorder does not respond to vitamin D.

The clinical manifestations (50) and the skeletal disorder as revealed radiologically (51), though similar in all these cases, may vary considerably in severity. In some cases the abnormalities in bone formation are obvious at birth or very shortly afterwards, and in at least one instance they have been recognised *in utero* by X-ray examination of the mother (52). In other cases the child has appeared to develop normally during the first few months, and it is only then that the generalised bone changes resembling rickets begin to appear. In still other instances the diagnosis may not be made until adult life, and although there is often a history of 'rickets' in childhood, the disability from this does not always appear to have been marked.

When the condition is seen in infancy the outstanding features have been a failure to thrive combined with the early development of rachitic-type bone deformities and a very poor calcification of the skeleton. A tense bulging fontanelle is a common feature, though the cause of this is obscure. The teeth when they appear are hypoplastic and tend to be shed prematurely. Although the prognosis is very poor in those cases where the disorder is clearly manifest at birth or shortly afterwards, the outlook in the cases where the condition does not become apparent till the child is six months or a year old is not unhopeful. The bones will slowly calcify, symptoms abate, and growth goes on, though ultimately there is usually some degree of bone deformity and the individual is rather short. One somewhat unexpected complication which can occur is premature craniostenosis, and this may require craniotomy (53). Despite the apparent spontaneous healing the low serum alkaline phosphatase level persists, so that the disease may be diagnosed for the first time in adult life when the patient may present with skeletal deformities and spontaneous fractures.

The low serum alkaline phosphatase present in these patients probably reflects a generalised defect in the formation of one of a group of enzymes which exhibit this kind of activity. Normally alkaline phosphatase activity is demonstrable not only in serum but also in a wide variety of different tissues, and it is particularly prominent in calcifying bone, small intestinal mucosa, renal cortex, and lactating breast. In several cases of hypophosphatasia various tissues obtained at post-mortem [49, 52] or by biopsy [54] have been found to show a significant reduction in alkaline phosphatase activity. These include liver, kidney, and small intestine, as well as bone itself.

The functional significance of the enzyme or group of enzymes which exhibit alkaline phosphatase activity is not understood. Certainly there is plenty of evidence which suggests that alkaline phosphatase activity is somehow concerned with bone formation. For example, the serum alkaline phosphatase is elevated in active rickets and in a variety of other bone diseases, such as Paget's disease and osteogenic sarcoma. It is also higher in the normal individual during the first fifteen years of life, when active growth is proceeding, than it is subsequently. Alkaline phosphatase activity may be demonstrated histochemically in cartilage just prior to ossification, and in mature bone it is found mainly in the periostial and endostial regions [55]. In the past it was generally believed that the main function of the enzyme in bone formation was concerned with the localised production of high concentrations of inorganic phosphate from phosphate esters so that insoluble calcium phosphate could be precipitated in the bone matrix. More recent work makes this hypothesis appear rather doubtful, but no completely satisfactory alternative theory has been developed [55]. While it is plausible to suppose that the peculiarities in bone formation seen in hypophosphatasia are the secondary consequence of a primary failure in alkaline phosphatase formation, there is no direct evidence for this and the details of the association remain to be worked out.

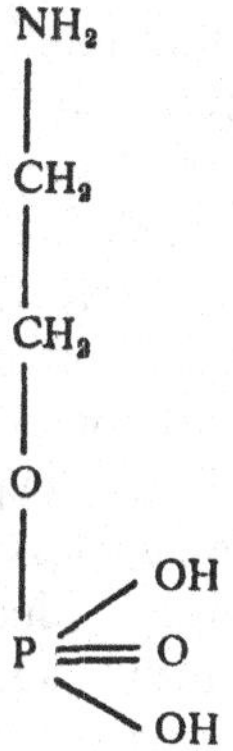

Apart from the alkaline phosphatase levels the only other characteristic biochemical peculiarity which has been observed in hypophosphatasia is an increased excretion of the substance ethanolamine phosphate (Fig. 65) in the urine [56, 57]. In hypophosphatasia quantities of the order of 100–200 mg. per l. of urine may be found, whereas normally it is present at most in traces. It has been detected in only very small amounts in the plasma and it is probable

$$NH_2 - CH_2 - CH_2 - O - P(=O)(OH)(OH)$$

Fig. 65.
Ethanolamine
phosphate.

that its renal clearance approximates to the rate of glomerular filtration [58]. The metabolic significance of ethanolamine phosphate is not known. It is normally present in the free state in a wide variety of tissue cells, including those of the liver, kidney and brain. It is possible that it may be a breakdown product of cephalin[59]. It also seems likely that it may be a natural substrate for alkaline phosphatase, and if so this could explain its increased excretion in hypophosphatasia where presumably its further hydrolysis to ethanolamine and inorganic phosphate would be very restricted. There is no evidence associating ethanolamine phosphate with bone formation.

Hypophosphatasia has in a number of instances been observed among more than one of a group of brothers and sisters, and the collected family data are consistent with the hypothesis that the affected individuals are homozygous for a rare abnormal gene[50]. It has also been noticed that among the apparently normal relatives of patients with hypophosphatasia individuals occur who have serum alkaline phosphatase levels which are slightly lower than what is believed to be the lower limit of the normal variation of this character. Others have borderline values. It has been suggested that these people are heterozygotes for the abnormal gene[50,51]. However, the normal variation in serum alkaline phosphatase activity is very wide and this test does not usually furnish a very certain method of detecting the heterozygotes, even among the relatives of known cases.

Another peculiarity which may be frequently observed among the healthy relatives of patients with hypophosphatasia is a significant increase in ethanolamine phosphate excretion. The quantities involved are quite small (about one-tenth of those found in the affected patients), but even quantities of this order of magnitude are only rarely found in random normal individuals. This increased excretion of ethanolamine phosphate has often been found in both parents of affected children and in relatives on both sides of the family[60]. Typical figures for the incidence of this peculiarity among different classes of relatives are shown in Table 46. It is probable that such individuals are heterozygotes for the abnormal gene, and if so the results suggest that about 60 per cent of heterozygotes may be detected in this way. There is, however, a significant irregularity about the distribution of the presumed heterozygotes who show an increased excretion of ethanolamine phosphate. This is seen if one considers the incidence of individuals with increased ethanolamine phosphate excretion among the sibs of parents of patients with hypophosphatasia, both of whom are presumably heterozygotes. Where the parent shows an increased ethanolamine phosphate excretion, the incidence of the same peculiarity in his or her sibs is significantly greater than its incidence among the sibs of those parents who do not have an increased ethanolamine phosphate excretion. This suggests that there are genetical factors which influence the manifestation of this character in heterozygotes, and further analysis indicates that this may depend on variations in the functional activity of the normal allele which is present.

Table 46. *Incidence of increased ethanolamine phosphate excretion among clinically normal relatives of patients with hypophosphatasia. (After Harris and Robson, 1958)*

Relationship	Number tested	Number with significantly increased excretion of ethanolamine phosphate	Expected number of heterozygotes
Sibs	11	6	7·3
Parents	27	18	27·0
Grandparents	35	11	17·5
Uncles and aunts	89	20	44·5
First cousins	83	11	20·7
Grandparents sibs	41	10	10·2
Children of grand-parents sibs	47	3	5·9
Totals	333	79	133·1

Proportion of heterozygotes detected $= \dfrac{79}{133} = 0.59$.

Another feature of the familial distribution of hypophosphatasia which emphasises the complexity of its genetical basis, is that when more than one patient with hypophosphatasia has been found in the same sibship, they have in most cases resembled each other rather closely in the severity and age of onset of the clinical manifestations of the disease. This sib-sib correlation suggests that several different genes can each give rise to this syndrome, and a great deal more work is required before the situation will be sorted out.

Diabetes insipidus

Something like 180 litres of water a day are filtered by the renal glomeruli in the normal subject. Only one to two litres of this usually appears as urine, the rest being reabsorbed by the renal tubules. About seven-eighths of the water is reabsorbed in the proximal renal tubules, the fluid here being maintained isotonic with the plasma. The remainder is thought to be actively reabsorbed, either in the Loops of Henle or in the distal tubules, and it is this process which leads to the formation of a hypertonic urine, and which is influenced by the antidiuretic hormone. Failure or partial failure of this process of active reabsorption results in the syndrome of diabetes insipidus, which is characterised by the excretion of large volumes of urine of low specific gravity. In adults the main features of the disorder are polyuria and polydipsia. In young infants there may be severe dehydration, and a marked increase in plasma electrolyte concentrations.

The formation of antidiuretic hormone (pitressin) depends on a complex functional unit which includes the posterior pituitary and its connections with certain neighbouring regions of the central nervous system. Damage to any part of this system may result in diabetes insipidus and it is known that this can follow from trauma, encephalitis, tumours, vascular accidents and so on. However, cases also occur in which there is no evidence of lesions of this kind in the neighbourhood of the neurohypophysis. Many of these cases appear to be genetically determined, and in some instances it has been possible to construct elaborate pedigrees showing the segregation of the disorder in several different generations over a long period of time.

Such apparently inherited examples of diabetes insipidus fall into two physiologically distinct classes. These have been called pitressin-sensitive diabetes insipidus and pitressin-insensitive, or nephrogenic, diabetes insipidus. In the former the defect appears to result from some defect in the elaboration of antidiuretic hormone, and in the latter in some defect in renal response to the hormone. They can be distinguished by studying the effect on the rate of formation and the concentration of the urine following the administration of pitressin.

Genetical studies indicate that inherited pitressin-sensitive diabetes insipidus is probably heterogeneous. In some families[61] the abnormality can be attributed to an abnormal autosomal gene for which the affected individuals are heterozygous. In others a sex-linked gene appears to be involved[62,63]. In the non-sex-linked variety a notable feature is the marked variation in the degree of severity of the disorder among heterozygotes in the same family. Thus Pender and Fraser found that among the adult cases in a large family which they investigated, the fluid requirements varied from about four to about twenty litres a day. Provided the fluid requirements were met the affected individuals appeared to remain in good health. In the sex-linked form of the condition the female heterozygotes usually appeared to be unaffected. However, some manifestations of diabetes insipidus often appeared in the last few months of their pregnancies. Nothing is known about the nature of the defect in antidiuretic hormone formation in either of these genetically distinct types of condition.

Pitressin-insensitive or nephrogenic diabetes insipidus presumably results from some abnormality in renal tubular function which interferes with the reabsorption of water by the distal parts of the tubules. Other aspects of renal function appear to be normal. The disorder has been found predominantly in males and the pedigrees suggest that it is determined by a sex-linked gene [63,64]. The disease, as it affects the males in these families, often appears to be rather more severe than in other types of diabetes insipidus, and complications in infancy due to dehydration and electrolyte disturbances are more common. The female heterozygotes while not usually showing the marked polyuria characteristic of the affected males nevertheless frequently exhibit diminished ability to form a concentrated urine under conditions of fluid restriction [64].

Haemochromatosis

Haemochromatosis is a rare disorder of metabolism characterised by a generalised accumulation of iron in the body. In the normal adult there is usually about 4–5 g. of iron present. In haemochromatosis the excess iron accumulated may be of the order of 25–50 g. [65]. Virtually all the tissues show some increase in iron content but the effect is particularly marked in the liver and pancreas [66]. Clinically the disease is characterised by enlargement and cirrhosis of the liver, diabetes mellitus, pigmentation of the skin and often cardiac failure. The clinical features of the disease do not usually become apparent until middle or late life (Fig. 66), though the progressive accumulation of iron has probably been going on at the rate of a few milligrams a day from birth. The hepatic cirrhosis and diabetes mellitus are usually attributed to local tissue damage produced in the liver and pancreas by the excessive deposition of iron [66].

In the normal individual about 60–70 per cent of iron in the body is present in haemoglobin, about 3–5 per cent in myoglobin, and about 0·2 per cent in haem proteins such as catalase and the cyto-chromes. Most of the rest is stored in the tissues closely associated with protein either in a soluble form known as ferritin, or in an insoluble form called haemosiderin. The exact relation between these two forms of storage iron is not understood. Both are present

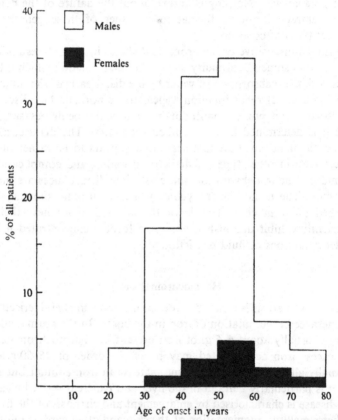

Fig. 66. Age of onset of idiopathic haemochromatosis in 787 patients.
(After Finch and Finch (66).)

normally and the iron in both of them is available for haem synthesis. However, whereas in the normal individual somewhat more ferritin than haemosiderin is present, when iron accumulates haemosiderin tends to preponderate (66), and in haemochromatosis it is this material which is notably present in great excess. Haemosiderin may be seen histologically as brownish granules which stain for iron.

Iron is transported in plasma bound to a specific process usually referred to as transferrin or siderophilin. This is an α-globulin and is normally less than one-half saturated with iron. In haemochromatosis the plasma iron is increased and the proportion of unsaturated siderophilin proportionately decreased [66,67].

Haemochromatosis is observed about ten times more frequently in males than in females. In normal males the excretion of iron from the body is very restricted [68] and the excessive accumulation of iron in haemochromatosis can only be explained in terms of an increased rate of absorption. The immediate cause of this increased rate of absorption of iron in this disease is, however, not understood. It has been variously attributed either to a defect in the complex regulating system in the intestinal mucosa which normally seems to restrict iron absorption more or less in accordance with physiological needs [69], or to the presence of some abnormal tissue protein with marked capacity for binding iron which in turn stimulates an increased rate of absorption from the gut [70]. There is little direct evidence bearing on this question.

The increased rate of absorption of iron is thought to be present throughout life in these patients, and the tissue accumulation is progressive. If it is true that the tissue damage is a direct consequence of the excessive local accumulation of iron, then presumably the delayed age of onset of the clinical signs and symptoms of the disease is a reflection of the time required for the necessary amount of iron to accumulate.

The occurrence of haemochromatosis in more than one member of the same family is not common, but it has been reported sufficiently frequently to make it unlikely that the association was fortuitous. It has been observed both in sibs and in parent-child combinations [66]. It has usually been supposed that the condition is genetically determined but that only a small proportion of genetically predisposed individuals develop frank clinical symptoms. There is no indication of sex linkage and it is thought, therefore, that the incidence of the predisposition is the same in the two sexes, but that the clinical manifestations of the disease are much more likely to occur in predisposed males than predisposed females. The obvious reason for such a sex difference is that women on the average excrete much more iron than men by menstruation, and transplacentally to the foetus during pregnancy. Assuming the rate of absorption of iron were much the same in predisposed individuals of either sex, then the rate of accumulation in the tissues would be on the average much less in women than in men. The average woman, for example, loses about 10–15 g. of iron in her lifetime from menstruation alone (66).

Further support for the idea that haemochromatosis is genetically determined is provided by recent studies of plasma iron concentrations among the apparently normal relatives of known cases. Finch and Finch (66) found that among the sibs of such patients a significant proportion had unusually high plasma iron levels. These presumably represent predisposed individuals in whom the clinical manifestations of the disease have not yet developed and may indeed never appear. Debre and his colleagues (67) have carried out an extensive study of some sixty-seven children of patients with haemochromatosis. Among the male children over the age of fifteen the mean plasma iron concentration was significantly different from that of the controls. It was in fact intermediate between the values found in the control population and those found in the series of patients with haemochromatosis (Table 47). Although the distribution among these sons was not obviously bimodal, the variance was significantly greater than in either the controls or the haemochromatosis patients. The distribution of plasma iron values in this population of sons was, indeed, much the same as would be expected if they were composed of two approximately equal groups, one with a distribution corresponding to that of normal individuals, and one with a distribution corresponding to that found in haemochromatosis patients. On the other hand, no significant elevation of plasma iron value was found in the daughters over the age of fifteen, or in either sex below the age of fifteen. Debré and his colleagues conclude that the increased rate of iron absorption characteristic of haemochromatosis may be determined by a single gene, for which the affected individuals are hetero-

Table 47. *Plasma iron concentration in patients with haemo-chromatosis and their sons. (After Debre et al. 1958)*

	Number	Mean plasma iron μg. %	Variance	Standard deviation	Standard error of mean
Male controls (over 15 years old)	38	139·9	1470·54	38·35	6·2
Patients with haemo-chromatosis	40	251·7	1463·50	38·26	6·0
Sons of patients (over 15 years old)	30	197·4	3029·21	55·04	10·0

zygous. The most sensitive indication of this functional defect which is available at the moment appears to be the plasma iron concentration, and even this will not usually reveal any abnormality in children or in young adult women. Presumably only a proportion of those individuals with detectably increased iron concentrations in the plasma actually develop frank clinical symptoms of the disease, and it is possible that various external factors may be important in precipitating these and influencing the clinical severity of the disorder.

Debre and his colleagues also draw attention to a peculiar and extremely uncommon form of haemochromatosis, in which the clinical signs appear in early adult life and which runs a very severe and fulminating course. They suggest that these patients may be homozygous for the gene which in heterozygotes produces the more usual milder and later-onset type of disorder. The parents of one such patient were both found to have high values of plasma iron (father 190, and mother $200\,\mu$g. per 100 ml.). It was also noted that, although in all cases of haemochromatosis taken together there is no apparent increase in parental consanguinity, it seemed probable from a review of the literature that parental consanguinity was in fact significantly increased in this rather rare and uncommon type of case.

Primary hyperoxaluria

This rare condition is characterised by the continuous excretion in the urine of unusually large amounts of oxalate. Quantities of the order of 150–300 mg. per day are excreted, compared with a normal output of the order of 20 mg. per day [71, 72]. Calcium oxalate is extremely insoluble and this continuous high oxalate excretion tends to result in the recurrent formation of calcium oxalate stones in the renal tract. Calcium oxalate deposition in the parenchyma and interstitial tissues of the kidney, and often in other organs, may also occur and this has sometimes been referred to as 'oxalosis' [73]. Death usually occurs in childhood or early adult life from renal failure. Diagnosis depends on the demonstration of the continuous high oxalate excretion, and it should be noted that calcium oxalate stones may also be found in individuals who do not exhibit this.

Occasional examples of what were probably familial cases of hyperoxaluria have been reported in the literature, but in most of these full biochemical investigations were not carried out on more than one affected individual in the family. More recently a series of families have been investigated in some detail by Scowen and his colleagues, and the preliminary results suggest that the condition is probably inherited as a rare Mendelian 'recessive' character [74]. No abnormal oxalate excretion was observed among the parents of affected patients, or among the many other apparently healthy relatives who were studied.

The nature of the metabolic lesion in these patients is uncertain. Variations in oxalate intake from the usual dietary sources do not provide an explanation for the unusually high levels of oxalate excreted [75]. When large doses of sodium oxalate were fed by mouth some increase in oxalate excretion in the urine was observed. This,

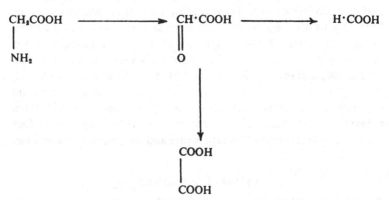

Fig. 67. Possible mode of formation of oxalic acid from glycine.

however, amounted to no more than 2–5 per cent of the dose administered and it was found that in normal subjects a similar increase in oxalate excretion occurred under the same conditions [75]. Thus it does not appear likely that an excessive rate of oxalate absorption from the gut is responsible. It also seems improbable that a failure in renal tubular reabsorption of oxalate is responsible, though this possibility cannot be absolutely excluded in the absence of satisfactory methods for determining serum oxalate concentrations.

Archer and his colleagues [75] direct attention to the possibility that oxalate may be formed from glycine and suggest that this may be the source of the excess oxalate excreted and deposited in the tissues in these patients. There is evidence from experiments in the rat that glycine may be converted to glyoxalate and that this may in turn yield formate and carbon dioxide (Fig. 67). It has also been shown that in the rat liver glyoxalate can, under certain conditions, give rise to oxalate. If these reactions go on in man, it is possible that hyper-oxaluria might result if the formation of formate from glyoxalate were blocked, or if, for some reason, a greater proportion of total glycine metabolism occurred via glyoxalate than normally. In general it is clear that only a very small fraction of the total daily glycine turnover need be involved in these pathways to result in the increased oxalate excretion which is observed.

Some evidence in favour of the idea that urinary oxalate in these patients may be derived from glycine has been provided by experiments in which large amounts of sodium benzoate were administered. Benzoate is conjugated with glycine and excreted as hippuric acid. It might be expected therefore to deplete the free glycine pool. In two patients with hyperoxaluria a significant depression in oxalate excretion was obtained by feeding sodium benzoate (75). In contrast to this no appreciable effect was observed in control subjects. It is possible that the small amounts of oxalate excreted normally may be derived from a different source from that of the excess oxalate excreted in hyperoxaluria.

Gout and hyperuricaemia

Gout is a disorder in which there is an abnormal tendency to deposit urate in certain connective tissues. The articular cartilages, synovial membranes and the capsules of joints are particularly affected, and inflammatory and degenerative tissue reactions occur which give rise to a form of chronic arthritis. Deposits of urates may also be found in the helix and antihelix of the ear, the olecranon and patella bursae, and the tendons of the hands and feet. Here they produce the characteristic gouty nodules or 'tophi'.

The clinical course of the disease is rather variable. Attacks of an extremely painful form of acute arthritis may occur at more or less regular intervals, in between which the patient usually feels reasonably well. The metatarso-phalangeal joints are most frequently involved in these acute episodes, the next most common being the small joints of the feet, ankles, hands and wrist. The first acute attack usually takes place in middle life, but there is much variation in this. In general, the earlier the clinical manifestation of the disease the more crippling does it tend to be.

Patients with clinical gout characteristically show a raised level of plasma urate. Typical values are given in Table 48. This increased concentration of urate in the blood is generally present whether the patient is having an acute attack of gouty arthritis or not, and the frequency of the acute attacks in any one patient does not appear to be closely correlated with the level of plasma urate.

Table 48. *Serum urate levels in normal and gouty individuals.*
(*After Jacobsen* [76], 1937)

Serum urate (mg./100 ml.)	Normal individuals		Individuals with gout	
	Males	Females	Males	Females
1– 1·9	—	1	—	—
2– 2·9	8	6	—	—
3– 3·9	13	7	—	—
4– 4·9	23	16	—	—
5– 5·9	16	7	—	—
6– 6·9	3	—	1	—
7– 7·9	—	—	5	—
8– 8·9	—	—	6	—
9– 9·9	—	—	4	—
10–10·9	—	—	1	1
11–11·9	—	—	1	—
12–12·9	—	—	2	—
13–13·9	—	—	—	—
Totals	63	37	20	1

Gout is about twenty times more common in men than in women. When it does occur in women the acute attacks do not usually appear before the menopause, and the clinical severity of the disease tends to be milder than in men.

The incidence of gout in the general population is difficult to determine, but the condition is by no means rare [77]. It is commonly believed that the disorder was at one time very much more frequent than it is today. Changes in diagnostic standards, and the absence of any satisfactory statistical data, however, make it difficult to reach any definite conclusion about this. It also used to be thought that alcoholism was a major predisposing factor to the development of the disease. This does not seem to be the situation nowadays.

It has been known for a long time that gout often affects several members of the same family, and many examples of this are quoted in the early literature [78]. There is indeed little doubt that the incidence of the disease among close relatives of affected patients is significantly raised (Table 49). The condition is often found in more than one generation of the same family, and it may be apparently transmitted by members of either sex who themselves may or may not have the condition. The pedigrees have always been found to be irregular in character and many apparently sporadic cases occur. Such irregularities can be partly accounted for by the fact that the disease is very variable in the age of onset, and often is not apparent until middle or late life. Some individuals who may subsequently develop the disease may at the time of the investigation appear normal. However, even allowing for this and also for the marked differences in the incidence of the disorder in the two sexes, the condition has a very patchy familial distribution.

Table 49. *Incidence of gout among relatives of a series of patients with gout. (After Hauge and Harvald, 1955)*

Relatives of patients with gout	Total number	Number of cases of gout
Brothers	73	11
Fathers	32	4
Sons	25	—
Sisters	76	—
Mothers	32	1
Daughters	23	—
Total	261	16

The explanation which has usually been advanced to account for this kind of 'irregularly dominant' familial pattern is that the affected individuals are heterozygous for a gene which predisposes them to the development of the clinical condition. It is thought that only a small proportion of these predisposed individuals actually develop the clinical signs and symptoms of the disorder. Consequently while there is a higher incidence of the disease among close relatives than in the general population, the pedigrees are irregular, generations are apparently 'skipped', and many cases are seemingly sporadic.

The assumption that the affected individuals are heterozygous rests on the fact that several generations of the same family are often affected, and the incidence of the disease in the parents of the patients is similar to the incidence among the sibs. It is, of course, necessary to assume on this hypothesis that the manifestation rate of the disorder is very much greater in male heterozygotes than in female heterozygotes. It is clear, however, that other alternative hypotheses could be constructed to explain the familial pattern observed. In general these would require the postulation of multiple genetical factors in the causation of the disease. In any case it would be

necessary to assume that clinically symptomless, but genetically predisposed, individuals exist, and this raises the question as to whether
such people can be identified by the presence of some peculiarity in
their metabolic processes. A number of studies of the blood urate
levels among the apparently healthy relatives of patients with gout
have been carried out with this object in view.

It has been found that the average level of plasma urate among the
sibs, parents and children of such patients is significantly greater than
in a comparable series of controls (77,79,80). Among such relatives of
affected patients there occur an appreciable number of individuals
who have what would usually be regarded as pathologically high
levels of plasma urate in the absence of any clinical signs or symptoms
of gout, or a history of such symptoms. Clinically such individuals
appear to be quite normal.

The distribution of urate values among the relatives of gouty
patients forms a continuous series and any sharp division into so-
called normal and so-called pathological values is necessarily rather
arbitrary. Nevertheless, the distributions do give some indication of
bimodality, and this has led Smyth, Cotterman and Freiberg (77) to
suggest that two genetically distinct classes of individuals occur,
'hyperuricaemics' and 'normals'. In each class it is thought that
there is a great deal of variation in plasma urate values, so that the
two distributions overlap considerably. The conclusion drawn by these
workers was that 'hyperuricaemia' was an inherited characteristic
and appeared in individuals heterozygous for an abnormal gene. This
condition predisposed the individuals concerned to the development
of clinical gout, although in practice only about 10 per cent of them
actually developed the condition. The absence of clinical symptoms
in most 'hyperuricaemics' would account for the apparent irregularity
of pedigrees of gout and the frequent occurrence of sporadic cases.
A similar conclusion has been drawn by Stecher and his colleagues (80).
However, Hauge and Harvald (79), in the analysis of their own
extensive data which was collected along similar lines, failed to
obtain a satisfactory fit on this hypothesis and concluded that the
genetical determination of hyperuricaemia and gout is likely to be
rather more complex. It is obvious, of course, that in its simplest
form the hypothesis leaves many things unexplained. For example,
even though symptomless hyperuricaemia and clinical gout may have
a similar genetical basis, there must be some good reason why one
person with the abnormality develops severe crippling arthritis and

another remains perfectly healthy. No doubt such problems will only be solved when a clearer picture of the underlying metabolic defect emerges.

It should be noted that the plasma urate level is far from being a fixed individual characteristic. Various environmental factors, in addition to errors introduced by technical difficulties, tend to produce fluctuations in plasma urate values, even when these are carried out on the same individual over relatively short periods of time. Furthermore, because of differences in technique, individual determinations can only be satisfactorily interpreted against norms obtained in the same laboratory. Another complication is introduced by the fact that the average plasma urate level in normal adults is higher in males than in females, so that different criteria of hyperuricaemia have to be adopted in the two sexes [81].

One of the interesting facts which has emerged from the family studies is the undoubted influence of sex and age on the development of hyperuricaemia. Among the male relatives of patients with gout, high values of plasma urate were not encountered until after puberty [77]. Among the female relatives hyperuricaemia was not usually apparent until much later in life, high values generally being found only after the menopause. While a significant correlation between urate level and age was observed in the adult female relatives of the gout patients, it was not observed in the adult male relatives [80]. It is tempting to suppose that the marked sex difference in the occurrence of clinical gout arises from the fact that a sufficiently high level of plasma urate is a necessary prerequisite for this to develop, and that such a situation is reached in genetically predisposed individuals at an earlier age in men than in women.

Uric acid in man is the end-product of purine metabolism. In gout there is characteristically an abnormally high concentration of circulating urate and a deposition of considerable quantities of urate in various tissues. Studies of the so-called 'miscible pool' of urate using isotopically labelled urate have shown that this pool is much larger in patients with gout than in normal individuals [82]. Thus there is a general accumulation of urate in the body and this might be attributed either to a diminished rate of excretion of urate, or to an excessive production of urate.

Although urate is believed to be an end-product of metabolism, and is excreted mainly by the kidney, nevertheless renal clearance studies indicate that a large proportion (90–95 per cent) of all the urate normally filtered by the glomerulus is reabsorbed by the renal tubules(83). A diminished rate of excretion of urate as the major factor in the causation of gout would necessitate that the kidney tubules in gout reabsorbed an even greater fraction of the filtered urate. In fact, clearance studies, both in young patients with no renal damage and in older patients with a moderate degree of renal damage, suggest that the fraction of urate reabsorbed from the glomerular filtrate is substantially the same in patients with gout(84,85,86) as in normal people.

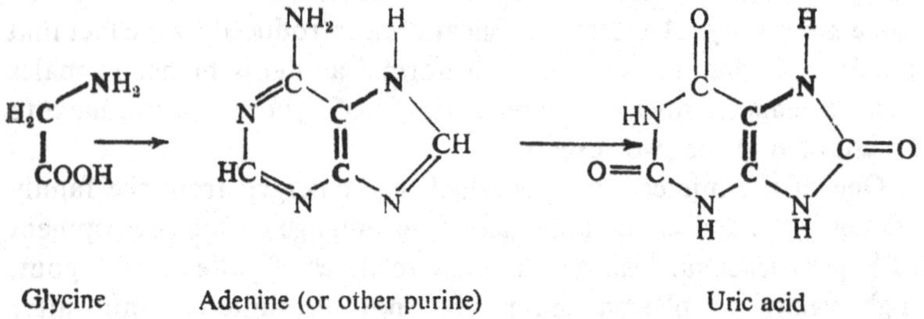

Glycine   Adenine (or other purine)   Uric acid

Fig. 68. Incorporation of glycine into uric acid.

It has, however, now been shown that in gout the formation of urate by the body is proceeding at an excessively high rate(86,87). This has been established by using isotopically labelled glycine in order to study urate formation in both gouty and normal individuals. Such studies became possible when it was found that the carbon and nitrogen skeleton of glycine becomes incorporated in purines and hence in uric acid in a characteristic manner (Fig. 68). Wyngaarden(87), using ^{14}C-labelled glycine in tracer doses, found that in six patients with gout and in one individual with symptomless hyperuricaemia there was a significantly greater rate of ^{14}C-incorporation into urinary urate than occurred in normal subjects.

These and other isotope studies using ^{15}N-labelled glycine(86,88) suggest that urate formation can occur by two pathways. One route is via the catabolism of nucleic acid. The other seems to be more direct. It may involve the early cleavage of nucleotides prior to their incorporation into nucleic acids, with the consequent liberation of purines and the formation of uric acid. The data suggest that in gout it is the second type of pathway which is involved in the excessive formation of urate. In contrast to this the hyperuricaemia which occurs in leukaemia and other conditions where increased cellular destruction is going on, is evidently due to an increased rate of nucleic acid breakdown.

Apart from establishing the precise nature of the metabolic defect, many other problems about gout require solution. For example, there is still no satisfactory explanation for the episodes of acute gouty arthritis which are a characteristic feature of the disease. They do not seem to be related directly to the level of the hyperuricaemia nor do they appear to be caused by urate deposits as such. One of the curious paradoxes about the disease is that the drug colchicine, which seems to have little or no direct effect on uric acid formation or excretion, aborts and often prevents attacks of acute gouty arthritis. On the other hand, uricosuric drugs such as salicylate or probenecid, which act by inhibiting tubular reabsorption of urate and are capable of greatly reducing the urate accumulation in the body, have little or no therapeutic effect on the episodes of acute arthralgia.

Further studies on the detailed mechanism of urate formation in hyperuricaemia may be expected to provide more precise criteria for identifying genetically predisposed but symptomless individuals than is possible at the moment using the plasma urate level as the sole indicator. Family studies might then provide a more coherent picture of the genetical basis of the condition.

REFERENCES

(1) Rimington, C. (1956). *Brit. Med. J.* **2**, 189.
(2) Shemin, D. and Rittenberg, D. (1945). *J. Biol. Chem.* **159**, 567.
(3) Westall, R. G. (1952). *Nature, Lond.* **170**, 614.
(4) Cookson, G. H. and Rimington, C. (1954). *Biochem. J.* **57**, 476.
(5) Rimington, C. and Miles, P. A. (1951). *Biochem J.* **50**, 202.
(6) Rimington, C. (1952). *Acta med. scand.* **143**, 161, 171.
(7) Schmid, R., Schwartz, S. and Sundberg, R. D. (1955). *Blood*, **10**, 416.
(8) Gray, C. H., Neuberger, A. and Sneath, P. H. A. (1950). *Biochem. J.* **47**, 87.
(9) Kench, J. E., Langley, F. A. and Wilkinson, J. F. (1953). *Quart. J. Med.* N.S. **22**, 285.
(10) Waldenström, J. (1957). *Amer. J. Med.* **22**, 758.
(11) Gibson, J. B. and Goldberg, A. (1956). *J. Path. Bact.* **71**, 495.
(12) Granick, S. and Schrieck, H. G. V. (1955). *Proc. Soc. Exp. Biol., N.Y.* **88**, 270.
(13) Waldenström, J. (1956). *Acta Genet.* **6**, 122.
(14) Schmid, R., Schwartz, S. and Watson, C. J. (1954). *Arch. Int. Med.* (1954), **93**, 167.

(15) Goldberg, A. and Rimington, C. (1954). *Lancet*, **2**, 172.
(16) Goldberg, A., Paton, W. D. M. and Thompson, J. W. (1954). *Brit. J. Pharmacol*. **9**, 91.
(17) Jarrett, A., Rimington, C. and Willoughby, D. A. (1956). *Lancet*, **1**, 125.
(18) Goldberg, A. (1954). *Biochem. J.* **57**, 55.
(19) Waldenström, J. (1937). *Acta med. scand.* Suppl. 82.
(20) Gray, C. H., Rimington, C. and Thompson, S. (1948). *Quart. J. Med.* N.S. **17**, 123.
(21) Mcgregor, A. G., Nicholas, R. E. H. and Rimington, C. (1952). *Arch. Int. Med.* **90**, 483.
(22) Holti, G., Rimington, C., Tate, B. C. and Thomas, G. (1958). *Quart. J. Med.* N.S. **27**, 1.
(23) Dean, G. and Barnes, H. D. (1955). *Brit. Med. J.* **2**, 89.
(24) Dean, G. and Barnes, H. D. (1958). *Brit. Med. J.* **1**, 298.
(25) Berger, H. and Goldberg, A. (1955). *Brit. Med. J.* **2**, 85.
(26) Kiese, M. (1944). *Biochem. Z.* **316**, 264.
(27) Gibson, Q. H. (1948). *Biochem. J.* **42**, 13.
(28) Barcroft, H., Gibson, Q. H., Harrison, D. C. and McMurray, J. (1945). *Clin. Sci.* **5**, 145.
(29) Hitzenberger, K. (1933). *Wien. Z. inn. Med.* **23**, 85.
(30) Worster-Drought, C., White, J. C. and Sargent, F. (1953). *Brit. Med. J.* **2**, 114.
(31) Darling, R. C. and Roughton, F. J. W. (1942). *Amer. J. Phys.* **137**, 56.
(32) Gibson, Q. H. (1943). *Biochem. J.* **37**, 615.
(33) Gibson, Q. H. and Harrison, D. C. (1947). *Lancet*, **2**, 941.
(34) Codounis, A. (1952). *Brit. Med. J.* **2**, 368.
(35) Hörlein, H. and Weber, G. (1948). *Dtsch. med. Wschr.* **73**, 476.
(36) Gerald, P. S., Cook, C. D. and Diamond, L. K. (1957). *Science*, **126**, 300.
(37) Crigler, J. F. and Najjar, V. A. (1952). *Pediatrics*, **10**, 169.
(38) Childs, B. and Najjar V. A. (1952). *Pediatrics*, **18**, 369.
(39) Rosenthal, I. M., Zimmerman, H. J. and Hardy, N. (1956). *Pediatrics*, **18**, 378.
(40) Childs, B. (1957). In *Etiologic Factors in Mental Retardation*. 23rd Ross Paediatric Research Conference. Ross Laboratories. Columbus, Ohio.
(41) Billing, B. H. and Lathe, G. H. (1958). *Amer. J. Med.* **24**, 111.
(42) Schmid, R., Axelrod, J., Hammaker, L. and Rosenthal, I. M. (1957). *J. Clin. Invest.* **36**, 927.
(43) Takahara, S. (1952). *Lancet*, **2**, 1101.
(44) Dent, C. E. (1952). *J. Bone Jt. Surg.* **34** B, 266.
(45) Dent, C. E. and Harris, H. (1956). *J. Bone Jt. Surg.* **38** B, 204.
(46) Pederson, H. E. and McCarroll, H. R. (1951). *J. Bone Jt. Surg.* **33** A, 203.
(47) Robertson, B. R., Harris, R. C. and McCune, D. J. (1942). *Amer. J. Dis. Child.* **64**, 948.

(48) Winters, R. W., Graham, J. B., Williams, F. T., McFalls, V. W. and Burnett, C. H. (1957). *Trans. Ass. Amer. Phycns*, **70**, 234.

(49) Rathbun, J. C. (1948). *J. Dis. Child.* **75**, 822.

(50) Fraser, D. (1957). *Amer. J. Med.* **22**, 730.

(51) Currarino, G., Neuhauser, E. B. D., Reyersbach, G. C. and Sobell, E. H. (1957). *Amer. J. Rœntgenol.* **128**, 392.

(52) McCance, R. A., Fairweather, D. V. I., Barrett, A. M. and Morrison, A. B. (1956). *Quart. J. Med.* **25**, 523.

(53) Schlesinger, B., Luder, J. and Bodiam, M. (1955). *Arch. Dis. Child.* **30**, 265.

(54) Sobell, E. H., Clark, L. C., Fox, R. P., Robinow, M. (1953). *Pediatrics*, **11**, 309.

(55) Bourne, G. H. (1956). *The Biochemistry and Physiology of Bone.* Academic Press, New York.

(56) McCance, R. A., Morrison, A. B. and Dent, C. E. (1955). *Lancet*, **1**, 131.

(57) Fraser, D., Yendt, E. R. and Christie, F. H. E. (1955). *Lancet*, **1**, 286.

(58) Cusworth, D. C. (1957). Ph.D. Thesis. London University.

(59) Chargaff, E. and Keston, A. S. (1940). *J. Biol. Chem.* **134**, 515.

(60) Harris, H. and Robson, E. B. (1958). *Ann. Hum. Genet.* (in press).

(61) Pender, C. B. and Fraser, F. C. (1953). *Pediatrics*, **11**, 246.

(62) Forssmann, H. (1945). *Acta med. scand.* Suppl. **159**.

(63) Forssmann, H. (1955). *Amer. J. Hum. Genet.* **7**, 21.

(64) Carter, C. O. and Simpkiss, M. (1956). *Lancet*, **2**, 1069.

(65) Granick, S. (1957). In *Biochemical Disorders in Human Disease*, ed. Thompson, R. H. S. and King, E. J. Churchill, London.

(66) Finch, S. C. and Finch, C. A. (1955). *Medicine, Baltimore*, **34**, 381.

(67) Debré, R., Dreyfus, J. C., Frezal, J., Labie, D., Lamy, M., Maroteaux, P., Schapira, F. and Schapira, G. (1958). *Ann. Hum. Genet.* **23**, 16.

(68) McCance, R. A. and Widdowson, E. M. (1937). *Lancet*, **2**, 682.

(69) Granick, S. (1949). *Bull N.Y. Acad. Med.* **25**, 403.

(70) Golberg, L. (1957). *Postgrad. Med.* **22**, 382.

(71) Archer, H. E., Dormer, A. E., Scowen, E. F. and Watts, R. W. E. (1957). *Lancet*, **2**, 320.

(72) Archer, H. E., Dormer, A. E., Scowen, E. F. and Watts, R. W. E. (1957). *Clin. Sci.* **16**, 405.

(73) Dunn, H. G. (1955). *Amer. J. Dis. Child.* **90**, 58.

(74) Scowen, E. F. (1958). Personal communication.

(75) Archer, H. E., Dormer, A. E., Scowen, E. F. and Watts, R. W. E. (1958). *Brit. Med. J.* **1**, 175.

(76) Jacobsen, B. M. (1937). *Ann. Int. Med.* **11**, 1277.

(77) Smyth, C. J., Cotterman, C. W. and Freyberg, R. H. (1948). *J. Clin. Invest.* **27**, 749.

(78) Hutchinson, J. (1876). *Med. Times, Lond.* **1**, 543.

(79) Hauge, M. and Harvald, B. (1955). *Acta med. scand.* **152**, 247.

(80) Stecher, R. M., Hirsch, A. H. and Solomons, W. M. (1949). *Ann. Int. Med.* **31**, 595.

(81) Wolfson, W. Q., Hunt, H. D., Levine, R., Guterman, H. S., Cohn, C., Rosenberg, E. F., Huddleston, B. and Kadota, K. (1949). *J. Clin. Endocrin.* **9**, 749.

(82) Stetten, de W. (1952). *Bull. N.Y. Acad. Med.* **28**, 664.

(83) Berliner, R. W., Hilton, J. G., Yu, T. F. and Kennedy, T. J. (1950). *J. Clin. Invest.* **29**, 396.

(84) Sirota, J. H., Yu, T. F. and Gutman, A. B. (1952). *J. Clin. Invest.* **31**, 692.

(85) Friedman, M. and Byers, S. O. (1950). *Amer. J. Med.* **9**, 31.

(86) Combined Staff Conference (1957). *Amer. J. Med.* **22**, 807.

(87) Wyngaarden, J. B. (1957). *J. Clin. Invest.* **36**, 1508.

(88) Benedict, J. D., Yu, T. F., Bien, E. J., Gutman, A. B., Stetten, de W. (1953). *J. Clin. Invest.* **32**, 775.

CHAPTER 10

THE PROBLEM OF GENE ACTION

Introduction

One of the central problems in genetics is that which is concerned
with the question of how genes act. What is the function of the gene
in the normal organism? How do abnormal genes produce their
particular effects?

The possibility of knowing anything about genes at all arises from
the fact that at any particular chromosomal locus a gene may occur
in more than one form, each with somewhat different properties.
Such alternative genes, or alleles, are thought to have arisen one
from another as a result of the sudden, rare, and rather unpredict-
able changes known as mutations. In somatic cells each gene locus
is in general represented twice, once in each of a pair of homologous
chromosomes. One member of each pair is ultimately derived from
one parent and one from the other. Thus when as a result of past
mutations, several allelic genes may exist at a particular locus,
individual people will differ from one another in the particular
combination they possess, and this will be reflected in some way in
the details of the metabolic processes. In the simplest situation where
there are two alleles A and a, three genetically distinct types of
individual can occur, AA, Aa, aa. Each of these three types of
individual may be expected to be biochemically different in some
respect from the other two, and our knowledge of this particular gene
difference ultimately rests on our ability to distinguish at least one
of these types from the others.

In human genetics any approach to the problem of the nature of
gene function is necessarily rather indirect. In practice what one
observes in the first place is some difference between people with
respect to a particular kind of character. By the analysis of the
manner in which the character is distributed in a population of
individuals, and more specifically within certain family groups, one
may be able to infer the existence of more than one allelic gene at
some chromosomal locus. A detailed investigation of the biochemistry of individuals presumed to carry the different allelic genes

in their various combinations may then enable one to obtain some idea of the primary and specific manner in which they differ from one another metabolically. From this one may ultimately expect to achieve some insight into the fundamental nature of the action of the genes concerned. In general the character or phenotypic difference which serves as a starting-point for such investigations is likely to be a somewhat remote consequence of the primary action of the genes concerned. The sequence of causal relationships connecting them is usually complex and can involve investigations aimed at elucidating phenomena at many different levels of biochemical and physiological functioning.

The kind of argument involved can be illustrated by a consideration of the metabolic disorder phenylketonuria. This is a typical example of an 'inborn error of metabolism', and it has been investigated from both the biochemical and genetical points of view perhaps more intensively than any other. Prior to the discovery of phenylketonuria by Fölling in 1934, it had been recognised that many forms of mental defect were genetically determined and certain of these, such as amaurotic family idiocy, had been characterised in clinical and morphological terms. However, Fölling's observation that some idiots and imbeciles characteristically excreted in their urine large amounts of phenylpyruvic acid represented the first instance where a clear-cut biochemical abnormality could be seen to be closely associated with a marked degree of mental impairment. Once the syndrome had been recognised it was relatively easy to identify further examples of the disorder by screening patients in mental deficiency institutions using the simple ferric chloride test for phenylpyruvic acid in urine. It emerged that the condition accounted for about $\frac{1}{2}$-1 per cent of all idiots and imbeciles; that it was quite sharply differentiated from all other forms of mental defect on the basis of the chemical findings in the urine; that the metabolic disorder was constant; and that the syndrome was genetically determined. Extensive studies of the relatives of such patients revealed that the disorder was distributed in families in the manner to be expected if it were inherited as a typical Mendelian recessive character. The observed incidence of the condition in the appropriate classes of relatives fitted the theoretical requirements of this hypothesis rather exactly, and so did the observed incidence of parental consanguinity. It could therefore be concluded with some confidence that the affected individuals must be homozygous for a rare abnormal gene, the frequency of which was estimated to be about 1 in 200 in most European populations.

The problem was thus posed as to how exactly this abnormal gene when present in double dose leads to the characteristic metabolic disturbance and to the mental defect. Another aspect of the same problem is the question as to what the function of the normal allele of the phenylketonuric gene is in unaffected individuals. In principle one would expect a comparison of the biochemistry of phenyl-ketonuric patients with that of normal individuals to indicate the character of the functional activity of the two alternative genes at this chromosomal locus. Furthermore, since both parents and a proportion of the unaffected sibs and other relatives should be hetero-zygous, that is possess both the normal and abnormal alleles each in single dose, a comparison of the biochemistry of such individuals with affected homozygotes on the one hand, and random normal individuals (the great majority of whom will be homozygous for the normal allele) on the other, may be expected to provide further information about the same question, and also throw light on the nature of the inter-action of the two alleles when present in the same individual.

It soon became clear that phenylketonuria represented a major disorder in the metabolism of the aromatic aminoacid phenylalanine. Phenylalanine itself was found in the blood plasma and in the cerebrospinal fluid in concentrations some thirty times those normally occurring, and phenylpyruvic acid was shown to be but one of several derivatives of phenylalanine which were excreted in grossly abnormal quantities in the urine. A consideration of these findings in terms of what was known of the metabolism of phenylalanine in the normal subject led to the hypothesis that they were the con-sequence of a block in metabolism at the point where normally phenylalanine is para-hydroxylated to form tyrosine, and the results of a variety of metabolic experiments in these patients fully sub-stantiated this hypothesis.

This concept of the metabolic lesion in phenylketonuria indicated that there was likely to be some kind of congenital defect in the enzyme system normally concerned with the conversion of phenyl-alanine to tyrosine. Direct assay for this enzyme activity in liver material obtained from a small number of phenylketonuric patients has shown that this enzyme system is indeed deficient, and that it is probably one specific component of the system normally occurring only in liver cells which is at fault.

Biochemical studies on the presumed heterozygotes have thrown further light on the problem. These individuals are not intellectually retarded and are clinically quite normal. Nevertheless it was found that they exhibit a disturbance in phenylalanine metabolism qualitatively similar though quantitatively very much less in degree to that encountered in the affected homozygotes. The phenomenon is seen most clearly when the heterozygous individuals are subjected to a phenylalanine tolerance test. When a relatively large dose of phenylalanine is fed under standard conditions the plasma phenylalanine levels in the next few hours are usually considerably higher than those obtaining in appropriate 'normal' controls. Even in the fasting state, however, the plasma phenylalanine concentration in the heterozygotes is on the average slightly higher than in normal homozygotes. One may conclude that the heterozygotes have a partial deficiency of the phenylalanine hydroxylation system, but that sufficient of the enzyme activity is present to cope with all normal requirements, so that no gross pathological consequences ensue.

Thus the effect of the phenylketonuric gene in double dose appears to result in the complete or almost complete absence of this specific enzyme activity, and in single dose in a partial deficiency of it. Put another way, this means that the normal allele of this gene must be present in at least single dose for adequate amounts of this enzyme activity to be exhibited. The obvious hypothesis that emerges from this is that there is a causal connection between the functional activity of these particular genes and the formation of this specific enzyme.

Genes and enzymes

Thus the genetical and biochemical analysis of phenylketonuria leads to the conclusion that a more or less direct relation exists between the presence of a certain gene and the presence of a particular enzyme. The investigation of a number of other examples of inherited metabolic disorders has led to similar conclusions. In each case the biochemical disturbances characteristic of the disease can be plausibly explained in terms of a block at some point in the normal course of the metabolic processes. This block can in turn be attributed to the deficiency of a single specific enzyme, and the enzyme deficiency itself explained in terms of a single gene substitution. Typical examples of conditions which fall into this classical pattern of 'inborn errors of metabolism' are galactosaemia where the particular enzyme concerned is galactose-

1-phosphate uridyl transferase, one form of glycogenosis in which there is a specific defect of glucose-6-phosphatase, and alkaptonuria where the enzyme normally concerned in the conversion of homogentisic acid to maleylacetoacetic acid is deficient. Other examples, or probable examples, of the same sort of thing are listed in Table 50.

Table 50. *Probable enzyme deficiencies in different conditions*

Condition	Deficient enzyme	Page reference
Phenylketonuria	L-Phenylalanine hydroxylase*	45
Alkaptonuria	Homogentisic acid oxidase*	51
Tyrosinosis	p-Hydroxy-phenylpyruvic acid oxidase	56
Albinism	Tyrosinase	64
Cystathioninuria	Cystathionine cleavage enzyme	96
Glycogen storage disease (a)	Glucose-6-phosphatase*	103
Glycogen storage disease (b)	Amylo-1:6-glucosidase*	106
Glycogen storage disease (c)	Amylo-(1:4 → 1:6)-trans-glucosidase	107
Galactosaemia	Galactose-1-phosphate uridyl transferase*	111
Primaquine sensitivity	Glucose-6-phosphate dehydrogenase*	128
Suxamethonium sensitivity	Serum cholinesterase (pseudo-cholinesterase)*	230
Methaemoglobinaemia (one type)	Diaphorase I (methaemoglobin reductase)*	248
Congenital hyperbilirubinaemia	Glucuronyl transferase	250
Acatalasaemia	Catalase*	252
Hypophosphatasia	Alkaline phosphatase*	255
Goitrous cretinism	Dehalogenase*	59

* Enzyme deficiencies demonstrated directly *in vitro*.

These examples suggest that many genes may act by controlling the synthesis of specific enzymes. There is, of course, a great deal of experimental evidence in the genetics of other organisms (notably the fungi), which leads to a similar kind of conclusion, and the results have been generalised in the form of the so-called one gene-one enzyme hypothesis. This suggests that genes—the units of inherited variation—bear a simple one to one relation with enzymes—the units of biochemical catalysis, and it implies that this forms the fundamental basis of inherited biochemical and morphological diversity. While it now seems likely that this hypothesis has not got quite the generality which it was once thought to possess, nevertheless there is little doubt that it provides a useful and unifying approach to the investigation of many different kinds of inherited metabolic variation.

As applied to the inborn errors of metabolism it may be formulated in the first instance in the following simple manner. One can suppose that in each case the normal allele of the particular mutant gene responsible for the disorder is somehow directly concerned in the synthesis of a single specific enzyme. The effect of the mutation is to alter the character of the gene in some way so that this function is inadequately performed. In consequence individuals who are homozygous for the mutant gene will fail to synthesise the enzyme or will do so in very inadequate amounts, and this will result in a characteristic disturbance of the normal metabolic pattern. What will happen in the heterozygote will depend on how much of the enzyme can be formed by the normal gene in single dose, and the actual quantities of the enzyme which are required to allow the particular metabolic process to go on normally.

The conclusion that in a particular inherited metabolic disorder there exists a relative deficiency of a certain enzyme, and that this is the cause of the various metabolic and clinical features of the condition, involves at least two different kinds of evidence. In the first place it is necessary to have a direct demonstration, using the techniques of enzymology *in vitro*, that the activity of a particular enzyme present in the normal organisms is absent or diminished, and that this is not due to the presence of inhibitors or some other alteration in the milieu in which the enzyme normally functions. Secondly, it is necessary to demonstrate that all the biochemical findings in the body fluids and tissues, and the changes that may occur in these as a result of fortuitous variation in the environment or the consequence of deliberate metabolic experiments, can be reasonably attributed to the consequences of the failure in the particular reactions which the enzyme normally catalyses. Furthermore, the various clinical and morphological features of the disease should be explicable in terms of the biochemical disturbances resulting from the enzyme deficiency.

The series of conditions listed in Table 50 represent disorders in which the situation has been analysed to a sufficient degree to make the hypothesis that a single enzyme deficiency is the underlying basis of the pathology seem highly plausible. In many of these examples, however, one or other facet of the evidence which would constitute a complete proof of this argument is to some extent incomplete. Consequently, although the information at present available is quite consistent with the simple gene enzyme hypothesis, other rather more complex possibilities cannot be satisfactorily excluded.

Some of the general problems and difficulties inherent in this kind of investigation are perhaps worth brief consideration. An important point in the argument, for example, turns on the direct demonstration of the specific enzyme defect *in vitro*. In practice this has been most readily achieved only in those conditions in which the appropriate enzyme is normally present in red cells or blood plasma. Conditions such as galactosaemia, acatalasaemia and hypophosphatasia are examples of this. In other conditions the relevant enzyme can only be examined in tissues, such as liver or kidney, and the appropriate material is much less readily come by. Even where blood can be used for such studies, analogous investigations on other tissues are clearly desirable. Such investigations necessitate the use of material obtained by biopsy in the living subject or at post-mortem. Its availability is very restricted and furthermore the time lag necessarily involved, particularly where post-mortem material is used, leads to extra difficulties in experimental control and interpretation. Thus, although in recent years several such investigations have been carried out in different conditions, using either biopsy or post-mortem material, the number of individual cases studied in each instance is relatively few, and the range of investigations possible in each subject somewhat limited.

Another difficulty which besets all such studies is deciding whether an enzyme defect is complete, or whether some residual activity remains. The answer to this kind of question has an obvious bearing on any conclusions drawn concerning the character of the functional activity of the mutant gene presumed to be concerned. In practice an unequivocal answer is often rather difficult to obtain. Where the enzyme system is being investigated directly *in vitro* it will depend both on the sensitivity and also on the specificity of the methods available. The preparation may contain more than one enzyme system capable of producing, as far as can be ascertained by available methods, similar end results. In such a situation, even if one such system were completely inactive, the overall activity would be only partially diminished. Where the evidence suggesting that the enzymic block is incomplete turns on the interpretation of metabolic data, the possibility of alternative pathways is always present and often difficult to exclude. This difficulty is seen in phenylketonuria, where there is some evidence that tyrosine formation may still go on to a limited extent, and in galactosaemia, where a small amount of the galactose in the diet does appear to be metabolised in some cases.

Another common problem in these conditions concerns the inter-relationships between the metabolic disorder as expressed in biochemical terms and the other pathological and clinical features of the disease. The simple gene-enzyme hypothesis implies that all the diverse manifestations of each of these conditions should be attributable to the metabolic consequences of a single enzyme deficiency. The analysis of the precise causal sequence involved is of significance therefore in validating the general hypothesis. In hypophosphatasia, for example, there is a generalised deficiency of alkaline phosphatase activity, and this is associated with a characteristic disturbance in bone development. The causal connections are, however, quite obscure. Until this has been sorted out the possibility cannot be excluded that the abnormality in bone formation depends on a biochemical disturbance not directly resulting from the known enzyme deficiency but nevertheless a consequence of the presence of the abnormal gene.

It has also to be remembered that the demonstration *in vitro* of a particular kind of enzymic activity by a protein does not necessarily mean that this corresponds to its normal metabolic function, or that the substrates used experimentally are those on which it acts under normal physiological conditions. In the same way the demonstration *in vitro* of the diminution or loss of a particular kind of enzymic activity in material from patients suffering from some inherited syndrome, does not necessarily imply that this loss of enzymic activity, as such, is the cause of the metabolic disorders present. These considerations are relevant, as an example, to the interpretation of the diminution of plasma oxidase activity in Wilson's disease. In this condition a characteristic finding is a marked reduction in the amounts of the copper-containing protein caeruloplasmin present in the plasma. Now caeruloplasmin has been shown to exhibit *in vitro* marked oxidase activity using a variety of different substrates such as *p*-phenylene diamine, dopa, and adrenaline. The oxidase activity of plasma is closely correlated with its caeruloplasmin content, and in Wilson's disease the plasma oxidase activity and the caeruloplasmin level are reduced in more or less proportionate amounts. But it is not known whether the oxidase activity of caeruloplasmin is of any significance physiologically, and one cannot assume that this activity is its main biological function. Furthermore, although it is possible that in Wilson's disease a defect in caeruloplasmin synthesis is the central lesion, there is nothing to suggest that the various other metabolic abnormalities found are due to the concomitant reduction in oxidase activity. Thus although there exists close correlation between the particular abnormal gene causing Wilson's disease and the deficiency of this particular enzyme activity as demonstrated *in vitro*, it remains uncertain whether this has any important place in the pathogenesis of the disorder.

One aspect of the analysis of biochemical disorders to which attention has been drawn in recent years concerns the problem of distinguishing between blocks in intermediary metabolism on the one hand and defects in cellular transport systems on the other. It has been shown, for instance, that the abnormal excretion of particular metabolites in the urine may arise because of some disorder in the process by which they are normally reabsorbed by the renal tubular cells from the glomerular filtrate, rather than, as had often been assumed without question in the past, from a defect in the processes of their intermediary metabolism. Typical examples of conditions where such abnormalities in renal tubule function have been observed are cystinuria, renal glycosuria, resistant rickets, and Hartnup disease. In each of these cases one is confronted with a highly specific disorder in the transport systems of the renal-tubule cells, and the elucidation of the nature of this disorder is of obvious significance in understanding the mode of action of the genes concerned. Very little is, however, known about the apparently rather complex processes which are involved in renal tubular reabsorptive function. Though it is reasonable to believe that these processes are enzymically controlled, and that deficiencies of particular enzymes might be the cause of the specific disturbances in reabsorption which are observed in these various conditions, there is in fact no direct information about this.

The recognition of these genetically determined peculiarities in the transport of substances across the renal tubule cells raises the question as to whether they may not represent only a special case of a much more general phenomenon. It seems quite possible that genetically determined peculiarities may occur in active transport processes going on elsewhere in the body. Such processes are essential for the maintenance of many different types of concentration gradients across cell membranes. Abnormalities in them might well result in unusual concentrations of particular metabolites in the body fluids which could easily mimic the changes arising from a block in intermediary metabolism of the classical type. Distinguishing between the two kinds of situation could prove a formidable problem.

Some questions arising from the gene-enzyme hypothesis

Despite the various difficulties involved in interpretation, and the incomplete nature of much of the evidence so far assembled, the simple unitary hypothesis that the manifold biochemical and clinical characteristics of many inherited metabolic disorders can be ultimately traced back to the effects of a single specific enzyme deficiency remains the most plausible and satisfactory general way of thinking about them. The simple concept that emerges from this—namely that genes may act by controlling the synthesis of enzymes, and the effect of a mutation is to alter the character of the gene in such a way that this function is not adequately performed—calls, however, for some comment.

In the first place it is clear that to say that the biochemical disturbances in a particular inherited condition are due to a failure in synthesis of a certain enzyme because the causative gene is unable to perform the function of its normal allele in enzyme formation, only throws the problem back to a deeper level. One still has to explain what the precise role of genes in enzyme formation really is. Most enzymes appear to be proteins, and the question here is probably part of the broader one of what role genes play in protein synthesis in general.

Another point is that the simple theory of the inborn errors of metabolism implies a rather negative role for the mutant gene. Its functional activity is characterised essentially by the absence or gross deficiency of a particular kind of enzyme activity in individuals who are homozygous for it. One wonders whether, in fact, one is really dealing with situations in which a protein with a particular kind of enzyme activity is not formed and nothing occurs in its place, or whether perhaps the synthesis may occur of a protein similar to that normally encountered but differing somewhat in its structure and hence in its enzymic properties. Slight modifications in protein structure might well lead to a considerable curtailment or indeed the complete loss of a particular kind of enzymic activity. Thus at first sight the situation could appear to represent a partial or complete failure in the formation of a certain protein, whereas in fact a protein qualitatively different might have been formed.

Very occasionally the protein formed by the mutant gene might possess new enzymic properties qualitatively different from those of its 'normal' counterpart, and indeed it is difficult to visualise the role of gene mutations in biochemical evolution unless some process along these lines is postulated. It is probable that the work of Kalow and his colleagues on the genetically determined variations in the inhibition characteristics of serum cholinesterase (see page 230) represents the first example in human genetics of just such a situation where two allelic genes each control the formation of functionally active enzymes with different properties. The search for further examples is obviously worth pursuing.

The genes controlling the A and B group specificities of the ABO blood-group system are of particular interest in this context. Mucopolysaccharides with A specificity are found in individuals of genotypes **AA** or **AO**, and similarly mucopolysaccharides with B specificity occur in individuals with genotypes **BB** and **BO**. Individuals of the genotype **AB** evidently form mucopolysaccharide molecules with both A and B specificities. It appears likely that the overall structure of these mucopolysaccharides is much the same in each case, and that the group-specific serological differences are determined by the presence of relatively short oligosaccharide sequences of different constitutions formed at a fairly late stage of the synthesis of the mucopolysaccharide molecules. It seems not unreasonable to suggest that this may depend on the presence of oligosaccharide-synthesising enzymes with somewhat different specificities. The enzyme in group A individuals might conceivably be concerned in forming a particular type of linkage in which acetyl-galactosamine was a necessary unit-sugar, while that in group B individuals was concerned in the formation of a different type of oligosaccharide sequence involving D-galactose. As yet little is known about the precise mode of formation of these group-specific substances, but if different enzymes are in fact involved these could presumably be regarded as the products of the activity of different allelic genes.

Genes and proteins

It is apparent that any discussion of the part played by genes in controlling the formation of enzymes must ultimately lead to questions concerning the nature of protein synthesis in general and the role that genes may play in this. In fact one of the most interesting developments in human genetics in recent years has been the recognition of a variety of inherited differences in which there occurs some obvious peculiarity in the synthesis of particular proteins or groups of proteins, and the analysis of such situations is turning out to have considerable theoretical significance in relation to the general problem of the nature of gene action. The particular proteins referred to here do not appear under normal circumstances to function as enzymes. There is, however, no reason to believe that their mode of synthesis differs in any fundamental way from the synthesis of enzyme proteins. In general they occur in considerably greater quantities than most enzyme proteins so that their direct investigation is considerably easier.

The proteins which are most accessible for study in human beings are those which occur in blood plasma and erythrocytes. It is relatively easy to obtain samples of blood for investigation and many different methods are now available for the fractionation and characterisation of the many proteins which are present. Tissue proteins, on the other hand, are much less easily obtained in a suitable form for such studies. It is not surprising, therefore, that most of the examples of inherited differences in non-enzymic proteins of which we are aware represent peculiarities either in the formation of the plasma proteins or of haemoglobin. Presumably the multiplicity of inherited protein differences which have so far been encountered are not peculiar to this fluid, and one may expect that analogous differences in proteins in other tissues occur, and will in due course be identified.

Two extreme and contrasting types of situation have been observed among these inherited variations in protein synthesis. In one type of situation, exemplified by such conditions as afibrinogenaemia and analbuminaemia, the presence of the particular abnormal gene in affected homozygotes seems to result in the complete, or very nearly complete, failure to synthesise one species of protein molecule. There is no indication that any alternative kind of protein is formed in its place. The other sort of situation is illustrated by the genetically determined variants in haemoglobin synthesis. Here the presence of the abnormal or mutant gene results in the synthesis of a qualitatively new form of haemoglobin similar in most respects to its normal counterpart but differing somewhat in certain of its physico-chemical properties. In heterozygotes where two different allelic genes are present, two different kinds of haemoglobin are formed.

It is easy to see how both these kinds of situation could serve as models to explain the various phenomena encountered in the meta-bolic disorders discussed earlier where the essential functions of the relevant genes seem to be concerned with the formation of specific enzyme proteins, but the activity of the mutant can be assessed in terms of only one sort of property of the particular protein under consideration, namely its enzymic activity.

A number of other inherited variations in protein formation have also been identified, where the findings so far cannot be readily formulated in terms of a simple hypothesis implying a more or less direct relationship between the presence of a particular gene and the synthesis of a single protein molecular species. In agammaglobulin-aemia, for example, the affected individuals exhibit a gross failure in the capacity to form the group of proteins normally classed as γ-globulins, and usually thought to include many different though related molecular types. There is also evidence that such individuals fail to synthesise a group of proteins normally present in the β-electrophoretic fraction of plasma and which can be distinguished immunochemically from the γ-globulins. Similar complexities have been encountered in the common variations which occur in haptoglobin synthesis. Here the character of a group of proteins or mucoproteins, which have the characteristic property of binding haemoglobin, is apparently determined by a pair of allelic genes. The individual haptoglobins differ from one another in their electrophoretic properties under certain conditions, and these differences appear to be largely a function of molecular size. Furthermore, the heterozygote evidently forms haptoglobins qualitatively different from those encountered in either sort of homozygote. In both these examples it may well be that the complexities arise because one is dealing with phenomena at a level somewhat more removed from the activity of the immediate product of gene action than are, say, the phenomena illustrated by the haemoglobin variants.

The discovery of the differences in haemoglobin synthesis and the demonstration of their relatively simple genetical causation opened up altogether new possibilities in the study of the nature of gene action. It was seen that alternative genes at a particular chromosomal locus could lead to the formation of alternative types of the same kind of protein, and the isolation and structural analysis of these alternative forms became an immediate possibility. Structural differences between such alternative proteins must reflect differences in their biosynthesis, and the magnitude and character of such differences would be expected to be a sensitive indication of the differences in functional activity of the alternative genes which controlled their formation.

Most of the haemoglobin variants that have been discovered so far appear to be alternative forms of normal adult haemoglobin. This has a molecular weight of about 67,000 and it is evidently made up of two identical half molecules. Each of the half molecules contains about 300 aminoacid residues and these are thought to be arranged in two distinct polypeptide chains with different sequences. The polypeptide chains are presumably linked together and organised spatially in a complex and characteristic manner. The structural peculiarities of the different haemoglobins might, then, be expected to lie either in modifications of the aminoacid sequences in the polypeptide chains or in alterations in the mode of linkage or spatial arrangement of the chains.

So far detailed studies have been reported only in the cases of haemoglobin S and haemoglobin C, the formation of which are controlled by genes which are probably allelic. Ingram has demonstrated that the essential difference between each of these haemoglobins and normal adult haemoglobin is that a single aminoacid residue, out of the 300 present in each haemoglobin half molecule, has been substituted by another. A particular glutamic acid residue in one of the polypeptide chains in haemoglobin A is replaced by a valine residue in haemoglobin S and by a lysine residue in haemoglobin C. The arrangement of all the other aminoacid residues in each of the three types of molecule is probably identical.

This result is quite remarkable for its simplicity. A single gene difference such as that between the sickle-cell gene and its normal allele is presumably the result of a single mutational step. This is the smallest unit of inherited variation. It may evidently lead to the smallest unit of structural difference in the haemoglobin formed, the substitution of a single aminoacid residue.

It is a salutary thought that such a subtle change in the structure of a single protein can have as its consequence the profound pathological and clinical disturbance characteristic of a condition such as sickle-cell anaemia. Most of these disturbances can be attributed to the relative insolubility of the abnormal haemoglobin in the deoxygenated state and this change in its physical properties must be due to the substitution of a valine residue for the normally occurring glutamic acid residue at one particular location in the molecule. It is tempting to speculate that an analogous alteration in the fine structure of an enzyme protein would lead to a drastic change in those of its physico-chemical properties which determined its enzymic activity.

This might well be the underlying basis of many of the inborn errors of metabolism.

Ingram's results represent the closest approach that has yet been made to the understanding of the precise way in which a mutation may modify the character of gene activity. It reinforces the conclusions reached from other lines of evidence that genes are somehow intimately concerned in protein synthesis.

Now proteins are complex macromolecules each of which is made up about twenty different types of aminoacid units. Their biological behaviour and specificity must ultimately depend to a great extent on the precise sequences of the constituent aminoacids in the polypeptide chains. It will also no doubt depend on the spatial configuration and interconnections of the polypeptide chains, though this may well, to a considerable degree, be a function of the sequential arrangement of the aminoacids in the chains themselves. Though knowledge of the processes concerned in protein synthesis is still in its infancy, it is difficult to avoid the conclusion that, for the formation of any given protein molecule by a cell, some model, template, or 'set of instructions' must already be present which enables the constituent aminoacids to be arranged in precisely the correct order for the formation of a protein of that specific type. The structural organisation of a particular kind of protein seems to be characteristic not only of the individual but also of the species. The template, or pre-existing code of information, must presumably, therefore, be transmissible from one generation to the next. It must also evidently be present in cells which do not at the particular time contain the protein itself. A single fertilised ovum has to contain within it all the necessary information for the production of proteins, many of which may not be formed till some cell generations later in the development of the individual. It seems necessary, therefore, to postulate that the structural organisation of large numbers of specific proteins formed by an organism must be represented in some way in the genetical determinants—the chromosomes and genes of classical genetics.

It is, then, appropriate at this stage to consider briefly some of the current ideas and speculations concerning the nature of gene structure and specificity.

The Watson-Crick hypothesis

Classical genetics led to the conclusion that the genes, the units of Mendelian heredity, were essentially small subdivisions of chromosomes arranged side by side along the length of these structures. Each gene was envisaged as being separable from the others in the same chromosome by the process of crossing over. The concept of the gene as the biological unit of inheritance necessitated that it should possess several remarkable properties. It had to play a specific functional role in cell metabolism; it had to be capable of exact self-duplication so that the functional specificity was preserved from one cell generation to the next; and although usually an extremely stable entity it had to be susceptible to occasional sudden change or mutation which would result in a new unit differing functionally from the original one, but self-reproducing in its new form.

The more refined genetical analysis which has become possible in the investigation of certain organisms in recent years has resulted in a further extension of these ideas. It appears that the gene defined as a unit of function is capable of further subdivision in terms of crossing over or of mutation. In effect a picture of intragenic structure is emerging. The chromosomal region which acts functionally as a single unit can evidently be altered by mutations occurring at different sites and also by crossing over occurring within its apparent limits.

Chromosomes, and presumably therefore genes, are composed largely, though not entirely, of desoxyribonucleic acid (DNA) and protein. For many years it was generally assumed that the characteristic properties of the gene were attributable to the particular structural organisation of the protein present. More recently the importance of the DNA has been emphasised and genetical specificity has been widely attributed to the inherent properties of this material. The evidence for the view that the DNA is of critical significance in this connection is largely based on the experimental results obtained in certain micro-organisms, where what appear to be inherited differences closely analogous to those occurring in higher forms have been shown to be directly determined by DNA in the absence of protein. The concept is supported, among other things, by finding that in more complex organisms the amount of DNA per set of chromosomes is a more or less fixed quantity in any given species, though in general it varies interspecifically.

Considerable impetus to the development of ideas in this complex and difficult field has been provided by the formulation of a chemical structure for DNA by Watson and Crick which goes some way towards accounting, in biochemical terms, for certain of the properties which are characteristic of genes and chromosomes (1,2). It presents for the first time a molecular model which provides a plausible basis for gene specificity, gene duplication, and gene mutation.

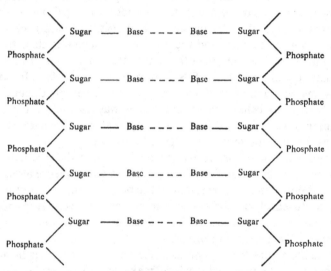

Fig. 69. Suggested arrangement of a pair of desoxyribosenucleic acid chains. The hydrogen bonding is symbolised by dotted lines. (After Watson and Crick, 1953b.)

The main features of the proposed structure of DNA may be outlined quite simply, though the details are rather more complex. The molecule is made up of two very long chains coiled round a common axis to form a double helix. The backbone of each chain consists of a regular alternation of phosphate and sugar groups (Fig. 69). The sugar is always desoxyribose, and to it is attached a nitrogenous base which may be one of four different types. The four bases are adenine and guanine which are purines, and thymine and cytosine which are pyrimidines. The two chains are thought to be held together by hydrogen bonding between the bases.

The bases are joined together in pairs, a single base from one chain being hydrogen-bonded to a single base from the other. However, there are certain restrictions on which bases can constitute a pair. In any pair, one base must be a purine and one base a pyrimidine, and of the possible combinations only two can occur. These are

> adenine with thymine,
> guanine with cytosine.

A given pair can be either way round, thymine, for example, can occur in either chain, but when it does its partner must be adenine.

The analytical data bear out this concept of base pairing. Thus in different sources of DNA the amount of adenine found is close to the amount of thymine, and the amount of guanine is close to the amount of cytosine. On the other hand, the cross-ratios of adenine to guanine vary widely in DNA from different species. In some cases smaller amounts of other bases have also been found, but these are thought to behave in an equivalent way to one of the four common ones. For example, 5-methyl cytosine behaves as an equivalent to cytosine in the proposed structure.

Now, while the phosphate-sugar backbones of the molecule are quite regular, the pairs of bases may occur in any sequence along the chain. Many different permutations are possible, and it is postulated that the genetical specificity is determined by the precise sequence of base pairs that is present. The sequence is, as it were, a code specifying the genetical information.

Since the nature of one base fixes the nature of the other member of each pair, the two chains which make up the molecule, though qualitatively different, are exactly complementary. The sequence of bases in one chain fixes the sequence of bases in the other. Duplication is envisaged as taking place by the breaking of the hydrogen bonds, the unwinding and separating of the two chains, and the reformation on each chain of its appropriate companion from an available pool of free nucleotides or polynucleotide precursors. Each chain is regarded as acting as a template for the formation of the other, so that from one molecule two precise replicates are formed each with exactly the same sequence of base pairs as in the original.

The functional specificity of a gene is determined according to this model by a long series of base pairs arranged in a definite sequence. A mutation presumably involves some change in this sequence. This might take place perhaps by substitution at one or more base pair levels, by rearrangement of the sequence, or possibly in other ways such as duplication or deletion of particular base pairs. Providing the general structure remains the same, however, duplication of the mutant form can then take place.

If the gene as a unit of functional activity is represented by a long sequence of such base pairs, mutational change may presumably occur at many different sites along this sequence. Similarly although no obvious physical basis suggests itself to explain the mode of crossing over and recombination, this can presumably be thought of as resulting in the formation of a new base pair sequence in which, on one side of the 'site' of crossing-over, a sequence derived from one of the original DNA chains occurs, and on the other side the sequence characteristic of the other chain which takes part in the recombination. Looked at in this way the idea derived from genetical experiments that the gene defined as a unit of function is subdivisible in terms of crossing over and mutation is perhaps not so mysterious.

While there is now much evidence in favour of the proposed structure of DNA, there are still many questions about it which are quite obscure. How, for example, is the genetical information which is supposed to be coded by the base pair sequence subsequently transferred in functional activity? What is the role of the protein normally closely associated with the DNA? How is the DNA chain organised in the very much larger chromosome structure? In the process of duplication how do the single chains unwind, and what is the mechanisms of resynthesis of the complementary chains? What exactly is involved in mutation and crossing over? These and many other questions must clearly be answered before a satisfactory synthesis of the results of genetical investigations on the one hand, and physico-chemical studies of the structure of DNA on the other, can be achieved.

If, however, the conclusion that the structural pattern of specific proteins is somehow defined by the genetical material is correct, and if the Watson-Crick hypothesis gives a satisfactory description of the manner in which such information is coded, it would seem that the sequence of base pairs in a particular region of DNA can determine the sequence in which a series of aminoacid residues is incorporated in a particular polypeptide chain. The hypothesis does not, however, necessitate that such polypeptide chains must be the immediate results of genic activity, the so-called primary gene products. In fact there is a great deal of evidence that protein synthesis mainly goes on in the cytoplasm of the cell and it appears more often to be closely associated with RNA rather than DNA. It is, therefore, a plausible elaboration of the hypothesis that the immediate function of chromosomal DNA is to serve as a template for the formation of RNA containing the same kind of information coded perhaps in a similar manner, and that it is the RNA which serves as the immediate template in protein synthesis.

It is easy to see how Ingram's results on the structures of haemo-globins S and C can be formulated in terms of postulates such as these. The normal allele of the mutant genes which result in the formation of these abnormal haemoglobins can be thought of as being represented by a long series of DNA base pairs whose sequence determines the order in which the aminoacid residues are arranged in one of the characteristic polypeptide chains in the haemoglobin molecule. The mutation in each case can be regarded as resulting in a specific alteration in the base-pair sequence at one point, with the consequence that the localised alteration in the coding leads to the incorporation of a different aminoacid at the equivalent point in the aminoacid sequence in the polypeptide chain whose structure it controls.

A somewhat unexpected conclusion emerges, however, when the matter is considered in this way. Such a polypeptide chain pre-sumably contains something of the order of 150 different places where a single aminoacid substitution could take place and each of these would evidently correspond on this hypothesis to different base-pair sites along the length of the relevant DNA chain. One might have expected that mutational change was more or less equally likely in all these positions. It is, therefore, surprising that the first two allelic mutants to be investigated should be found to differ by a single aminoacid substitution in exactly the same place in the polypeptide chain. Perhaps the significance of this will emerge when the structural examination of the other haemoglobin variants provides a somewhat wider perspective.

The extension of this work to the other haemoglobin variants is also of importance in the interpretation of the genetical evidence that mutant genes at at least two independent chromosomal loci can determine the formation of different types of adult haemoglobin. For the moment the simplest hypothesis is that the base-pair sequences at two separate loci determine the aminoacid sequences in the two different polypeptide chains which are thought to occur in the protein molecule. It will be interesting to see how far this hypothesis will stand up to the tests of further structural analyses, and of further genetical studies of the number of loci involved.

While the hypothesis provides an elegant explanation of the synthesis of alternative proteins as a result of gene mutations, it is perhaps not immediately obvious how it can accommodate situations where a complete or almost complete failure in the synthesis of a particular protein seems to occur. One might speculate perhaps that the new protein structure prescribed by the character of the gene mutation is such that it is relatively much more unstable than its normal counterpart and consequently has no more than a transient existence. Another possibility, however, is that the deficiency of the protein may in these cases not be a direct consequence of a mutation of the gene which normally determines the structural organisation of the particular protein, but may be secondary to the effects of a mutant gene concerned in the formation of some other protein (possibly an enzyme) which in turn is necessary for the synthesis of the protein whose deficiency was directly observed. The underlying abnormality may be more subtle and less easily detected than its more obvious secondary consequences.

In this connection it is perhaps worth making the rather obvious point that although a particular gene may have to be present to allow of the synthesis of a particular kind of protein, other factors must also be important in deciding whether the synthesis of the protein should occur in a given cell at a certain time. It is generally believed that with a few exceptions each somatic cell in the body contains in its nucleus a full complement of genes identical with those present in the original fertilised ovum from which the organism developed. However, it is clear that the influence of any one of these genes on the metabolic processes going on in the cell which contains it varies very widely from one cell type to another.

Haemoglobin A and its various genetically determined variants, for example, are only elaborated in quantity in certain red-cell precursors, and they are apparently not formed in appreciable amounts by other cells in the body, even though these cells presumably contain the same genes. The change-over from the predominant formation of foetal haemoglobin to the predominant formation of adult haemoglobin or one of its variants at birth illustrates another aspect of the matter. Presumably in the foetus the cells which are making foetal haemoglobin carry the same set of genes as the cells which in adult life make the adult haemoglobins, but the detailed characters of the synthetic processes going on are clearly very different.

Similarly many of the enzymes whose formation is believed to be genetically determined occur normally only in certain types of tissue cells and not in others. For example, the particular component of the enzyme system phenylalanine hydroxylase, a deficiency of which occurs in phenylketonuria, is normally only present in cells of the liver.

The essential point is that a gene does not exist *in vacuo*, but in a particular intracellular milieu, the nature of which must influence the character of the gene's activity. Many things will be involved in this. They include the cell's previous history, the nature of its immediate environment, and the functional properties of all the other genes which are present. The complete picture is clearly extremely complex and in the multicellular organism it is necessarily tied up with the whole problem of the biochemistry of development and tissue differentiation.

How far current ideas about the role of genes in protein synthesis will stand the test of time remains to be seen. It must be remembered that they are based on a very restricted number of detailed examples and no doubt present concepts and working hypotheses will have to be modified considerably as investigations of a wider range of phenomena at the appropriate level of analysis become possible.

In conclusion it may be said that such work as that of Ingram on the structural differences between haemoglobins A, S and C, and of Morgan and Watkins on the structural differences between the A, B, H and Le^a blood-group substances, has opened up an entirely new chapter in human genetics. It has become possible for the first time to consider inherited differences between human beings in terms of the chemical structures of particular macromolecules and the significance of this for future work can hardly be overemphasised. The application of such approaches to other types of genetically determined biochemical variation will undoubtedly reveal many new perspectives, and we may expect exciting developments in the coming years.

REFERENCES

(1) Watson, J. D. and Crick, F. H. C. (1953*a*). *Nature, Lond.* **171**, 737.
(2) Watson, J. D. and Crick, F. H. C. (1953*b*). *Nature, Lond.* **171**, 964.

GENERAL REFERENCE

The Chemical Basis of Heredity, ed. McElroy, W. D. and Glass, B. Johns Hopkins Press, Baltimore, 1957.

INDEX

Bold type indicates principal place of reference.